# Critical acclaim for *Tale*

"Fascinating . . . [Plotkin] ex⎸
charismatic and mysterious powers of the shamans . . . He has a gift for evoking a sense of place, and the characters he meets come alive on the page." —*Los Angeles Times*

"Intriguing, engaging, exciting, and disturbing—a rare accomplishment in a botanical work . . . In their richness and diversity, these pages recall Amazonia itself." —*American Horticulturist*

"*Tales of a Shaman's Apprentice* combines high adventure, scientific insight, and a treasure trove of fascinating information." —*Zoogoer* magazine

"*Tales of a Shaman's Apprentice* teaches a great deal, while reading like a marvelously exotic travelogue. Most importantly, it re-excites our sense of wonder." —Juliet Wittman, editor of *Discovery*

"Plotkin's tales permit the reader who has never ventured into any rain forest . . . to experience almost firsthand the hazards, as well as the pleasures, of studies with witch doctors. His accounts of hacking his way through lianas thick and thin, of being soaked in sweat and rain, of avoiding large crocodilians, and of being bitten by vampire bats, are the stuff of adventure movies." —J. Worth Estes, *Natural History* magazine

"This is a lot more than ethnobotany—it's an adventure story. . . . Plotkin is not just some fashionable rain forest *Angst* meister; he's been there and knows whereof he speaks." —*Men's Journal*

"A compelling, insightful narrative that whisks the reader into a time and place where plants, animals, and indigenous societies coexist . . . A skillful blend of travel adventure, botanical and cultural history, and Amazonian research." —*Library Journal*

"Plotkin reminds us often of the intimate connections we still have with the rainforest. . . . This book *will* help save the forest and hopefully the children of the forest, as it reminds us why we should become involved." —*Audubon*

PENGUIN BOOKS

## TALES OF A SHAMAN'S APPRENTICE

Trained as an ethnobotanist at Harvard, Yale, and Tufts, Mark J. Plotkin has done extensive research throughout South America. Formerly director of the plant program at the World Wildlife Fund, he currently serves as research associate at the department of botany at the Smithsonian Institution. Along with various awards (including the San Diego Zoo Gold Medal for Conservation), Plotkin has been featured in a PBS *Nova* documentary, CBS's *48 Hours*, and he plays a leading role in the IMAX film *Amazon*, which was nominated for a 1997 Academy Award in the Best Short Documentary category. He was named as a "Hero for the Planet" by *Time* magazine in 1998, and is also the author of *Medicine Quest: In Search of Nature's Healing Secrets*, available from Penguin.

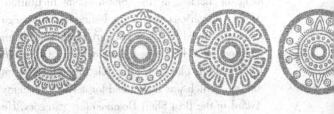

# TALES OF A SHAMAN'S APPRENTICE

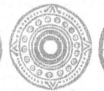

An Ethnobotanist
Searches for New Medicines
in the Amazon Rain Forest

## MARK J. PLOTKIN, PH. D.

PENGUIN BOOKS

*For my friends in the forest*

PENGUIN BOOKS
Published by the Penguin Group
Penguin Group (USA) LLC
375 Hudson Street
New York, New York 10014

USA | Canada | UK | Ireland | Australia | New Zealand | India | South Africa | China
penguin.com
A Penguin Random House Company

First published in the United States of America by
Viking Penguin, a division of Penguin Books USA Inc., 1993
Published in Penguin Books 1994

Photographs from the author's collection

THE LIBRARY OF CONGRESS HAS CATALOGUED THE HARDCOVER AS FOLLOWS:
Plotkin, Mark J.
Tales of a shaman's apprentice: an ethnobotanist searches for new
medicines in the Amazon rain forest/Mark Plotkin.
p.   cm.
Includes bibliograhical references and index.
ISBN 0-670-83137-9 (hc.)
ISBN 978-0-14-012991-5 (pbk.)
1. Indians of South America—Amazon River Region—Ethnobotany.
2. Indians of South America—Amazon River Region—Medicine.   3. Plotkin,
Mark J.   4. Amazon River Region—Description and travel.   I. Title.
F2230.1.B7P56   1993
581.6'34'09811—dc20      92-50768

Printed in the United States of America
ScoutAutomatedPrintCode

Set in Bodoni Book
Designed by Francesca Belanger
Map by David Julian

# Foreword

. . . . . . . . . . . . . . . . .

When I first traveled to the Amazon in 1941, the world was a different place. Most people thought of the rain forest—if they thought of it at all—as a green dungeon to be avoided at all costs. This erroneous idea permeated literature, as the famous Colombian novelist José Eustacio Rivera wrote in his book *The Vortex* (1924):

> Deformed trees . . . held imprisoned by creepers. Lianas bound together in a death grip. Stretched from tree to palm in long elastic curves . . . they caught falling leaves, branches and fruits, held them for years, until they sagged and burst like rotten bags, scattering blind reptiles, rusty salamanders, hairy spiders and decayed vegetable matter over the underbrush.

Contrast that with the first impression of a rain forest by the British scientist Richard Spruce, one of the greatest plant explorers of all time, who in 1849 wrote from the Amazon:

> I first realized my idea of a primeval forest. There were enormous trees, crowned with magnificent foliage, decked with fantastic parasites and hung over with lianas which varied in thickness from slender threads to huge python-like masses, were now round, now flattened, now knotted and now twisted with the regularity of a cable. Intermixed with the trees, and often equal to them in altitude, grew noble palms; while other and far lovelier species of the same family, their ringed stems sometimes scarcely exceeding a

finger's thickness but bearing plume-like fronds and pendulous bunches of black or red berries, quite like those of their loftier allies, formed, along with shrubs and arbuscles of many types, a bushy undergrowth, not usually very dense or difficult to penetrate.

Having lived in the Amazon almost permanently for thirteen years (1941–1953), and having made shorter visits almost annually since 1954, I have dedicated a good part of my professional life to the rain forest and its peoples. I believe that I realize what a uniquely fascinating and complex world it is—and what a beautiful part of our planet. One of the many aspects of the Amazon that are difficult to comprehend is the intimate relationship between the forest Indian and his ambient vegetation. But the unacculturated native is usually interested in, and more than willing to cooperate with, true scientific research. The widespread belief that his "secrets," especially his uncanny knowledge of the plants and animals, must be pried from him is, in general, a falsehood.

The essence of what makes *Tales of a Shaman's Apprentice* such a special work is precisely Mark Plotkin's gentlemanly approach to the natives and his ability to work with Indians as a trusted friend. When Mark first headed south to the Amazon in the late 1970s, he had no intention of writing a book. I had sent him to the northeast Amazon to conduct ethnobotanical research: to document how rain forest tribes were using rain forest plants. Because he went there to learn from the Indians, he was able to collect plants, participate in ceremonies and rituals, and share other experiences as few outsiders have been able to do. One of Mark's outstanding qualities as a field ethnobotanist is his conviction that among the Indians, he is the student and they are the teachers.

Two aspects of the book merit special mention. Mark Plotkin is a member of the last generation of ethnobotanists who will be able to see the Amazonian Indians living a life not all that different from their ancestors of thousands of years before. To hunt with breechcloth-clad men carrying arrows tipped with vegetal poison, to see shamans curing the sick in palm-thatched huts, to hear the rasping sound of cassava being grated by women of the village—these scenes and sounds predominate in the classic accounts of the nineteenth-century explorer-naturalists like Charles Waterton, Alfred Russel Wallace, and the Schomburgk brothers, Robert and Richard. Mark has beautifully captured these experiences for the reader of today.

The other facet of this book that makes it so intriguing is the author's exceptional grasp of history. I have often felt that the history of civilization could be written in terms of economic plants, something all too often ignored by (or unknown to) modern historians. In *The Wonders of Instinct*, the nineteenth-century French entomologist J. H. Fabre wrote:

> History celebrates the battle-fields whereon we meet our death, but scorns to speak of the ploughed fields whereby we thrive; it knows the names of the kings' bastards, but cannot tell the origin of wheat.

*Tales of a Shaman's Apprentice* could not appear at a better time. With the rampant environmental destruction and vertiginous population growth, the end of this decade is probably our time limit to protect the world's rain forests and the fragile cultures that inhabit them. This book represents an outstanding contribution, an enthralling account by a talented writer and discerning scientist. Mark is able to express the importance of rain forest plants and peoples in terms that are compelling and poignant. As a consequence, his book is destined to become a classic and, as such, deserves to be read by everyone interested in botany, ethnobotany, anthropology, tropical medicine, shamanism, and environmental conservation in the humid tropics.

In 1963, I wrote:

> Civilization is on the march in many, if not most, primitive regions. It has long been on the advance, but its pace is now accelerated as the result of world wars, extended commercial interest, increased missionary activity, widened tourism. The rapid divorcement of primitive peoples from dependence upon their immediate environment for the necessities and amenities of life has been set in motion, and nothing will check it now. One of the first aspects of primitive culture to fall before the onslaught of civilization is knowledge and use of plants for medicines. The rapidity of this disintegration is frightening. Our challenge is to salvage some of

the native medico-botanical lore before it becomes forever entombed with the cultures that gave it birth.

Eleven years after the publication of this article, Mark Plotkin enrolled in one of my courses at Harvard. *Tales of a Shaman's Apprentice* shows that he took this advice to heart.

RICHARD EVANS SCHULTES, Ph.D., F.M.L.S.
Botanical Museum of Harvard University
Cambridge, Massachusetts

# Acknowledgments

I am indebted to many people whose assistance and encouragement made this book possible. My primary debt of gratitude is to the Indians with whom I lived and worked. My friends and teachers Koita, Kamainja, Fritz von Troon, and the Jaguar Shaman merit special mention.

The kindness and the inspiration of Dr. Russell Mittermeier and Dr. Richard E. Schultes helped get me started.

I would also like to thank the following friends, family, colleagues, institutions, and organizations: Dr. Stephen Altschul, Audubon Park Zoo, Gerard Brunings, Janet Cave, Dr. Napoleon Chagnon, Conservation International, Dr. Gordon Cragg, Dr. Edwin Corey, Dr. P. Cox, Wesley DeRooy, Dr. Jim Duke, Lisa Di Mona, Dr. Louise Emmons, Dr. Norman Farnsworth, Dr. Adrian Forsyth, the late Dr. Al Gentry, Dr. Michael Goulding, Nan Graham, Kathryn Harrison, Harvard University Extension, Christopher Healy, Courtney Hodell, Phil Johnson, Dave Julian, Bill Kurtis, Stephen Lemann, Dr. Jacques Lizot, Liliana Madrigal (especially!), Stanley Malone, Dr. John McIlhenny, Dr. Dennis McKenna, Dr. Gary Nabhan, Dr. Norton Nickerson, Doris Omi, Dr. Tom Palley, the late Dr. Ted Parker, Dr. Rob Peters, Gabrielle Plotkin, Helene Plotkin, Norman Plotkin, Tim Reiser, Abbe Reis, Rafe Sagalyn, Lindley Schutz, Gillian Silverman, Dr. Doel Soejarto, Amy Schenkenberg, Dr. Joshua Sherman, Dr. Les Sponsel, Jeremy Tarcher, Pam Trejos, Dr. Ernest E. Williams, World Wildlife Fund, and Yale School of Forestry.

Special thanks to Conservation International, whose support makes the Shaman's Apprentice Program possible.

# Contents

# Contents

# Tales of a Shaman's Apprentice

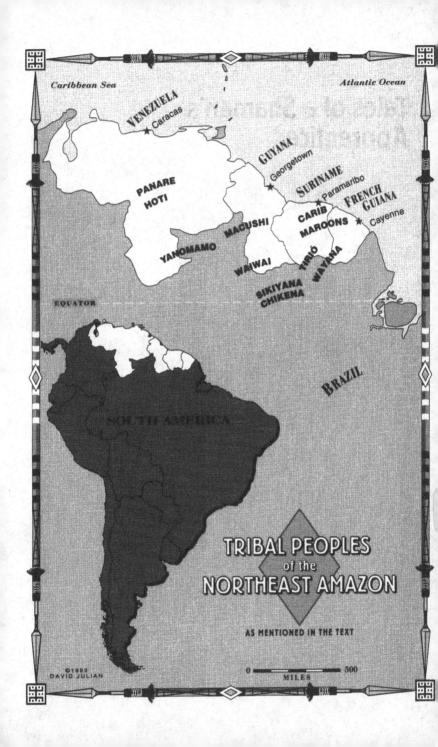

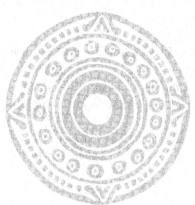

## CHAPTER 1

# Through the Emerald Door

The tropical rain forest is the greatest expression of life on earth.

—Thomas Lovejoy, 1983

● ● ● ● ● ● ● ● ● ● ● ● ● ● ● ● ● ● ●

*I had followed the old shaman through the jungle for three days and, over the course of our trek, we had developed an enigmatic relationship. The medicine man obviously resented my desire to learn the secrets of the forest plants that he knew and used for healing purposes. Still, he seemed pleased that I had come from so far away—he called me the* pananakiri *("the alien")—to acquire the botanical wisdom that the children of his tribe had no interest in learning.*

*I did not yet speak his language; an Indian from a neighboring tribe served as our translator. At the end of the third day, the old shaman turned to the other Indian and said, "Tell the* pananakiri *that I have taught him all that I am going to teach him. Tomorrow I am going hunting." I had no objections; there were other shamans in the village with whom I wished to work, and I returned to my hut with the medicinal plants I had collected.*

*That night, I had a terrifying dream. An enormous jaguar strode into my hut and stared deeply into my eyes, as if trying to divine my thoughts. Powerful muscles tensed in its back as it arched its body to spring.*

*So vivid was the apparition that I awoke with a scream. I sat upright in my hammock, trembling, my body soaked in a cold sweat. Carefully, I looked around the hut: I saw nothing—no footprints on the dirt floor, nothing disturbed or overturned, nothing to indicate the presence of an unwanted visitor. The only sound was the rustling of palm fronds as a gentle breeze blew through the village.*

*The next morning, just after sunrise, the young Indian who had served as our translator came to my hut. "Shall we go into the forest and look for more plants?" he asked.*

*"Before we do," I said, "find the old shaman and tell him that last night I saw the jaguar." I gave no details, and the Indian left. He returned a few minutes later.*

*"Did you tell him?" I asked.*

*"Yes."*

*"What did he say?" I asked.*

*"He broke into a big smile and said, 'That was me!' "*

Few people can recall the particular moment when they decided how to spend the rest of their lives. Mine came during a Harvard University night school lecture on a chilly September evening in 1974. That one moment opened the door to the fulfillment of a dream and to an adventure that is still unfolding.

The classroom where the lecture was held was like an ethnographic museum. One wall was covered with huge green maps of the Amazon, the flat terrain fractured by the blue lines of rivers whose names were familiar to few outside that region. Another wall pulsated with the red and black, crazy-quilt patterns of South Pacific bark cloths, laboriously crafted by islanders who had pounded brown paper mulberry bark until it was soft and malleable and then colored it with natural dyes from the forest around them. From the rafters hung Amazonian Indian dance costumes—straw-yellow grass skirts and mahogany-brown bark-cloth masks painted with glistening black demon faces, announcing an element of the macabre. Two long display cases flanked the room, filled to overflowing with botanical booty from around the world: shiny silver marijuana pipes from India, hallucinogenic snuff tubes from Brazil, black palm blowguns from Colombia, tiny bows and arrows from the Congo, and bamboo opium pipes from Burma. Lying among these objects were dried specimens of the plants that gave them purpose: marijuana, curare, and opium, among others. Other curiosities covered scarred wooden tables: coils of Manila hemp rope from the Philippines, elongated cassava tubers from the Amazon, coconut palm-leaf mats from the South Seas, tiny grinning skulls carved from ivory palm nuts from the Andes, and little-known tropical fruits shaped like everything from hand grenades to candles to stars.

Richard Evans Schultes, professor, explorer, presided over this jungle tableau. The world's preeminent authority on ethnobotany, the systematic study of how the people of a particular region use the local plants, Schultes had lived for more than thirteen years while a young man with Amazonian tribes, some of whom had never seen another white man. He spoke their dialects, ate their foods—including beetle grubs, alligator tails, and jungle rats—took part in religious ceremonies, and consumed their hallucinogenic plants. He was said to know as much about healing plants as any Amazonian witch doctor, and his work influenced personalities as diverse as writer Aldous Huxley, sixties drug guru Timothy Leary, and Pulitzer Prize–winning Harvard biologist Edward O. Wilson.

Schultes called the class to order, turned off the lights, and began his magic. He showed us no mathematical models or abstruse ecological theories, but timeless photographs of another world. We saw witch doctors, chiefs, hunters, matriarchs, and princesses performing sacred ceremonies, carving weapons, cultivating gardens, and preparing food. Makuna Indians in cotton breechcloths hunted fish from canoes with bows and arrows, and Barasana shamans sat around their cooking fires telling stories of past hunts and drinking hallucinogenic drafts of the caapi vine. Young Kubeo women, their black hair shining in the tropical sun, grated cassava roots and carried calabashes of river water to their huts. Little boys of the Taiwano tribe stalked and impaled lizards with arrows deftly shot from their little bows.

Interspersed with these images were slides of the plants that made possible the culture of northwest Amazonia: the foodstuffs, medicines, fibers, poisons, and sacred hallucinogens. These plants—clinging vines with massive blossoms, spiked bromeliads, graceful palms, giant canopy trees with roots like flying buttresses—were unlike anything I had ever seen before. One picture in particular changed my life forever: a scene in which three figures, dressed in grass skirts and bark-cloth masks, danced at the edge of a jungle clearing.

"Here you see three Indians of the Yukuna tribe doing the sacred *kai-yah-ree* dance under the influence of a hallucinogenic potion made from the *Banisteriopsis* liana to keep away the forces of darkness. The one on the left has a Harvard degree. Next slide please."

From that moment on I was hooked—hooked on plants, hooked on Indians, hooked on the Amazon.

My infatuation with the jungle had actually begun years earlier, when I was a child growing up in Louisiana. One hot summer night when I was about four years old, I was playing in the kitchen of my grandmother's house. I looked up and saw a green anole lizard—an American chameleon—crawling up the screen door. I ran into the living room screaming, "A dinosaur, a dinosaur!" Everyone thought I was frightened and tried to calm me down, insisting that it couldn't be a dinosaur; they were extinct, gone forever. I was heartbroken at the news. But lizards weren't extinct, so with that resilience peculiar to children, I focused my rapt attention on them and their dinosaurlike relatives—the snakes and turtles that inhabited the sleepy swamps surrounding my hometown of New Orleans.

When we were kids, all of my friends shared my interest in reptiles, but as we grew into adolescence most of the other boys trained their sights on more traditional southern pursuits—football, liquor, and the opposite sex. They anxiously awaited their sixteenth birthdays so they could get their driver's licenses and go out on dates; I longed to drive so I could go farther afield in my search for black rat snakes and cottonmouth water moccasins. Once I snared my prey, I would weigh and measure them, photograph and study them, and eventually let them go —just the kind of backyard science project that gave many professional biologists their start.

In 1973, at the age of eighteen, I set off for the University of Pennsylvania and its outstanding cellular and molecular biology department, but within a semester I discovered I had no interest in that discipline. Later that year, I visited a high-school classmate who attended Harvard. I stopped at the university's zoology museum and wandered through the exhibits of tropical nature; I realized immediately that the equatorial rain forest was where I wanted to be, not studying in the sterile laboratories in Philadelphia.

As a well-intentioned but penniless college dropout, I figured my most likely ticket to the tropics would be to take a job as a manual laborer at the museum that so intrigued me. I knew that the Harvard Zoology Museum was home to many scientist-explorers; I hoped that someday one of them would invite me to go along on an expedition to the rain forest in search of some elusive exotic quarry.

I joined the museum's staff in September 1974 and spent my days building specimen cabinets and carting huge dinosaur bones from one corner of the building to another. A few days after I started, a co-worker suggested that I enter night school to amass a few college credits while I worked. There was one course, he said, that, if I didn't immediately enroll in, I would spend the rest of my life regretting it.

Professor Schultes imbued his students with a sense of the value, the beauty, and the fragility of the rain forest ecosystem and the indigenous peoples who are so much a part of it. A leading authority on Amazonian botany, medicinal plants, coca and cocaine, hallucinogens, Mexican mushroom cults, natural rubber, palms, orchids, and arrow poisons, he is often called the father of ethnobotany. During his years in the remote northwest Amazon, Schultes found close to two thousand plant species that the Indians used for medicinal purposes; he was convinced that thousands more awaited discovery. He returned from the jungle determined to inspire a new generation of ethnobotanists, to usher them through the emerald door into lives devoted to the study of rain forest plants and peoples.

Even though rain forests occur in three major regions—Asia, Africa, and the Neotropics (South America, Central America, and the Caribbean)—Schultes encouraged his students to focus on the Amazon. While it is usually associated with Brazil, the Amazon jungle's leafy tentacles reach into eight other South American countries, covering an area almost as large as the continental United States. A land of superlatives, a forest without equal, the Amazon teems with more varieties of plants and animals than any other place on earth. A single Amazonian river may harbor more types of fish than are found in all the rivers of Europe combined. In just one Amazonian national park—Manu in southeastern Peru—there are more bird species to be found than in the entire United States. Amazonia is home to the world's largest eagle, snake, anteater, armadillo, spider, freshwater turtle, and freshwater fish. It also boasts several animals of truly mind-bending proportions—a toad (the *cururú*) that weighs as much as 7 pounds, a rodent (the capybara) that weighs over 120 pounds, and a catfish (the *piraíba*) that tips the scale at almost a quarter of a ton.

Plant life in the Amazon is also unimaginably diverse: One of every four plants on earth—about sixty thousand of the world's approximately two hundred fifty thousand species—grows there, and many of these species remain unseen, and unstudied, by Western eyes. A majority of the world's insects live in the Amazon rain forest, and the fact that the forest has not been devoured by this entomological onslaught is testament to these plants' abilities as chemical warriors. Plants protect themselves by producing an astonishing array of chemicals that are toxic to insects, thereby deterring predation. When ingested by humans, these same plants—and their chemical weapons—may act in a variety of ways on the body: they may be nutritious, poisonous, or even hallucinogenic. And in some cases, they are therapeutic.

Many of the human body's powerful reactions are a direct response to plant alkaloids, a class of chemical compounds most common in tropical plants. Alkaloids, which are characterized by a molecular structure that must include a nitrogen atom and at least two carbon atoms, have had a major impact on every culture—if not every person—on the planet. They provide everything from the kick in our morning coffee (caffeine) to the addictive compounds in our most dangerous drugs (cocaine, heroin, and nicotine), the toxic principles in some of the deadliest poisons (strychnine and batrachotoxin), the analgesic effects in our most potent painkillers (codeine and morphine), and the mental pyrotechnics in some of the most powerful hallucinogens (mescaline and psilocybin).

The alkaline properties of alkaloids often give them a bitter taste, and this astringent tang was frequently a clue for people the world over that a plant had therapeutic properties. The concept of "bitters"—just about any concoction that contained bitter-tasting plants and was said to have healing properties—is found in medicinal systems from ancient Israel to the colonial East Indies to modern Amazonia.

Quinine, an alkaloid from the bark of the cinchona tree and one of the bitterest substances known, was first discovered thousands of years ago by South American Indians in what is now Peru and Ecuador. Since then it has been widely used throughout the tropics and much of the temperate world to cure malaria, a disease caused by a parasite, transmitted by mosquitoes, that destroys red blood cells. Although thought of by many as a jungle disease, this illness does not discriminate based on geography: malaria has been and still is a world-ranging disease. At one time or another, cities as diverse as London, Madrid, Paris, Rome, and Washington, D.C., were gripped by the often fatal disease. It is said to have killed Alexander the Great and Oliver Cromwell, as well as tens of millions of people whose names history never recorded. Malaria has been and continues to be responsible for more deaths than any other disease in the world.

Yet a single plant alkaloid revealed to us by South American Indians has helped eradicate malaria in the temperate zone and reduce the prevalence of the disease in the lowland tropics. Although cinchona contains more than thirty alkaloids, the most important is quinine, which functions something like a therapeutic "smart bomb," rapidly seeking out and selectively destroying malaria parasites hiding in the human bloodstream. Although quinine served as the antimalarial drug of choice for hundreds of years, it began to be replaced by synthetic analogues as early as 1959; the United States wanted to reduce its reliance on "strategic commodities" that could not be grown within its borders. As sometimes happens with synthetic drug treatments, new, resistant strains of malaria developed; to defeat severe cases of the disease, physicians often prescribe medicines containing the natural compound.

There exists no shortage of "wonder drugs" waiting to be found in the rain forests, yet we in the industrialized world are woefully ignorant about the chemical—and, therefore, medicinal—potential of most tropical plants. Brazil is home to more plant species than almost any other country in the world, yet according to Dr. Otto Gottlieb, that country's leading plant chemist, "we know little or nothing about the chemical composition of 98.6% of the Brazilian flora." In fact, only about 5,000 of the world's 250,000 species have been extensively screened in the laboratory to determine their therapeutic potential, and the approximately 120 plant-based prescription drugs on the market today are derived from only 95 species. A quarter of all prescription drugs sold in the United States have plant chemicals as active ingredients. About half of those drugs contain compounds from temperate plants, while the other half have chemicals from tropical species. According to one recent study, the value of medicines derived from tropical plants—that is, the amount consumers in the United States spend on them—is more than $6 billion a year.

One powerful "new" medicine derived from a plant used in ancient folk medicine is ginkgo extract. Called a "living fossil" by Charles Darwin (its relatives have been found in the fossil record from 280 million years ago), the ginkgo is the oldest living tree species on earth. Long extinct in the wild, it has survived and flourished in temple gardens in both China and Japan, where ginkgo leaf extract has been used for more than five thousand years to treat illnesses ranging from asthma to severe allergic inflammations. Today, ginkgo extract is sold widely in Europe and generates revenues of more than $700 million annually. Because it acts as a vasodilator, increasing blood flow throughout the body, it is primarily used to treat conditions in the elderly that are thought to be caused by diminished blood flow to the brain. The extract also appears to be effective in the treatment of asthma: ginkgo interferes with a compound in the human body known as platelet activating factor, a bronchoconstrictor that diminishes oxygen intake into the lungs. In addition, ginkgo extract offers promise for the treatment of certain kidney disorders, toxic shock, and the rejection of transplanted organs.

Of all the therapeutic compounds brought from the world's living pharmacy into our modern drugstores for uses as varied as contraceptives to cancer treatments, few, if any, were truly discovered by university-trained botanists. These plants were "discovered" by botanists much as America was "discovered" by Columbus—in both cases, the Indians got there first.

A good example is taxol, a drug approved in December 1992 for the treatment of advanced ovarian cancer. An alkaloid found in the bark and needles of the Pacific yew tree in the American Northwest, taxol selectively interferes with the division of cancer cells by attacking the microtubules—the threads that pull chromosomes apart—during cell division. Taxol was discovered through a screening program operated by the National Cancer Institute, which since 1960 has been randomly collecting plants and testing them for therapeutic effectiveness. Yet early ethnographic accounts unearthed by Dr. James Duke, an ethnobotanist with the USDA, show that Indians had long used the yew tree

for a variety of medicinal purposes: the Potawatomi tribe treated venereal diseases by crushing the leaves and applying them directly to the
sores, and the Chippewa, Iroquois, and Menominee tribes eased the pain
of arthritis and rheumatism by boiling the branches and leaves of the
yew and bathing in the steam.

This is not to minimize NCI's impressive efforts and its success in
quickly bringing taxol to market. Since 1968, when the screening program was refined to focus specifically on cancer and, later, on AIDS,
the institute has tested more than fifty thousand specimens (including
bark, stems, and flowers) from twenty-five thousand plant species. They
have found promising research leads (but not cures) in the fight against
AIDS, including a woody vine in Cameroon that produces an alkaloid
that has broad spectrum effects killing both HIV-1 and HIV-2 in a test
tube. But so much of the compound is needed to kill the virus that the
drug would likely prove toxic to humans. In another instance, Dr. Doel
Soejarto of the University of Illinois, who was collecting specimens for
NCI, gathered a promising sample from a tree in Sarawak, in northern
Borneo: it produced a nonalkaloid chemical compound effective in the
laboratory against HIV-1. Scientists were unable to find more of the
substance in other trees of the same species, so Soejarto went back to
collect more specimens from the original site. Unfortunately, he found
that the area—including the tree—had been cleared by local peasants
to make a garden.

At this point, there is no official ethnobotanical component to NCI's
research. But Dr. Paul Cox of Brigham Young University, a leading
authority on the ethnobotany of the South Pacific, did submit samples
of a rubber tree relative used by Samoan healers for treatment of back
pain, diarrhea, abdominal swelling, and yellow fever. NCI found that it
contained a novel compound, which they call prostratin; in a test tube,
it appears to protect healthy cells from contracting the AIDS virus.
While this, too, is an important research lead for better understanding
how the virus invades cells, it is *not*, at this point, either a vaccine
against the disease or a cure.

NCI has done extraordinary work under demanding circumstances
and within a limited budget; nonetheless, most ethnobotanists believe
that a greater emphasis on useful plants employed by indigenous peo-

ples and a cooperative relationship with ethnobotanists and tribal healers might lead to more finds like prostratin in the future.

Over thousands of years, through a method of trial and error, indigenous
tribes have built up a storehouse of knowledge about the native vegetation. That first class with Professor Schultes almost twenty years ago
was the beginning of my career in ethnobotany, and of a lifelong commitment to documenting medicinal plant lore among tribal peoples of
the rain forest.

In the field, an ethnobotanist takes notes on uses of a particular plant,
then collects what is called a voucher specimen. In the case of a small
shrub or herb (which, to a botanist, is any plant with a fleshy stem
instead of a woody one), this can be the entire plant; if the plant to be
collected is a large shrub or a tree, the voucher specimen can be a
branch. In either case, the specimen preferably includes any fruit or
flowers, since in the Linnaean system of classification, you usually need
to see a plant's reproductive parts to identify the species.

Once the specimen has been collected, it is pressed between two
sheets of newspaper, which helps draw out excess moisture. Next the
specimens, as many as thirty at a time, are placed between two pieces
of plywood about the size of an elongated photo album; these are then
bound together with rope or straps and placed twelve to eighteen inches
above a small fire. This dries the plants, which are then ready for
transport to a herbarium; there, each specimen is glued to a twelve-by-
eighteen-inch piece of paper, on which is recorded the plant's name
(both in Latin and in the indigenous language), when and where it was
collected and by whom, and how the local people use it. The voucher
specimen then stands as a benchmark against which future collections
can be compared.

Botanists use herbaria much as scholars use a library—to conduct
background research on a particular plant and to identify plants collected in the field. Identification begins with a taxonomic key, a written
set of instructions that allows you to determine the correct family, genus,
and species of each specimen. To double-check the identification made
with the key or to find the correct scientific names when no key is
available, you compare your specimens with the dried voucher specimens in the herbarium.

Voucher specimens are seldom analyzed in the laboratory; there is little plant material to analyze without completely destroying the specimen. In addition, while many plant alkaloids remain intact in herbarium specimens for hundreds of years, other compounds undergo significant changes as soon as the plant dies. Therefore, a scientist collecting plants for chemical analysis gathers at least a kilogram—just over two pounds—of dried plant specimens and a kilogram of fresh material that is stored in alcohol to preserve the active compounds. Most ethnobotanists tend to collect voucher specimens rather than bulk samples; we have traditionally been more committed to preserving ethnobotanical knowledge than working with pharmaceutical firms, who have shown limited interest in this avenue of research.

The focus of my ethnobotanical work during the past twelve years has been the plants and peoples of the northeast Amazon, an area that straddles the borders of Brazil, French Guiana, Guyana, Suriname, and Venezuela. This is one of the last places on the planet where rain forests flourish undisturbed from horizon to horizon; it is home to mountains that have never been climbed and cut by rivers that have yet to be named by Western cartographers. Here, until relatively recently, tribal peoples lived undisturbed by—indeed, unaware of—the outside world.

Known to early European explorers as the "Wild Coast of Guiana," the region between the mouths of the Orinoco and Amazon rivers held little appeal for explorers who came in search of gold and silver, rumored to be abundant in the interior. The shores were patrolled by black clouds of voracious mosquitoes and tribes of cannibalistic Carib Indians, who filed their teeth to points to emphasize their fierceness. Further inland, the region was said to be populated with an assortment of odd and dangerous creatures: two-headed snakes, dragons, female warriors, and men with heads like dogs or without heads at all, peering from eyes in their shoulders and speaking from mouths in their chests.

Explorers of the Amazon never encountered these fantastic beings, but they did find hundreds of Indian tribes, which modern anthropologists divide into several major language groups, including Arawakan, Panoan, Tukanoan, Tupi-Guarani, and Carib; they constitute the majority of the lowland tribes. Their ancestors—like those of all Amerindians—crossed the Bering Strait from eastern Asia twenty thousand to fifty thousand years ago and, in so doing, discovered the New

World. In one of the most awe-inspiring migrations since the origin of
our species, the people who would eventually settle Amazonia made
their way from Alaska to South America. Along the way, they developed
the means to survive and thrive in a range of challenging environments,
from the frozen ice floes above the Arctic Circle to the burning desert
sands of Sonora. Through splits, migrations, wars, and intermarriage,
the language groups separated into tribes. Most of the tribes with which
I have worked—the Tiriós, Wayanas, Akuriyos, Waiwais, and Macushis—are all Carib groups. The Yanomamo tribe of the Brazil-
Venezuela border regions, with whom I spent time studying their use
of hallucinogenic snuff, are what is known as an isolate—a tribe whose
affinity to other groups is unclear. Some experts believe that this tribe
may have been part of the first group to cross the Bering Strait and
settle in the Amazon.

When a Westerner looks at the jungle, he sees green—herbs, vines,
shrubs, trees. When an Indian looks at the jungle, he sees the basics
of life—food, medicines, and raw materials from which to build shelters,
weave hammocks, and carve a hunting bow. But life among the Indians
is changing. Those seeking to "help" the Indians, to educate them in
the ways of Western civilization, have succeeded in shattering a culture
that has thrived in the interior reaches of the Amazon basin for tens of
thousands of years.

From the arrival of Christopher Columbus and other early explorers
who came to subjugate the natives and plunder their riches, to the
modern-day visits of well-intentioned but misguided missionaries who
seek to replace the Indians' long-held religious beliefs with the Westerners' God, the indigenous peoples have been on a collision course
with the outside world. They have been pressured to forsake the
traditions of their forbears and accept the ways of other, so-called advanced societies. To a people living nearly naked in the forest—some
of whom, until recently, still made fire by rubbing sticks together and
cut down trees with simple stone axes, and even now hunt game with
bow and arrow—the white man with his clothes, matches, machetes,
axes, and shotguns appears to be a superior creature. But the Indians
who give up their homes, beliefs, life-style, and language in exchange
for the white man's religion, moral code, and material goods often pay
a terrible price, as they have from the very first contact between Eu-

ropeans and Amerindians. On Friday, October 12, 1492, Christopher Columbus unsheathed his sword to impress the Indians of the Caribbean island then known as Guanahani. The Indians, having never seen metal before, marveled at the strange pointed object that glinted in the morning sun. One bold fellow grabbed the blade, then howled in bewilderment and pain as the metal sliced into his flesh and his blood dripped onto the sand—a perfect metaphor for much of what has transpired between the two cultures ever since. The Indians' understandable eagerness to grasp the fruits of Western technology has cost them dearly in terms of introduced diseases (through increased contact), denigration of their religion (through missionary activity), and the loss of ancestral lands (stolen or traded away for material goods).

Professor Schultes constantly reminded his students that over ninety tribes had become extinct in Brazil alone since the turn of the century. He believed ours would be the last generation fortunate enough to be able to live and work among these tribes as he had, to experience their traditional way of life firsthand, and to record their vast ethnobotanical knowledge before the plant species—or the people who used them—succumbed to the march of progress.

His was not an unfounded fear. Rain forests are shrinking—some experts believe at a rate of one hundred acres a minute—and it is estimated that 10 percent of the world's plant species will be extinct by the year 2000. In addition, the medicine men and women—or shamans, as they are also known—who have traditionally guarded and passed on the tribal lore of healing plants, are finding few in the younger generation who will continue the tradition. Thus it has become the goal of most ethnobotanists—myself included—to record and preserve the plant knowledge of forest peoples. It is our hope that this wisdom might someday benefit the tribes in their dealings with the outside world and at the same time, perhaps, uncover new, potentially useful plant-based medicines.

Over the last decade, I set out to learn as much as I could about the way the Amazonian Indians use forest plants before that knowledge disappeared. And I aimed to learn from the shamans, who serve as the repositories of the most detailed tribal lore of curative plants. Heirs to an oral tradition that stretches back deep into the mists of prehistory, the shamans are not only the crucial link between the tropical rain forest and our neighborhood pharmacy; I believe they are our greatest hope for finding cures to currently incurable diseases (cancer, AIDS, the common cold), as well as diseases that will undoubtedly appear in the future.

The plant kingdom has long served as humankind's primary source of therapeutic compounds. This began to change in the 1930s, with the advent of synthetic chemistry, and was cemented in the 1950s with the introduction of laboratory-bred "wonder drugs," such as the antibacterial sulfonamides, or sulfa drugs. Predictably, the American pharmaceutical industry quickly lost interest in natural products as sources of potential new medicines. When Schultes returned to Harvard in 1939, after completing ethnobotanical research among the Indians of southern Mexico, he was unable to find an American drug firm or even a single American chemist willing to work with him; they dismissed him, saying they didn't want to waste their time looking at his folk medicines. Crestfallen, he had to send his materials to a sympathetic young Swiss chemist for analysis. This chemist, Albert Hofmann, later became famous as the inventor of LSD. Less widely known, however, is that he isolated the hallucinogenic alkaloid psilocybin from mushrooms in Schultes's Mexican collections; from this natural model, he synthesized the cardiac beta-blocker visken, which has improved the quality of life for millions of people with heart problems.

Powerful laboratory drugs like the sulfonamides and the sedative diazepam (better known as Valium) have given some chemists the illusion that synthetic chemistry is the sole future of new drug discovery. Smug scientists congratulating themselves on "inventing" new drugs led the anthropologist Robert de Ropp to wryly observe that "some chemists, having synthesized a few compounds, believe themselves to be better chemists than nature which, in addition to synthesizing compounds too numerous to mention, synthesized those chemists as well." In fact, nature had conceived of diazepam long before modern-day chemists. Several years ago scientists found that tiny amounts of the drug occur naturally in wheat and potatoes, albeit in quantities too small to have an effect on people or to warrant harvesting. Similarly, Dr. Norman Farnsworth of the University of Illinois, a leading figure in natural product chemistry, enjoys pointing out how proud chemists were thirty years ago when they synthesized an antidote for accidental poisoning by organophosphorus insecticides. Later it was found that the substance occurred naturally in electric eels.

I knew from Schultes's teachings that new medicines were probably just waiting to be found in the rain forest plants, but one of the issues that troubled me as I began my research is what has come to be called "intellectual property rights." Briefly stated, no matter what disease an ethnobotanist might find a cure for during the course of his research, the indigenous peoples who taught him the cure would not benefit from the sales of the new drug. A classic example of this is the case of the rosy periwinkle.

Although native to southeastern Madagascar, the pink-flowered periwinkle, a member of the dogbane family, was transported throughout the tropical and subtropical world by early European explorers who prized it for its beautiful foliage. But the plant is also valued for its therapeutic properties and has been used as a folk medicine in Madagascar, Asia, Africa, Central America, South America, and the Caribbean to treat such ills as inflamed eyes, sore throat, wasp stings, fevers, and hemorrhages. But it was the plant's use by black peasants in Jamaica to treat diabetes that led scientists to investigate further in 1957.

At the University of West Ontario, researchers R. L. Noble and C. T. Beer extracted the active compounds of the rosy periwinkle by grinding up the entire plant and soaking it in alcohol. They then injected this extract into rats, which had the effect of drastically reducing the rodents' white blood cell counts. Since leukemia is characterized by an abnormally high white blood cell count, the researchers next tested the extract against leukemia cells in vitro; again, the white blood cell count was dramatically lowered. This led to the isolation of the alkaloid vinblastine, a cancer treatment widely used today to combat lymphoma, solid tumors, and Hodgkin's disease.

Independently of the Canadian team, a scientist named Gordon Svoboda at the Eli Lilly Company in Indianapolis tested an extract of the rosy periwinkle in a broad-based anticancer screening program. He found that the extract had a strong inhibitory effect on a type of leukemia known in the lab as P-1534. From this study, the alkaloid vincristine was isolated, and is used today to treat acute Hodgkin's disease, lymphocytic leukemia, and other childhood cancers.

The rosy periwinkle was eventually found to harbor more than seventy different alkaloids, six of which have antitumor properties. The two isolated by the researchers at the University of West Ontario and at Eli Lilly—vinblastine and vincristine—function as mitotic spindle poisons. During cell division (mitosis), chromosomes split in two and attach themselves to spindles that help pull the halves apart. The alkaloids selectively attack cancerous cells, poisoning the spindles and thus interfering with reproduction of the malignant cells.

Annual sales of these two drugs exceed $100 million, yet not a penny goes back to Madagascar, the country of origin for the rosy periwinkle and one of the poorest countries in the world.

I believe that the country of origin should reap some monetary benefits from the sales of drugs made from its plants. To that end, I decided that before I would have the plants I collected in the forest analyzed in the laboratory, I would wait for two things to happen: for the drug companies to regain their interest in natural products and for some company, some mechanism, some law to appear that would help me channel profits from the potential drugs back into the hands of the Indians themselves. Until then, I would just store my plant specimens in the herbarium and keep the data I collected on ethnobotanical usage to myself.

The tribal healers hold the key to unlocking one of the great mysteries of our day and age—how to demonstrate the value of the rain forest in concrete economic terms and, in so doing, provide the rationale for protecting Mother Nature's ultimate creation. For through our ignorance, greed, and religious zeal, we have set off a chain of events that is destroying both the ecosystem and the only cultures that know how to preserve it. Through ill-planned logging schemes and culturally insensitive missionary activity, by failing to help reduce population growth spiraling out of control and by encouraging the ruling elites in tropical countries to incur mountains of debt that are squeezing the life out of their economies, we have helped create a situation that works against the world's ecological and socioeconomic self-interest. If the rain forests are to survive, their future depends on cooperation between the countries in which the forests occur and those companies desiring the plants. First, the tropical countries must allow only the sustainable harvesting of their natural resources—a method that allows raw plant material to be collected without endangering the life of the species. Currently, such destructive methods as cutting trees down or completely stripping them of their bark are sometimes used to harvest medicinal species. These methods could be replaced by only removing a certain percentage of the leaves or peeling small strips of bark from each tree. The companies buying the plants must offer financial incentives for those countries using only ecologically sound methods to harvest plants. The communities would benefit not only from the preservation of their most valuable resources, but from the jobs created by the demand for trained harvesters. Second, a percentage of the profits from any new product must flow back to the country of origin. Once an economic incentive for rain forest conservation has been achieved, the continued existence of these forests can be guaranteed.

After working for a decade with the Indians of the Amazon, spending anywhere from two weeks to two months per visit, I have gathered more than three hundred plant samples and written reams of notes on the ethnobotanical knowledge of four tribes. I've learned that the botanical genius of these peoples is not limited to medicines but includes extraordinary agricultural knowledge as well. Pre-Columbian farmers, without benefit of the wheel or draft animals, discovered and domesticated more than half of the modern world's seven major food crops—corn, potatoes, sweet potatoes, and cassava—as well as tomatoes, peanuts, chile peppers, chocolate, vanilla, pineapples, papayas, passion fruit, and avocados. The annual global market value of corn alone is worth $12 billion—more than the value of all the gold and silver stolen by the rapacious conquistadores. And the Indians' agricultural systems are as impressive as their crops. When Dr. Alan Kolata, an anthropologist with the University of Chicago, worked with Amerindians in Bolivia to resurrect pre-Columbian farming systems, the crops' yield increased sevenfold.

Ironically, if the American farmer had to grow only species native to the United States, we would be living off of Jerusalem artichokes, pecans, black walnuts, sunflower seeds, blueberries, cranberries, raspberries, and gooseberries. To paraphrase the contemporary Kenyan economist Calestous Juma, the exploitation of tropical plant resources by the United States has turned a continent of berries into a global agricultural power.

Early on, I realized that I would never be able to record more than a fraction of the ethnobotanical information possessed by the shamans throughout the Amazon. Moreover, it soon became increasingly obvious to me that it was at least as important that the ethnobotanical wisdom be perpetuated within the tribes themselves. To accomplish this, the Indians and I developed a methodology we call the Shaman's Apprentice Program, a process by which my notes—the invaluable information supplied by the tribes—are translated back into the local language and studied by a young tribe member who is designated a shaman's apprentice. That individual then teaches the accumulated wisdom to other young members of the tribe, acting in essence as a bridge between the preliterate tradition and a literate future for the tribe. In this way, the indigenous people can control their own destiny, choosing to hold on to a part of their culture that would otherwise slip away.

If, as Pasteur says, "chance favors the prepared mind," I had been waiting for mine. It came one cold Cambridge afternoon in late 1978; I was in the Harvard museum basement feeding white mice to the department's pet boa constrictor and watching snow eddies swirl outside the window. Russ Mittermeier, one of the toughest and most knowledgeable Amazonian field biologists in the business, stopped by and did forty chin-ups on the doorjamb, then casually said he was setting off again for the Amazon, this time to search for endangered crocodilians. He needed a field assistant to help capture, measure, and weigh some of the larger specimens. Was I was interested in going with him?

His quarry wasn't medicinal plants, but the trip was the realization of a dream I'd had since childhood and the start of a career dedicated to the rain forest. I jumped at the chance, and six months later I was in the jungle.

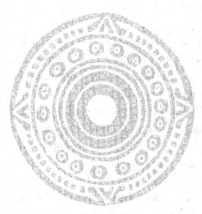

# CHAPTER 2

# The Search for the Black Caiman

A number of the bigger crocodilians are perversely unable to see the special nature of the human animal, and absent-mindedly eat him from time to time.  —Archie Carr, 1940

• • • • • • • • • • • • • • • • • •

Traveling up the remote jungle river was like moving back through the millennia: our little canoe became a time machine and the compass was set for the Age of Reptiles. Only a thin shell of wood separated us from the man-eating crocodilians that swarmed in the watery depths below our canoe. And as the sun rose higher in the sky, the mist rising off the water, the hoots, whistles, and howls of creatures in the surrounding forest and the sweet and enticing smell of a strange and luxuriant vegetation reminded us that we had left behind the land where humans ruled and we were now entering another dominion.

It was my first trip to South America, and the goal of this expedition, led by Russ Mittermeier, was to look for the black caiman, a highly endangered crocodilian. Thirty years old and already a legend at Harvard, Mittermeier was born in the South Bronx and raised in Manhattan. After finishing his graduate coursework in biological anthropology at Harvard, he had set off for a brief trip to Brazil to choose a study site for his dissertation research. He returned two years later speaking fluent Spanish, Portuguese, and Surinamese, and carrying a steamer trunk crammed with lizards, frogs, feather headdresses, and poison-tipped blowdarts. Subsequent expeditions to carry out primate research in Brazil, Colombia, French Guiana, Peru, and Suriname gave him an overview possessed by few biologists, before or since. To the employees of the Harvard Museum, Russ Mittermeier, with his office full of blowguns, turtle shells, monkey skulls, sloth skeletons, and curare-tipped arrows, was the archetypal jungle explorer minus the fedora.

I met Mittermeier not long after I joined the museum staff. I was told there was a special treat in store for me—a fellow was returning after a year and a half in the Amazon and I could help him unpack his collection, the "privilege" of a junior staff member; nobody likes to unpack dead animals preserved in formaldehyde. But I was intrigued by the specimens and by Mittermeier's tales of his exploits. The fact was, he told of his adventures in a way that made them sound very ordinary. This had the effect of making his exploits, and him, seem all the more fascinating. When he asked me to be his field assistant, I immediately applied for an unpaid leave of absence for the month of July 1979 and spent part of each remaining day for the next six months plying Mittermeier with questions about the Amazon.

The little plane banked left over the choppy gray Atlantic, then circled back to begin the approach to the capital city of Cayenne. We were landing in French Guiana, a forgotten corner of the world. Visiting remote regions is a great thrill, but they can be difficult to reach: when we finally disembarked in French Guiana, we had spent fourteen hours traveling and had changed planes four times. We were jolted out of our bleary-eyed stupor by the intense tropical heat and by the sight of a flaming red sun dropping behind the jungle at the edge of the airstrip. In the trees overhead, blue and gold macaws began to settle down for the night. Their clamorous calls and vivid plumage seemed to embody the vitality of tropical nature.

The abundance and variety of life overwhelmed me. As darkness fell, a chorus of screams, whistles, snorts, roars, squawks, squeaks, hoots, and hollers erupted from the forest that encircled us. Mittermeier was able to identify the source of each call—birds, monkeys, bats, frogs, insects. A dusky brown moth the size of a salad plate clumsily swooped past my head as we entered the customs building at the airport. After a cursory wave through customs, we boarded what looked like a converted school bus for the ride into town. The driver found a radio station with a Caribbean beat, cranked up the volume, and hit the gas.

As we drove, Mittermeier explained the history of French Guiana. Although it was the Spanish who first explored the northeast coast of South America, it was the French who built the first permanent settlements, in the early 1600s. Plantations were established and shortly thereafter slaves were imported from West Africa to provide labor for the colonists. The country remained a typical colonial backwater for most of its history. Unlike Guyana and Suriname, French Guiana never gained its independence and has remained a department (essentially a state) of France. Because of its proximity to the equator, French Guiana is an optimal site for tracking spacecraft. In 1968 the European Space Agency built a facility near the town of Kourou from which to launch the Ariane satellites. This space-age techno-industry contrasts sharply with most of the rest of the country. Though French Guiana is about the size of Austria, it supports a population of only seventy-five thousand people, predominantly black descendants of slaves imported during the colonial era. Over 95 percent of the country's inhabitants live on the coast, which constitutes only about 20 percent of the landmass. The other 80 percent of the country is virgin rain forest, sparsely inhabited by indigenous Indian tribes and blacks.

By the time we arrived at the Hotel Montabo, an elegant inn on a hill overlooking Cayenne, night had fallen. We entered the lobby, threading our way around fashionably dressed French tourists to reach the desk clerk. We had made no reservations—Mittermeier had sworn reservations weren't necessary, but the clerk now shook his head. The employees of the space agency were on holiday, he announced, and the hotel was completely full. Not only were we out of luck at the Montabo, he said, but the only two other hotels in town were also completely booked.

Just then someone tapped Mittermeier on the shoulder. Behind us stood a short, barrel-chested Guianese wearing a red T-shirt and white cotton pants. His skin was so black it was almost blue and his mouth was filled with gold teeth that glinted each time he flashed his wide, rather cold smile. His eyes were hidden behind reflector shades. "My name is Gerard," he said in heavily accented English, "and I drive the taxi. Why don't I take you to the Hotel Imperial?" We were tired, hungry, dirty, and had no place to sleep; I considered Gerard a godsend. Mittermeier, on the other hand, had never heard of the Hotel Imperial and was a little suspicious. But since we had no alternatives, we climbed into the cab.

Gerard drove us into the city and down by the waterfront. He pulled up in front of an old building; faded white letters on the tired facade spelled out HOTEL IMPERIAL. "*Monsieurs, nous arrivons!*" the driver announced with an air of dignity. We paid Gerard, unloaded our backpacks, and went up to the hotel desk. An old yellow electric fan with mahogany blades swirled lazily overhead, slicing through the hot, sticky air. Outdated calendars featuring photos of scantily clad young women papered the walls behind the desk. Several tall, thin black men sat in the lobby, smoking unfiltered cigarettes.

Finally, a stout black man pulled aside a hanging curtain and stepped behind the desk from a room in the back. Another broad smile. "Welcome, gentlemen!" he exclaimed. "I have two excellent rooms for you!" We thanked him, but explained that we were two students traveling on a budget and could only afford one room for the two of us. The smile was immediately replaced with a stern, inhospitable expression. "Listen, monsieurs," he said, "we have two excellent rooms for you. We do not want any trouble or funny stuff here." This went back and forth a few times, with him offering us two luxury suites and we insisting that we could only pay for one room. Finally, Mittermeier pulled some money out of his pocket and put it on the counter, announcing that we were going upstairs for the evening and would leave the next day. The clerk, looking disgusted and a little uncertain, reluctantly gave us the key to a room.

We woke early and headed down to the village green—the Place des Palmistes—to get some breakfast. Sitting there in a small café, we could have been in any seaside village in France. A beautiful French waitress named Monique served us buttery croissants, fresh baguettes, Camembert cheese, and strong coffee with chicory. Signs on the wall advertised Kronenbourg beer and the latest French movies while the jukebox played Edith Piaf. Satellite engineers sat at a table next to us, computing with hand calculators and arguing loudly in Parisian French. On the other side sat several stone-faced, sunburned men dressed in the uniform of the French Foreign Legion. "The coast is basically France," explained Mittermeier, "but don't worry, the interior is the Amazon." We paid our check and headed into the marketplace to buy supplies.

Cayenne was built mostly in the 1700s. The narrow streets, thick gray stone walls, black wrought-iron balconies, and hidden patios with their gurgling fountains are strikingly reminiscent of the French Quarter in my hometown of New Orleans. The market, however, could only have been found in the tropics. Sturdy black women in calico dresses and colorful bandannas peddled everything from wood carvings to machetes to magical charms. Forest Indians sold squawking baby toucans as pets and Portuguese-speaking fishermen from Brazil were vending the morning's catch. But the most overwhelming aspect of the market was the panoply of extraordinary fruits: bittersweet *maracujas*, creamy Brazil nuts, the honey-sweet *inga* pods, and tart guavas.

In the far corner of the market I caught up with Mittermeier, who had somehow managed to find a guide for our upcoming excursion and was now buying hammocks. He told me to be sure to have a look at what they were selling in the next stall.

I turned to see the wildlife souvenir section of the market: ashtrays made of cobalt blue *Morpho* butterfly wings; artificial flowers fashioned from the feathers of the endangered scarlet ibis; bookmarks of boa constrictor hide; dried piranhas on little wooden stands; and stuffed baby caimans standing on their hind feet, dressed in bright pink pajamas and carrying pink parasols. What was most offensive was not seeing nature's creatures made into objets d'art—some carved elephant tusks rank among the world's greatest art treasures—but seeing so much of it done so pathetically. Then I saw the waist-high paper bags filled with dead parrots. The death toll was in the hundreds, and that was one day's harvest. "What are these for?" I asked incredulously. An enormous black woman who sat nearby replied, "I will stuff them and sell them to French tourists. If you come back early tomorrow, I will do a great big scarlet macaw just for you!"

By the time we finished buying hammocks, machetes, mosquito nets, a cooking pot, and food, including rice, crackers, and salted fish, it was after midday. Cayenne had begun to withdraw behind its shutters for the siesta hours; many of the stores had closed and few people were on the street. The heat and humidity began to take its toll on us and we ducked into a café for a couple of cold beers.

We drained the first round and were ready to order another. But the waitress's curt manner signaled she wanted to close the place up and head home until the heat of the day had passed. Most of the other patrons had already taken their leave. At the corner of the bar, however, sat a shriveled old Frenchman who showed no intention of leaving. Dressed in black and wearing a filthy gray beret, he was nursing a shot glass of liquor.

We called for the check. The waitress caught us staring at the old gentleman and said in a hushed voice, "*Le bagne, monsieur*"—the penal colony. What we were seeing was one of the last survivors of the hellhole that was known as Devil's Island.

In the mid-nineteenth century, the French were faced with the dilemma of what to do with French Guiana, their underpopulated, underdeveloped colony on the South American mainland. They hit upon a solution similar to that devised by the English for Australia: prisoners would be sent there. This would rid the mother country of undesirables and at the same time provide a steady influx of Frenchmen to increase the colony's population and thus ensure that the land would not be overtaken by the Brazilians to the south. Between 1852 and 1938, seventy thousand prisoners were shipped to the colony in cages aboard an old German freighter. In order to prevent riots and mutinies, the cages were fitted with steam valves to scald defiant prisoners, an ominous foreshadowing of the living hell for which they were destined.

In French Guiana, the prisoners were denied access to basic medical care and died slow, miserable deaths from dysentery, parasites, malaria, beriberi, elephantiasis, and other tropical diseases. Ruthless guards answered to no one and their knifings, torture, and murder of prisoners went unreported. So few men incarcerated on French Guiana survived the ordeal that Victor Hugo termed the place the "Dry Guillotine."

Although prisoners served their sentences in several different locations throughout the colony, the most hardened criminals were sent to three small islands ten miles off the northeast coast. Ile Royale was designated for the incorrigibles, St. Joseph housed those sentenced to solitary confinement, and Devil's Island was for political prisoners and those prone to escape attempts. Devil's Island is the smallest of the islands—only 1,300 by 440 yards—and is isolated from the others by treacherous currents. To deter escapes as much as to dispose of the dead, corpses of convicts were thrown into the channels around Devil's Island to keep the sharks in a near constant feeding frenzy. The island served as home to Alfred Dreyfus, unjustly accused of treason, and to Henri Charrière (better known as Papillon), who was sent to French Guiana for murdering a pimp. He claimed to have eventually escaped on a coconut raft.

The wretched souls serving time in French Guiana sometimes received a double sentence. If a person was condemned to serve ten years for manslaughter, he often had to spend an *extra* decade in French Guiana to prove that he was fully rehabilitated and ready to return to France. The end result, of course, was that by the time most of these sentences expired, the majority of the prisoners were either dead or so estranged from their families—physically and emotionally—that they elected to remain in French Guiana. The years of suffering and loneliness were deeply etched on the wizened face of our drinking companion.

We walked back to the hotel carrying our provisions for the voyage upriver. Mittermeier told the desk clerk that we planned to stay one more night, paid him in full, and we headed up to our room to pack for the upcoming departure. As we laid out our belongings to decide how best to consolidate the load, the door swung open. Leaning against the door frame was a beautiful mulatto woman, probably the descendant of black, Chinese, and French parentage. She had high cheekbones, straight black hair, and skin the color of café au lait. She was naked under an open silk robe that drifted over the curves of her body. She extended an invitation for us to visit her and her friends in the other rooms on the floor; they wished to welcome the American visitors to their country. Smiling mischievously, she shut the door behind her.

Mittermeier and I looked at each other and burst out laughing. The harder we laughed, the funnier it seemed, and we laughed until tears rolled down our faces. Finally Mittermeier asked, "Do you think Harvard will reimburse us when they find out we stayed in a bordello?"

The sun had not yet risen when we shouldered our backpacks and walked down to the waterfront. We were to rendezvous there with the guide Mittermeier had met in the market. The stalls that had bustled the day before were empty of all life, except for several vultures who fought noisily for a few pieces of offal.

At the edge of the market we saw Georges, our boatman. An immense black man, he wore only a small pair of red swimming trunks that all but disappeared under his enormous potbelly. An Australian bush hat was cocked at a jaunty angle on his head. *"Bonjour,"* said Georges, giving me a shy smile and a strong handshake. He said he was glad we both spoke some French, since he didn't speak any English, as he pointed us toward a boat slip at the edge of the market. Our transportation was a ten-foot dugout canoe with a nine-horsepower motor on the stern. When I realized that we were taking this little thing out into the Atlantic and then up the Kaw River to look for giant crocodilians, I looked at Mittermeier in dismay. "Are you nuts?"

He just smiled reassuringly and said, "Sorry, chief, the *Queen Mary* was all booked up. Get in!"

We loaded the canoe, untied the bowline, and Georges pushed us off with a broken wooden paddle. Once the water had deepened beneath us, he pulled the ignition cord several times until the engine turned over, and we putt-putted out into the ocean. The smell of salt filled our nostrils and a cold rain began to fall. Three-foot waves broke over the bow and water filled the boat. The little canoe was about as maneuverable as a cork in the rough waters. I leaned over the side, horribly seasick, and momentarily quit worrying about the crocodilians; sharks were a more immediate concern.

After about two hours, Georges tacked hard to the right and we entered the mouth of the Kaw River. The water was calm and the rain had ceased, yet an eerie mist shrouded everything around us. *"Bienvenue à la terre du caiman noir,"* said Georges. "Welcome to the land of the black caiman!"

When the fog lifted, I could see that the river was full of tiny eyes scanning the surface like little submarine periscopes. They belonged to four-eye fish, so named because their eyes are divided horizontally into upper and lower sections: the upper for vision above the water, the lower for seeing underwater. These curious eyes are the perfect adaptation for life in the muddy estuaries where the four-eye fish thrives, constantly searching for floating insects. So buoyant are their eyes, according to Georges, that the fish cannot swim underwater for long without popping to the surface. And when they are frightened (as he demonstrated by throwing a stick overboard), the four-eyes frantically skitter along atop the water, like inept flying fish who never quite manage a takeoff.

The trees lining the riverbank slowly emerged from the vapor; short ones, tall ones, massive ones, skinny ones, flowering ones, and dead ones wrestled and tangled in a silent struggle to reach the life-giving sunlight denied them on the shadowy forest floor. The vegetation was dense and unimaginably diverse—trees, herbs, fungi, stranglers, orchids, ferns, climbers, bushes, lichens, and mosses. All this, and we had not yet been inside the jungle.

It is the warm and wet conditions of the rain forest that spawn so many different forms of life. In this natural greenhouse of high rainfall and high humidity, plants and animals can grow and reproduce all year long; there is no winter to brutally disrupt the life cycle. In the temperate zone, animals and plants not only have to compete against each other for survival, but must also struggle against a cold season in which they forgo growth, reproduction, and sometimes even feeding.

Another factor contributing to the abundance of tropical life-forms is the age of the rain forest ecosystem. Rain forests have thrived for millions of years, allowing new species to constantly evolve. Over time, the climate has undergone changes, including extended periods of wet and dry weather. During dry periods, the rain forests split from a single extended forest into forest islands separated by savannas; new species evolved on these islands. When the wet periods came, the rain forest islands rejoined, and the net result was more plant and animal species.

The great diversity of what biologists refer to as microhabitats also plays a part in the rapid creation of new species. Microhabitats are small, specialized environments, usually isolated from other, similar environments. In a tall forest tree, for example, you might find five microhabitats. The very top of the tree, which is exposed to weather and wind, may support a small number of tiny epiphytes (the so-called "air plants" that derive nutrients and moisture from air, rain, and debris). Just below this is a zone protected from the elements; it might be dominated by larger epiphytes. Below this area is the driest part of the tree trunk, which would be covered with gray and green lichens. Below that, the next microhabitat typically features lush growth of mosses and lichens. The final area, at the base of the trunk (especially if the tree has large, planklike buttress roots, which typically help anchor the larger trees in the rain forest), would support luxuriant moss growth, particularly in the shady recesses between the buttresses themselves.

Each of these five microhabitats is home to a different group of insects, amphibians, or other creatures. And, like the proverbial Chinese boxes, each species within a microhabitat may harbor its own micro-microhabitat. For example, some mites thrive only in the nasal passages of a single species of jungle parrot and occur nowhere else in the world. In this manner, diversity begets diversity.

Mittermeier asked Georges to steer the boat over to where a huge fig tree grew out over the river. As we glided underneath, Mittermeier pulled out his machete and lopped off a low-hanging branch. Growing on the end of the branch, in what had been the elbow where the branch met the trunk, was a plant that looked like the top of a pineapple. Mittermeier explained that this was known as a "tank bromeliad" because of the constantly water-filled, cup-shaped depression in the center of the plant. This "tank" served as the centerpiece of an entire miniature ecosystem. In the pool I could see tiny white wriggling mosquito larvae and little gray-black tadpoles.

Mittermeier pointed out that in addition to the two species we were seeing, these tanks were known to support algae, protozoans, dragonfly larvae, and numerous other insects. These microhabitats also serve as home to salamanders, snakes, and frogs, some of which are unique to this habitat. In return, the bromeliads derive their nutrition from the excretions and decomposing remains of the species that live within the tank. One study in Costa Rica found that animals living in or dependent on one type of bromeliad totaled over 250 species! I was gaining a new appreciation for the interdependence of tropical plants and animals.

We rounded a bend in the river, setting off a tremendous commotion—screeching and flapping unlike anything I had ever heard before. We looked up to see three large birds about the size of pheasants sitting on the branches of a dead tree. They were clumsy, smelly, and looked like a cross between a chicken and a pterodactyl.

Known as hoatzins, these birds have long brown and orange tail feathers, brownish white chests, and a crest of scraggly brown and orange feathers. Most striking, though, are their tiny heads, highlighted by smooth, bright blue facial skin and luminous red eyes. Extremely awkward fliers, the birds responded to our approach by screeching and halfheartedly attempting to hop into the nearby bushes.

Just then Mittermeier pointed out several baby hoatzins who had

dived into the river at our approach. As they returned to their parents'
tree, they climbed up using not only their feet but also a bizarre pair
of claws near the end of each wing! They looked like living versions of
archaeopteryx, the earliest known bird, which arose during the late Ju-
rassic almost 200 million years ago and also possessed wing claws.
Mittermeier assured me that we were not seeing a living archaeopteryx
but rather an odd and distant relative of the cuckoo. Nevertheless, the
hoatzin is one of the world's most ancient birds, believed to have evolved
originally somewhere between 26 million and 54 million years ago. Our
encounter with the hoatzins only added to the antediluvian air that permeated the ecosystem surrounding us.

Once we had passed the hoatzins, Mittermeier detailed the less en-
dearing aspects of the object of our search, the black caiman. One of
the largest predators in the Amazon basin, the black caiman reaches a
length of over thirty feet and is known to eat human flesh. When the
great British naturalist Henry Walter Bates was traveling in the Brazilian Amazon in the mid-1800s, he witnessed a particularly grisly epi-
sode:

A large trading canoe arrived at [the town of Caicara] and the crew,
as usual, spent the first day or two after their coming into port, in
drunkenness and debauchery ashore. One of the men, during the
greatest heat of the day, when almost everyone was enjoying his
afternoon's nap, took it into his head whilst in a tipsy state to go
down alone to bathe. He was seen only by . . . a feeble old man
who was lying in his hammock . . . who shouted to the besotted
Indian to beware of the black caiman. Before he could repeat his
warning, the man stumbled, and a pair of gaping jaws, appearing
suddenly above the surface, seized him around the waist and drew
him under the water. A cry of agony "Ai Jesus!" was the last sign
made by the wretched victim. The village was aroused: the young
men with praiseworthy readiness seized their harpoons and hurried
down to the bank; but of course it was too late, a winding track of
blood on the surface of the water was all that could be seen. They
embarked, however, in canoes, determined on vengeance: the monster was traced, and when, after a short lapse of time, he came up

to breathe—one leg of the man sticking out from his jaws—he was dispatched with bitter curses.

We had come to French Guiana to learn whether the black caiman lived in this area. According to the current zoological thinking, these crocodilians flourished only in the Amazon basin proper, south of the Guianas (Guyana, Suriname, and French Guiana), which are at least partially separated from the Amazon by the Tumuc-Humac Mountain Range. Although the Guianas are considered to be part of Greater Amazonia by most scientific authorities, there are species of both plants and animals that occur in the Amazon basin but are not found in the Guianas. Because the black caiman is all but extinct in many parts of its original range, finding a healthy population that could be protected by establishing a wildlife sanctuary would be an excellent way to ensure the survival of the species.

During previous expeditions to French Guiana, Mittermeier heard tales that "*le caiman noir*" had been sighted in an isolated part of the interior. He had managed to track down the source of these rumors—an ex-hunter turned conservationist. While purists might disdain ex-hunters who have seen the light and decided to protect the animals they once ardently pursued, history has shown that these individuals sometimes evolve into the most impassioned and effective conservationists (Theodore Roosevelt and his contemporary William Hornaday, who became director of the Bronx Zoo, being notable examples). Furthermore, professional hunters, by economic necessity, tend to know their animals, so when Mittermeier heard that it was a "great white hunter" claiming that the caimans occurred in French Guiana, he felt an exploratory trip was worthwhile.

Some find it difficult to understand why anyone would want to study and protect endangered crocodilians, which are hated and feared in many parts of the world. These creatures are reptiles, after all, symbols of evil, the cause of our fall from grace in the Garden of Eden. They are huge, violent machines, programmed to kill. They maim or slaughter without fear of retribution.

The attitudes of nineteenth-century European settlers in the Amazon reflected this antireptile bias. Henry Walter Bates described how this feeling manifested itself on a boat trip in Brazil:

> During a journey of five days which I once made on the upper
> Amazon steamer . . . [black caiman] were seen along the coast
> almost every step of the way, and the passengers amused them-
> selves, from morning till night, by firing at them with rifle and ball.

In the 1860s, Bates wrote that in the Amazon black caimans were as
common as tadpoles in an English pond. But because of the excellent
quality of its hide, the black caiman was hunted to the brink of extinction by commercial interests. As recently as 1950, the Brazilian state
of Pará exported 5 million black caiman skins. The scale of the slaughter was best described in the early 1970s by the late Colombian her-
petologist Federico Medem, who wrote that overhunting "resulted in
such a wholesale slaughter that the lower reaches of the river stank for
weeks. . . . A single caiman hunter obtained some 5,000 skins."

The result of this overexploitation has been the near disappearance
of the species. When Mittermeier traveled throughout the Brazilian Amazon in the 1970s, he saw only *one* black caiman in eight years.

As conservationists, our particular interest in this species stemmed
from the belief that the decline in the black caiman population has had
a deleterious effect on the people of the Amazon. Fish serves as the
major source of protein for the Amazonian people. Paradoxically, after
most of the black caimans had been exterminated in Brazil, there was
a serious decline in the populations of edible fish. Much of the Amazon
is nutrient-poor, and the German ecologist E. J. Fittkau hypothesized
that black caimans originally played the role of "nutrient-concentra-
tors." The reptiles made their homes in the lakes and swamps off the
main body of the river and great concentrations of their excrement represented the major food source for plankton at the base of the food
chain. These backwaters also served as egg-laying sites for fishes whose
hatchlings preyed on the microorganisms feeding on the caimans' waste.
When the caimans were wiped out, these natural fish hatcheries also
disappeared. This proved to be yet another vivid example of the extraordinary interrelationships of tropical nature, and how human inter-
vention not only had a negative impact on the ecosystem as a whole but
on human welfare as well.

As our boat pressed on, I began to realize how much I had under-
estimated our Creole boatman. Georges had originally struck me as a

good-natured, roly-poly city boy who had borrowed a friend's boat to play tour guide and earn some pocket money. To the contrary, in the course of our journey he proved to be an excellent naturalist. He was able to identify all of the animals by their calls. At one point Georges told us to be sure to get a look at the scarlet ibis that liked to nest in the dead tree around the next bend in the river. We made the turn, and there they were—the reddest birds I had ever seen, sitting among the branches of a gray laurel tree, looking like ornaments in a Christmas pine. Their feathers were such a vivid and intense red that they seemed unreal.

And then the silence of the river was torn by two deafening explosions right behind us. Mittermeier and I pitched forward in fright, our hands covering our ears. Turning around, we saw our boatman with a shotgun at his shoulder. He smiled and pointed at a spot slightly in front of the canoe. Two scarlet ibis, blasted out of the tree, were making a futile effort to stay afloat. The magnificent animals, who only moments before were part of the most beautiful scene I had ever witnessed, now looked like broken and discarded toys encircled by feathers and blood.

Mittermeier and I were speechless. But Georges cut the engine, paddled the canoe closer to the birds, and dropped them into the boat at his feet. "My dinner!" he said with a sheepish smile, and we continued up the river.

As we chugged along, Mittermeier sat in the bow on the lookout for a black caiman. Suddenly he motioned back to Georges to cut the engine. Mittermeier looked over the bow, his eyes widened, and then he dove into the river. I remember thinking that he had lost his mind. Up to this point we both had had our doubts about the existence of the black caiman in French Guiana, but I thought that he chose far too personal a method for testing this hypothesis.

Mittermeier broke the surface of the river with a howl of glee and tossed a huge turtle into the boat. I recognized it as a matamata, a grotesque species native to the Amazon basin. It had a flattened head, an elongated snorkellike proboscis, tiny eyes, a seemingly jolly smile, three ridges that ran the length of its shell, and long flaps of skin hanging off its head.

Peacefully entrenched on the bottom of a river, baby matamatas look like dead leaves and the adults resemble old automobile tires. The turtle's diet consists almost entirely of fish, which it catches in an extraordinary manner. The turtle's lower jaw is a thin bar of cartilage. When a fish approaches to feed on what it believes to be a piece of decomposing vegetation, the matamata drops its jaw, creating a powerful vacuum that sucks the unsuspecting victim down the turtle's throat.

It was easy to understand Mittermeier's joy in finding the matamata. Like the black caiman, the matamata is an Amazonian species that is not supposed to occur in French Guiana. Mittermeier hypothesized that there had been a sort of "leakage" of Amazonian flora and fauna into eastern French Guiana. The easternmost range of the Tumuc-Humac Mountains did not extend all the way to the coast, and perhaps allowed a northern migration of Amazonian creatures into the region. We headed upriver with a growing sense of anticipation.

By now the sun was directly overhead. The heat and humidity were oppressive; we could take off our shirts and fry in the sun or leave them on and bake. We emptied our canteens over our heads to cool off, all the while scanning the river's edge for signs of the giant reptiles. From sitting through endless Tarzan movies as a child, I had expected to see these animals slyly sunning themselves on the riverbank, ready to plunge into the water and attack our boat.

After navigating a sharp turn in the river, Georges beached the canoe on a small sandy shelf and tied the bowline to the stump of a dead guava tree. Inviting us to follow, he hiked up a trail into a patch of riverine forest to check several bird traps that he had set earlier in the week. Still slightly traumatized by our encounter with the scarlet ibis, I declined the invitation and stayed with the boat. Mittermeier went with him.

One of the best ways to observe wildlife is to remain perfectly still. Nature is a constantly changing mosaic and animals are always on the move. But the sighting of a potential predator will cause many animals to freeze until the intruder has been evaluated and judged nonthreatening. Silence and stillness can convince hidden creatures that they are not in danger and they will then go about their business.

I sat on the sand, savoring a gentle breeze that blew across the river and rippled the surface of the water. Green dragonflies played tag on the sand and a huge bumblebee buzzed past. Dark tadpoles swarmed in the shallows. A flock of yellow-headed vultures flew lazy figure-eights to the south, marking the presence of carrion. As I watched the vultures soar, I picked up a blurry movement out of the corner of my eye on the other side of the river. Something was moving in my direction through the waist-high grass.

My first thought was that it might be a caiman and I should find a tree and head skyward. Before I could move, the vegetation parted and a tapir stepped onto the beach and began to drink, totally unaware of my presence across the river.

With the body of a pig, the hooves of a horse, the ears of a hippo, and the snout of a rhinoceros, the tapir looks like it was pieced together from spare parts found in a taxidermist's attic. An adult tapir may weigh over a quarter of a ton, making it the largest mammal in the South American rain forest. Considered a delicacy by the Indians, this gentle—and usually nocturnal—animal has been exterminated in many areas. Consequently, tapirs are very shy and it is rare to see them come into an open area. I felt I had traveled through a wrinkle in time, watching nature before it had been spoiled by the hand of humankind.

Again the grass on the riverbank parted and the tapir's baby trotted down to the water's edge. Adult tapirs are a buff-gray color, but the youngsters are a warm brown with whitish yellow spots and stripes down their sides. I was glad that Georges and his shotgun were elsewhere.

About twenty minutes later, Mittermeier and Georges returned. Having found his traps empty, Georges was singing a vivid and profane set of curses in his lilting Creole patois. With one look at the smirk on Mittermeier's face, I could see that he shared my secret glee that Georges had come up empty-handed. We climbed into the boat and set off.

Hour after hour, we continued upriver. The sun was merciless, and the boat was too slow to generate enough of a breeze to keep us cool. I tied my kerchief into a headband to keep the pouring sweat out of my eyes. The pace and relentless heat made us feel as if we had been traveling for days, even though we had left Cayenne less than eight hours before. Suddenly Georges cut the engine to neutral. Ahead, a large and mysterious object was slowly floating toward us. "*Voyez la,*" said Georges softly. "Look there!"

"What is it? What's there?" I asked in my halting French.

*"C'est un caiman noir!"*

Our adrenaline was pumping as the crocodilian drifted closer and closer. The animal was dead, floating belly-up, and its magnitude—it was almost twice the length of the boat—was such that it looked more like a deceased dinosaur than an extant species. Georges paddled the boat alongside and we looked for a spear or gunshot wound, since an animal this size has no natural enemies. The smooth, pearly white scales of the belly skin were unmarked, as were the glistening, thick ebony scales that covered the head, sides, and back. Since no wound was evident, we concluded that we were witnessing something rare in nature—an animal that had died of natural causes. We were so awed by the sight of the beast that all we could do was stare. Even the birds stopped calling, as if in deference to the demise of this king of the jungle river.

The squawking of a striated heron broke the silence. Remembering that we were there to collect scientific data instead of gawk, Mittermeier pulled out our tape measure. But it was so small and the reptile so large and unmaneuverable, it proved all but impossible to measure the caiman from inside the boat. Neither one of us wanted to jump into the river and we were puzzling over what to do next when Georges came to the rescue.

Taking the little tape measure, the boatman used it to measure his paddle, which was exactly four and a half feet long. We now had a yardstick with which to measure our find from inside the boat. Putting the paddle next to the crocodilian was like holding a pencil against the side of a barn; only then did the dimensions of the beast begin to fully register. The Age of Reptiles was supposed to have ended over 100 million years ago but, looking at the twenty-foot behemoth floating next to our boat, we were not so sure. A black caiman that size could have risen up out of the river, pulled any one of us out of the canoe, and in the blink of an eye set off for its lair—something that we knew had happened to a hapless Indian fisherman in Peru the year before.

Mittermeier informed Georges that we wanted to remove the skull as a specimen for our museum. This process, especially with an animal this size, is a difficult and unpleasant task at best, and the flooded grasslands were an inconvenient laboratory. Georges rolled his eyes both to indicate his opinion of our dim-wittedness and to say that he did not want any part of this foul-smelling creature in his boat. Faced with the prospect of a clash with the captain, we reluctantly abandoned our prize. Looking back over my shoulder, I could see the corpse of the great caiman continuing its journey to the sea, fodder for the sharks waiting hungrily at the mouth of the Kaw River.

We continued on, exhilarated by our find. The primary purpose of the expedition was to determine whether the black caiman occurred in the Guianas; we had confirmed the rumor. Just as we started to relax a bit, Georges, as seemed to be his wont, jolted us out of our lethargy. We came to a sharp bend in the river, and the boatman cut the engine and pointed ahead. "There is a huge *caiman noir* that lives nearby. Keep a sharp lookout!" When Georges said huge, he meant that the animal was well over twenty feet—he had not been impressed with the monster we had just encountered. As we rounded the bend, we heard a loud splash and watched a wave break along the bank. But despite our efforts, we never caught sight of the beast.

Several hours later we reached Georges's village, which sat on a slightly elevated patch of riverbank at the edge of a forested hill. The village of Kaw consists of approximately twenty buildings and is home to about sixty Creoles, black descendants of slaves freed in the latter part of the nineteenth century. The architecture struck me as an odd mixture of the primitive and the modern—thatched huts with aluminum roofs mingled with wooden buildings with thatched roofs. I later learned that such blending is not uncommon where the jungle meets up with our "civilization."

Georges beached the canoe on the sandy riverbank and we unloaded our gear. Our guide pointed us to a hut, and it seemed we were given the best accommodations—a wooden building with an aluminum roof. What we found, though, was that this modern edifice soaked up the sun's heat during the day and radiated it into the hut all night. And when it rained, the noise level exceeded that of a hailstorm.

Georges unloaded his paraphernalia from the canoe; the most highly prized item was a sack of salt to be divided carefully among the villagers. Once the cargo had been removed, he reached under his seat in the canoe and pulled out a round aluminum canister about the size of a tuna fish can. Opening the container, he poured a thick ebony liquid into his cupped palm and quickly snorted it up his right nostril.

Georges's eyes rolled back in his head and he seemed on the verge of going into convulsions. A few minutes later, he smiled sweetly, adjusted his cap, and began to carry the last of his supplies up to the village.

"Georges," I asked, trotting after him, "what was that?"

"Oh," he replied matter-of-factly, "that was from the *mahot cochon* plant."

"But what does it do?"

"It makes you go nuts for three minutes!" With that cryptic reply, punctuated by a lopsided grin, he headed off to his hut.

Back in the hut, Mittermeier and I unpacked our equipment, slung our hammocks, and dined on stale crackers and canned sardines. As darkness fell, Georges came over to make sure we were comfortable and to tell us that if we wanted to see really *big* caimans—not like the adolescent we had seen that afternoon—the *best* way would be to go looking for them under the full moon. I remember feeling that the *safest* way to search for them would be in a nuclear submarine, but I kept the thought to myself.

Exhausted by a long, hot, productive day, we crawled into our hammocks and, although the sun had just begun to set, within minutes we fell asleep. We did not wake up until late the next morning, and the village was already bustling with activity. Most of the men (including Georges) had gone fishing, something they did three or four days a week, since fish was their major source of protein. The children were washing and playing at the river's edge. The women were stoking their cooking fires and several of the older girls sat in a circle, weaving baskets and singing a beautiful song in a call-and-response pattern. A few of the older men had decided to forgo the fishing trip and divided their time between caulking their canoes and telling hunting stories.

I was happy to remain in the village and absorb this completely alien culture, but Mittermeier said his Teutonic ancestry did not allow him the luxury of "laying about and doing nothing" and insisted on hiking into the jungle to look for monkeys. Delighted by the prospect of seeing the rain forest from the inside, I readily agreed and off we went.

In their personal accounts, the early explorer-naturalists invariably compare entering the great rain forests to stepping into a cathedral. The enormous tree trunks resemble nothing so much as great stone pillars and the thick green canopy arches high overhead like a vaulted ceiling.

The enormity of it all emphasizes the insignificance of human beings. The forest is not as dark as some accounts led me to believe; the shafts of light that penetrate the thatching of leaves at the forest top are like the beams that stream through stained-glass windows on a sunny afternoon. The forest glows a warm, luminous green. Perhaps the emotions it evokes were best summed up by Prussian explorer Richard Schomburgk in 1867:

> All the pictures my imagination had painted in anticipation of the impression of a virgin forest would make on me sank like faded shadows into insignificance before the sublime reality that discloses itself on entering it!

The forest floor was covered with moist, decaying brown and black leaves, and here and there I saw pieces of dead wood, covered with white, wood-rotting fungi. Small and sporadic patches of tiny, feathery selaginella moss made the only greenery; obviously most of the life-giving direct sunlight was being absorbed by the leaves in the canopy high above our heads.

Lianas, woody vines as thick as my wrist that ran from the canopy down to the ground and sometimes back up again, crept everywhere like giant threads that somehow wove the forest together. Mittermeier pointed out how poor the soil was—in some places it seemed to be little more than white sand—and noted that the luxuriance of the vegetation had fooled some of the early explorers into believing that these must be among the richest soils on earth. In fact, the opposite is often the case. "Rain forests," Mittermeier observed, "are sometimes literally castles built on sand." The secret of the jungle, he explained, is that it is a closed ecosystem. Instead of rich mineral soils, the ground here is ancient and weathered and the minerals are almost all locked in the vegetation itself. When leaves fall or plants die, the decomposition is incredibly rapid and the nutrients are sucked right back up into the ecosystem. This is the major reason why a large tract of rain forest, once cleared, never regenerates. The nutrients are released into this dreadful soil and, instead of being absorbed by the vegetation, they are soon washed away by heavy tropical rains. Even when the rain forest is felled on a small scale, it may never return to its original form with a full complement of species. The jungles around Angkor Wat in Cambodia were cut down over five hundred years ago and today the existing forest is still not as species-rich as the original, primary forest.

As we moved on, a certain stillness seemed to permeate the forest. Little happens at midday because of the heat. Most of the movement—hunting, foraging, and feeding—takes place in the early morning or late afternoon hours. Apparently the siesta is enjoyed by all creatures of the tropics.

One exception was a column of reddish brown ants on the march at the edge of the trail. Clasped tightly in each of their mandibles and held high above their heads was a fragment of green leaf, a practice that earned them their common names: leaf-cutter or parasol ants. These industrious insects collect leaves throughout the forest and carry them back to their underground nests. There the ants chew the leaf fragments into a pulp on which they cultivate a fungus; this fungus serves as their dietary staple. To manage their fungal gardens, the ants weed out undesirable species of fungi, fertilize their crops with fecal material, and are believed to produce antibiotics to keep out undesirable bacteria and hormones to accelerate fungal growth. A single colony may be home to well over a million ants and may entail displacement of over twenty cubic meters of soil. Apparently the ants cannot live without the fungi; nor can the fungi survive without the ants.

Mittermeier explained that this type of plant-animal interdependency is more the rule than the exception in the rain forest. Pollination, for example, which is simply the movement of pollen from the male to the female part of the flower, usually involves an external agent such as wind or insects. There is, however, little wind inside the rain forest and the tropical plants often rely on animals to move things around for them. Rain forest species do not just depend on bees for this assistance but also manage to entice flies, beetles, bats, lemurs, moths, birds, butterflies, and even rodents.

This mutually beneficial collaboration between a species of plant and a species of animal, called a pollination relationship, almost belongs in the realm of science fiction. The brown-and-white-mottled Amazonian *Gongora* orchid produces an intoxicating substance that attracts and befuddles the bee that visits the flower. The orchid is shaped so that the inebriated bee then falls onto a part of the flower, where it both deposits the pollen it carried from another *Gongora* and picks up new pollen.

The *Gongora*'s knockout drop by no means represents the most manipulative nor the most perverse approach to pollination. In the 1984 classic *Tropical Nature*, entomologist Adrian Forsyth writes that some orchids "play on the indiscriminate lust of male tachinid flies by mimicking females." From a certain angle, the color patterns of the orchid and its leaf shape resemble the female fly and, according to Forsyth, "when the male attempts to copulate with the pseudofemale, he actually pollinates the orchid."

Some of the compounds produced by both temperate and tropical plants to attract pollinators have been used by humans for tens of thousands of years. An excellent example is the essential oils, also known as volatile oils, that are often produced by a plant to attract animal pollinators and that serve humankind as perfumes and spices.

There is no way of knowing exactly when people first began using spices and perfumes. The earliest records date back to the dawn of the Old Kingdom (2575 B.C.) in the Egypt of the pharaohs. The ancient Egyptians used perfumes for aesthetic purposes, such as masking body odor; as offerings to the gods, in the form of burning incense; and in embalming their dead in the process of mummification. Spices and perfumes were considered commodities of paramount importance to the ancients, as evidenced by the numerous references to them in the Bible, the Torah, *The Iliad*, and *The Odyssey*. In ancient Greece, wealthy denizens were said to have a different perfume for each part of the body. The Romans also made wide use of perfumes, incenses, and scented oils, while introducing their spices to the conquered peoples of Germany and Great Britain. New perfumes and spices were brought to Europe when the knights returned from the Crusades in the eleventh and twelfth centuries. One of their most popular introductions was rose water, which proved highly desirable among the nobility for rinsing the hands after eating. (Soap was still considered a luxury and forks would not be invented for another three hundred years.)

Spices played a more utilitarian role in the ancient world, being used to prevent food from spoiling, to improve the taste of food that had already started to putrefy, and to add zest to monotonous diets. And like perfumes, spices were used in the embalming process in ancient

Egypt. So great was the demand for spices among the ancients that it was a powerful motivation for opening trade routes to other parts of the world. The discovery of America was not the result of intellectual curiosity but rather Columbus's search for a shorter route to the Spice Islands. Vasco da Gama's pioneering voyage around the southern tip of Africa sprang from a similar desire. Although much of the spice trade between Europe and tropical Asia was first established by the Portuguese, the Dutch proved the more adept capitalists and took control of this business from the seventeenth century until the late eighteenth century. The development of the British navy, and in some ways the rise of the British Empire, grew out of Great Britain's attempt to break the Dutch monopoly of the spice trade. As a result of all this exploration and commercial one-upmanship, we now commonly use numerous spices derived from tropical plant compounds, including allspice, chile pepper, cardamom, cinnamon, cloves, nutmeg, mace, turmeric, vanilla, and paprika.

By now it was late afternoon; the forest was just starting to cool down from the midday heat and the ecosystem was waking up. A noisy flock of brown-throated parakeets passed high over our heads. Mittermeier pointed out fresh tracks that had been made by capybaras, giant rodents that weigh in at over a hundred pounds and are usually found in or near the water. "If we keep walking, we may find these capybaras," he said, "but if we're going to look for caimans tonight, we should probably return to the village and wait for Georges."

When we arrived, we found Georges waiting for us on an old tree stump. He wore gym shorts and, as always, was shirtless. In a moment of sartorial panache, he had placed a red parrot feather in the brim of his hat.

"I caught some *ayumara* fish," he said, "and my wife will cook them for us. Do you want to look for caimans or would you rather wait until tomorrow night?"

Ever the Teuton, Mittermeier said, "Let's go!"

We walked down to the river and climbed into the canoe. I almost sat on George's shotgun. "What are you going to need this for?" I asked. "It'll be dark soon and you won't see any birds."

"It is not for birds, *mon cher*," he responded. "It is for *le caiman noir*."

Mittermeier said, "Hey, Georges, I thought you said you didn't hunt black caiman."

"It is not to hunt them. It is to—how do you say?—*discourage* them!" With that he gunned the engine and we turned upriver.

Ahead of us, several small silvery fish were jumping out of the water. Turning a bend in the river, we spooked a white heron standing on the bank and it flew along just in front of us, then veered off into the vegetation. As the sun set, the croaking of unseen frogs became so loud it all but drowned out the noise made by the little engine.

I leaned back and asked Georges, "Do you know if any of these plants we see along the river here can be used as medicines?"

"I don't think so," he replied. "But the person you really need to ask is my grandmother."

Georges cut the engine and we drifted toward the starboard shore. "What's up? What do you see?" asked Mittermeier. I craned my neck forward, looking for some new zoological peculiarity.

"Look!" said Georges. "A *wapa!*"

Thinking he was describing some animal, I kept scanning the bank. "Where?" I asked.

"There!" he said, pointing to a dark brown tree with an odd, bumpy bark. From the tips of the branches hung elongated, flattened fruits characteristic of the legume family.

"What's that?" I asked.

"I already told you!" said Georges. "It's a *wapa* tree!"

"Is it used for something?"

"Yes. When I was a little boy and got a toothache, my grandmother would make tea from the bark and it would stop the pain."

I took out a little notepad and recorded this tidbit of ethnobotanical lore, figuring that I should try to meet his grandmother if I decided to come back and focus on collecting plants.

"I tied up to this tree to fish today," said Georges.

"Why's that?"

"Because when the fish hear the fruit explode, they come to eat the seeds," he replied.

"He must be kidding," I said to Mittermeier in English. But apparently he wasn't. Mittermeier replied that although there is an audible *pop* when certain fruits explode and scatter the seeds, he felt the fish were responding to vibrations that resulted from fruit striking the surface of the water. "In Brazil," he said, "I have seen fishermen using a lure called a *gaponga*, which is a weight tied to the end of a line and pole. The weight is repeatedly dropped on the surface of the river in imitation of the sound of falling fruit, and the fishermen spear the fish that surface expecting to find—rather than be turned into—a meal."

Plants must find some means of moving their fruits and seeds away from the parent plant to maintain a healthy distribution of the species. As they do with pollination, plants often rely on animals to disperse their seeds and fruits—animals such as ants, birds, bats, monkeys, turtles, and even elephants. Although some animals defy the plants' intentions and digest the seed, thus eliminating the possibility of the plant reproducing itself, many fruits are designed so that the animal devours the fruit whole, digests the nutritious pulp, and expels the seed unharmed. The seed then generates, often in a pile of fertilizer. So intricately linked are the lives of some plants and animals that in some cases a seed will not germinate until it has been passed through the gut of a particular animal!

From my seat in the bow, I could see the blue-gray river ahead of us and the flooded green and yellow grasslands that stretched for miles on both sides, alternating with areas of verdant forest. On the far horizons rose the Kaw Mountains, covered with unexplored rain forest. Darkness was falling quickly now, and a full moon soon shone overhead. Within a few minutes we were in the dead of night and the light of the moon cast ghostly shadows as it filtered through the leaves of the arching trees. The forest that lined the riverbanks, raucous and vital during the day, now gave off a slight air of mystery. Most of the animals had already gone to sleep; the howler monkeys had long ceased calling to each other to mark their nesting trees. But other creatures were in the middle of their day. Fish-eating bats hovered above the river's surface, ready to dive-bomb their prey. Luminous insects flew lazy patterns at the forest's edge. Frogs hooted and honked. The night sky was spectacularly clear and entire galaxies seemed to hang just above our heads. The smells of the jungle wafted across the river, and I felt like we were on a timeless boat ride through an earthly paradise.

Georges cut the engine and pointed his flashlight at the water just ahead of the boat. A golden eye reflected the beam. We coasted forward and, just when it seemed we would float past the animal, Georges's hand shot into the river, grabbed the creature, and threw it into the boat. It was a spectacled caiman, a crocodilian found throughout tropical America and so named because of a protrusion on its snout thought to resemble pince-nez. Although some caimans reach a length of six feet, most are considerably smaller—this one was only about two feet long. He made a great show of snapping his jaws and leaping about, but the little creature was relatively harmless. Mittermeier expertly grabbed the animal behind the head, measured and weighed it with equipment he carried in his backpack, recorded the data, and then released the reptile into the river unharmed.

Four species of crocodilian inhabit the Kaw River: the black caiman, the spectacled caiman, and two varieties of dwarf forest caimans that are red in hue. Besides their skin color and size, the species are distinguishable by the color their eyes reflect in the glare of a flashlight. The spectacled caiman has a yellow iris, the dwarf forest caimans have orange irises, and the black caiman has a ruby-red iris, giving it a malevolent look. When we saw a yellow or orange iris gleaming back at us in the glare of the flashlight, we knew the animal was smaller than we were; when we saw that red glow, I secretly hoped the beast would sink out of sight before the boat got too close.

This night we spotted seven crocodilians, including two black caimans. Once we learned how to find the animals in the glare of our flashlight, the routine was set: locate a white, orange, or small red eye, motor over and pick up the animal for measurement, then release it; see a big red eye, motor toward it . . . and watch it slowly sink out of sight. Georges explained that it was this shyness that allowed the black caimans to get so big; animals that remained afloat as boats approached soon fell prey to the skin merchant. Nonetheless, he said, large black caimans were known to snatch the unwary out of canoes, although this happened only rarely. Usually, a large black caiman will retreat rather than attack.

At one point, we rounded a bend in the river and saw a huge red eye in the distance. We headed toward it, waiting for it to submerge. The eye remained still in the glare of my flashlight, fixing me with a baleful stare. I concluded that it must have been a juvenile, since it stubbornly ignored my unspoken desire for it to sink. It began to move straight toward me. Precariously perched in the bow of the boat, I let out a terrified yell and scrambled for the shotgun behind me. In my mind I could see a pair of huge black jaws rising out of the river to pull me down into the cold and muddy depths.

My mad scramble almost turned the boat over, but Georges's only response was a loud peal of laughter. A soft humming filled my ears as the red eye continued to approach, but now I could discern the soft patois of the fishermen whose boat was headed in our direction. On the bow of their canoe they had hung a red lantern to attract the fish they sought that night.

We were out so late that night, we slept through much of the next day. We were awakened by a knock at the door; outside stood Georges's wife, a short, squat Creole woman in a faded blue cotton dress. She smiled shyly and silently handed us an aluminum pot full of boiled fish. Having lived off of canned sardines for two days, we devoured this gift and then wandered down to the river for a wash. It was already midday and most of the villagers were taking their siestas; the little bathing beach formed by a sandbank was empty when we arrived. I was not particularly anxious to get into the water, given the reptiles that we knew existed there, so I stuck to the shallows. Once done with my bath, I walked to the edge of the sandbank and plunked myself down at the foot of a beautiful tree. It was about sixty feet tall with smooth greenish gray bark and high, narrow buttresses. At the end of the branches hung long white bunches of pale green flowers.

Mittermeier squatted at the edge of the river, busily washing a filthy pair of socks. He looked over his shoulder to tell me something and an alarmed look spread across his face. "Don't lean against that!" he said.

"What?" I asked, drowsy in the midday heat.

"Don't lean against that tree!"

I sat up with a start and looked around, expecting to see a giant black caiman sunning itself behind the trunk.

Mittermeier walked over and pointed to a horde of little brown ants running down from the crown of the tree to investigate the intruder—me!

"I don't know what they call this species here, but it's one of those damn ant trees," said Mittermeier.

"What's an ant tree?" I asked as I scrambled to my feet.

"These are plants that have coevolved with species of ants for their mutual benefit. The trees often have hollow stems in which the ants live and raise their young. Some plants go so far as to have developed specialized structures that produce nutrient-rich solutions on which the ants feed. In return, the ants viciously attack insects or other intruders that might damage the tree," Mittermeier explained. "Some ants also devour vines, stranglers, and lianas that climb onto their host plant. In the most extreme cases, the insects clear away all vegetation within a several-foot radius. Debris from the ant nests inside the tree fertilize the plant. Some of these ants and trees rely on each other to such a great degree that one cannot survive without the other."

The explorer Robert Schomburgk recalled in his journal his encounter with the same species of tree I almost leaned against:

Being unacquainted . . . with the tree and its formidable [ant] inhabitants, and ignoring the warning gesticulations of my [Indian guide], I was trying to break off one of its boughs, when thousands of these insects rushed out of the small round openings in the internodes, completely covered me and in the greatest fury seized my skin with their jaws and, vomiting a white liquid, buried their terrible stings in my muscles. But not only had the ants from the severed portion of the bough fallen into our [canoe] but thousands more poured out of the openings in the stump and rained down into the boat since the whole colony had been aroused by the shaking of the tree. A few powerful strokes of the oars carried the boat out of the neighborhood of the tree and in the twinkling of an eye the whole crew was in the water, for only thus could we escape from the savage onslaught of the ants. Even a few tame [monkeys] and parrots were not spared. The former with wild leaps freed themselves from their tethers and jumped into the river after us, although few animals are more averse to water. . . . I must confess that thereafter a secret horror crept over me whenever we passed one of the trees.

Georges wanted to get an early start that afternoon so he could check several traps before sunset. We climbed into the boat and headed upriver for an hour before he beached the boat on a little sandbank formed by a bend in the river. We got out and Georges heaved the boat onto the shore. He grabbed his machete and followed a narrow trail into the jungle.

As we entered the forest, I let out a loud curse as something stung my right forearm. Jumping quickly to the other side of the trail, I first inspected my arm and then looked back where I had walked to see if I could find the culprit. No caterpillar or other stinging insect was anywhere in evidence and Mittermeier gave a low chuckle as he examined the scene. "This is probably what did it right here," he said, pointing with his machete to a liana growing at the edge of the trail. "In Brazil it is called *cipó do fogo*, which means 'fire liana,' because of the burn it inflicts on the skin. Don't worry," he said with a smile, "it wasn't meant for you!"

"What do you mean?" I asked.

"You have to remember," he began, "humans are a relatively recent arrival in the Amazon forest. The Indians themselves probably didn't arrive in the Amazon until twenty thousand years ago. The *cipó do fogo* evolved that caustic chemical not to repel Indians or Creoles or even a clumsy biologist, but in all probability to repel insects." Whenever you're in the rain forest, you are in the middle of chemical warfare that has been ongoing for hundreds of thousands, if not millions of years.

"Well," I recalled, "Professor Schultes always says, 'Plants live by their chemical wits!'"

Georges had continued down the path and we began to follow. Mittermeier resumed his lecture on chemical defenses as we walked down the trail. "The thing to keep in mind is that there are many types of insects and other plant eaters here. Tropical plant species are thought to be twice as likely to contain alkaloids as temperate plants, and they use many other types of chemicals as well, such as tannins. We use tannins to convert animal skins into leather. Imagine what happens if an insect bites into a plant full of tannins. It may kill him, it may tan him, and, if the bug survives, he isn't likely to repeat the mistake. Here, this is what I was looking for."

Reaching down, he picked up a slim green vine with palm-shaped leaves and long, dangling tendrils—a member of the passion fruit family. He explained that butterflies tend to specialize in a particular group of plants—monarch butterfly caterpillars live mostly on milkweeds, for example, and a group of beautiful black, orange, and yellow butterflies called heliconids feed mostly on passion fruit vines. What makes this so interesting is that the vines themselves are often crawling with toxic chemicals that the plant has produced to deter predation, but the heliconid butterflies have gone it one better—they have developed the means not only to detoxify these chemicals, but sometimes even to store them in their own bodies, thereby rendering themselves toxic to birds! The battle rages on, as passion fruit vines continue to evolve new chemical defenses while the butterflies develop into new species with the ability to break down or otherwise utilize these poisons. It is a never-ending cycle that results not only in new species of plants and animals, but new chemical compounds of the kind so useful to native peoples, and to us.

While the combatants in this chemical war are not restricted to plants and insects, insects are the major players, due in part to their large numbers. Of the 30 million species of organisms alive today, somewhere between 27 million and 29 million are insects. When the great British biologist J. B. S. Haldane was asked, near the end of a long life devoted to studying nature, if he had learned anything about the Creator, he replied, "Yes, he seems to have an inordinate fondness for beetles!" In addition, most of the world's insects are found in the tropics and more than half of them are herbivorous. Yet there are other animals involved in coevolution. In tropical Asia, *Strychnos* trees produce fruits with enough strychnine to kill large mammals, but some local bats manage to thrive on them.

"Then is it safe to say that most of the useful products that come out of the rain forest resulted from this type of chemical warfare?" I asked.

"Not really," Mittermeier replied. "Maybe most of the *medicinal* compounds, but when you start thinking of things like fibers or waxes, probably not. Although, in the case of natural rubber, I can't imagine that the trees had in mind producing a compound that would make the industrial revolution possible when they evolved their latex! Any insect that drills into the bark of a rubber tree will get a face full of an adhesive material that may not kill it but certainly will discourage it from further attacks. So this plant-animal antagonism has produced important non-medicinal compounds as well."

We were so caught up in the local ecology that Georges had forged on ahead without us and checked his traps. Finding them empty, he returned while we were in mid-discussion on animal-insect coevolution. Apparently annoyed at the lack of something to bring home for the cooking pot, Georges strode past us and growled, "If you want to see caiman, it is time to leave." Softening a bit as he saw me carrying the passion fruit vine Mittermeier had handed me, he said, "You should talk to my grandmother back in the village. She knows plants better than anyone else."

We climbed back into the canoe and headed upstream to continue our caiman search. That night the giant black caimans once again eluded us.

The next morning we were awakened by Georges, his ever-present shotgun slung over his shoulder. He wore a green baseball cap, a tiny pair of green bikini shorts, and black rubber boots.

"I am going after tapir today," he announced. "I'll be back in time to go out on the river tonight. Let me show you where my grandmother lives so you can talk to her about plants." Mittermeier noted that this exchange had nothing to do with either monkeys or crocodilians, so he went back to sleep.

Climbing out of my hammock, I slipped on some shorts and a pair of sandals and hurried after Georges. There was no sign of the other men in the village—they were already off hunting or fishing. The women, in their timeless fashion, sat in small groups weaving baskets and peeling what looked like yams. As we approached the far side of the village, away from the river, Georges pointed to a ramshackle hut made of wood and red clay, with a thatched roof. "That's hers!" he said, and turned and walked off. So much for a formal introduction.

I must confess I was feeling a bit like Hansel, minus Gretel, heading to the witch's cottage. The many works I had read in Schultes's course that emphasized the vital link between herbalism and witchcraft flooded my memory and made this feel like anything but a mere plant-collecting exercise. Licking my lips to relieve a sudden case of dry mouth, I walked slowly to the little hut. Just as I raised my hand to knock on the door a deep voice said, in French, "Come in!"

I pushed the door open and stood there blinking, trying to adjust my eyes to the dark interior. I could make out an old Creole woman seated in a rocking chair, smoking what appeared to be a large meerschaum pipe. Her skin was as black as coal and her white hair made it look even darker. Cataracts were forming over her alert brown eyes. Wearing a tattered white cotton dress, she was small and thin, but more wiry than frail. Calmly rocking back and forth, puffing on her pipe, she asked what I wanted.

In my halting French I tried to explain that although I had come to her village to look for the great caiman, I was also interested in plants. Feeling that a little flattery might prove helpful, I claimed that everyone in the village had agreed she was the expert on medicinal plants. I wondered if she would show me a few samples of her most powerful species.

Grumbling that she was too old to collect healing herbs for a white boy with a funny accent, she got up out of her chair, put on an old straw hat, and was out of the door before I knew it. I rushed after her.

What she called her garden looked to me like a weed patch. Nevertheless, the vegetation growing helter-skelter behind her house was a source of pride. She pointed out the cacao trees and the papaya trees, claiming that both provided medicinal compounds as well as edible fruits. These trees were surrounded by a variety of herbs and bushes with little to distinguish them to my untrained eye. But it soon became apparent that I was standing in the middle of a green pharmacy.

With a tea brewed of leaves from the *montjoly* bush, she treated fevers. A cold-water infusion of the leaves of the *maveve* shrub cured liver ailments. To stanch bleeding from a cut, the old woman instructed, apply the sap of the *mokomoko* plant. The sap of the bloodwood tree healed skin lesions, and the *jeajeamadoe* tree sap relieved toothache. The list went on and on. After an hour or so, the old woman's interest began to flag and she mumbled something about her siesta being overdue. She headed back into her house, leaving me alone in her garden with a growing sense of wonder and respect for the botanical riches that encircled me.

That night was the last of the expedition and we were on the river until daybreak, recording data about the small caimans we were able to catch. Georges beached the canoe and we wearily scratched our mosquito bites as the sun rose a soft but fiery red over the rain forest–covered mountains to the east. When he finished unloading the equipment, Georges reached under his seat and pulled out his little aluminum can. Using his right thumb to push off the tightly capped lid, he poured the viscous black liquid into his left palm and then noisily snorted it up. His eyes rolled back and his right leg began to twitch.

When Georges returned to reality several minutes later, I was still standing there watching him. He smiled, adjusted the angle of his hat, and passed me the can. "Your turn," he said.

This was the moment of truth. To decline would be rude; to accept, foolhardy. A thousand questions raced through my mind. Never in a classroom had I been taught what to do in such a situation. In the years that followed, I would have witch doctors swing machetes at my neck, treat my various illnesses with jungle plants, and blow hallucinogenic snuff into my nostrils. But I knew nothing yet. In this moment of indecision, I remembered an inspirational passage from a paper of Schultes's that I had read the night before my departure. It described his participation in a native ritual in the northwest Amazon:

The mask for the *Cha-vee-nai-yo* dance is weird: a human face fashioned of blackened pitch painted with yellow and white geometric designs, with eye-holes through which the dancer peers, a wedge-shaped wooden nose and a leering, toothless mouth. The eerie sight of so many hideously unreal devil masks and the weirdly monotonous minor chant with its far-off, hollow sound, as it is sung through the mask and hood, had an almost hypnotic effect upon me as I watched the dance. And, as I took part in this dance and joined in the chant myself, it was not hard for me to imagine that such an unearthly ritual must be placating some unearthly force.

Schultes had never refused to participate and it was this openness to other cultures and other realities that made his research and his insights so unusual and so successful. I stuck out my hand.

With a slight grin, Georges slowly poured the thick black liquid into my palm. I rapidly snorted the dark potion. In the back of my throat I tasted a bitter substance, but this was soon forgotten. I felt the blood coursing through my veins and felt increasingly omniscient and all-powerful. I was a rocket blasting off and with each passing second I felt higher, faster, stronger, and more alive. But after a short voyage, I ran out of jet fuel. First, I felt weak, then slow, then queasy, then outright nauseous. I broke out in a sweat, collapsed onto the ground, and vomited three times.

Half an hour later, I had made enough of a recovery to stagger back to my hut and stumble into my hammock. Despite persistent nausea and a slight ringing in my ears, I fell into a deep yet restless sleep. When I awoke several hours later, Mittermeier had already packed our things for the return trip. Georges came by and gave a hearty laugh when he saw my still-green complexion. "What the hell was in that?" I asked, somewhat uncertainly.

"My secret recipe!" he replied. "The leaves of the wild tobacco and the ashes of the *mahot cochon*, a cousin of the cacao tree. Would you like some more?" Georges pulled the can out of a packet in his shorts.

Before I could vehemently decline, he burst out laughing. Nevertheless, I sensed something of a bond between us, a solidarity formed by my willingness to try something important to him, which, I later learned, previous visitors had spurned.

As I stood by the canoe, ready to board for the voyage back to Cayenne, Georges put his hand on my shoulder and gave me some advice. "We here know some things about how to use the plants of the forest. If you really wish to learn more, you must be prepared to travel deeper into the jungle. There you will find the Maroons. They are the true people of the forest and will teach you things that I cannot. Good luck, and do not be afraid of canoes with red lanterns. *Au revoir!*"

A year later, I set out for the land of the Maroons.

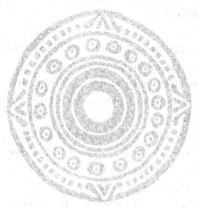

# CHAPTER 3
# Among the Maroons

The runaway slaves fought with a spirit which could not be matched by the Dutch mercenaries or the faithful slaves. . . . In the forest the bush-negro reorganized his life on the African pattern.

—V. S. Naipaul, 1962

● ● ● ● ● ● ● ● ● ● ● ● ● ● ● ● ● ● ●

Suriname holds a special fascination for even the casual visitor. Embedded in the northeast shoulder of South America between Guyana (formerly British Guiana) and French Guiana, Suriname is a cultural mosaic without equal, a microcosm of South America, Africa, Asia, and Europe. It is also one of the world's least populated countries. Less than four hundred thousand people—about the population of Oklahoma City—make their home in Suriname, and 95 percent of them live on the seacoast, scratching out a living as rice farmers, fishermen, and shopkeepers. The northern portion of the country, along the Atlantic Ocean, is a coastal plain covered mostly by swamp and mangrove forest. South of the coastal plain lies the savanna belt, grasslands occasionally punctuated by shrubs and small trees. Lush tropical rain forest blankets the rest of the country, from the savanna belt in the north, south to the Brazilian border. In fact, Suriname has a higher proportion of tropical forest cover than any other country in the world.

As was the case in the rest of the Americas, Suriname was first discovered and settled tens of thousand of years ago by Paleo-Indian tribes, who wandered south after crossing the Bering Strait. Although Christopher Columbus caught sight of the area's coast on his third voyage to the New World, in 1498, the first serious European exploration of the region did not occur until the end of the sixteenth century.

Sir Walter Raleigh, the British explorer and courtier to Queen Elizabeth I, led an expedition to South America in 1595. Mistaking a piece of marcasite for gold, he entered what was then known as Guiana in search of the precious metal. Mines rumored to be located at a golden city called Manoa, next to a lake named Parima, were said to have supplied the golden walls and ornaments of the Incas' Palace of the Sun in Peru. Raleigh wanted to find those mines.

To show the local Indians what he was searching for, the explorer passed around many gold coins from England, but to no avail. Not only did he never find the vast quantities of gold he expected, he is said to have remarked that he left more gold in Guiana than he ever took out. And the fabled Lake Parima that lured him to the area was most likely what is today called Lake Amuku, a body of water that forms only in the wet season in the Rupununi savannas of southwestern Guyana.

Nevertheless, Raleigh was interested in colonizing the area, but he could garner no support for the project. It would be more than fifty years before his countrymen settled the first permanent colonies in Suriname, establishing sugar cane plantations there in 1651. Sixteen years later, the country was conquered by the Dutch and then formally ceded to them in the Treaty of Breda. In return, the British received the rights to a small parcel of land in the north called Nieuw Amsterdam—a Dutch colony better known today as New York.

The British had enslaved the local Indians to work on their sugar plantations, and the Dutch continued the brutal tradition. But the tribal peoples made for an unsatisfactory work force: they knew the terrain and escaped whenever the opportunity arose; many others died in droves from diseases the colonists brought with them and against which the Indians had no immunity. Soon the plantation owners began importing slaves from western Africa, from Sierra Leone down to Congo-Brazzaville, to provide the necessary muscle. By all accounts, the slavery system in colonial Suriname was extraordinarily savage—slaves who had been caught stealing or running away were hung alive from meat hooks, hacked to death with axes, burned at the stake, or broken on the rack. Dr. Richard Price, an anthropologist at Johns Hopkins University and a leading authority on the history of Suriname, has estimated that between three hundred thousand and three hundred twenty-five thousand slaves were brought into the colony between 1668 and 1823, yet the total black population by 1823 numbered no more than fifty thousand.

Many blacks escaped into the uncharted rain forests of the Surinamese interior, where they established tribal cultures not unlike those of their African homelands. The colonists sent out search parties to kill or capture the runaway slaves, but most of these expeditions returned empty-handed—if they returned at all. The blacks fiercely defended their settlements and in turn organized raids on the plantations. The colonists were frustrated by their inability to subjugate the black groups. By the mid-eighteenth century, the whites decided to end the costly guerrilla warfare and negotiated a peace treaty with the black tribes. Descendants of these proud ex-slaves continue to live in the Suriname rain forest, where they maintain their tribal traditions.

Although traditionally known in Suriname as Bushnegroes, as early as the sixteenth century this group of blacks has been called Maroons. According to Dr. Price, the term comes from the Spanish word *cimarrón*, meaning "fierce, proud, and untamed," and originally referred to domestic cattle that had reverted to the wild. It soon became associated with Indian slaves who had escaped the Spanish, and then, by the early 1500s, with escaped African-American slaves.

It was with these people that I decided to conduct my research. In December 1979, I left America to spend two weeks in the Suriname bush.

While the largest segment of Suriname's population is black, the country is also home to the descendants of the original Indian inhabitants and the kin of the British and Dutch colonists. In addition, there has historically been a sizable community of Jews living in Suriname. In the mid-seventeenth century, the Inquisition forced many Spanish and Portuguese Jews to flee their homelands. Some went first to Brazil, at that time a Portuguese colony, and then into Suriname. There they established the first synagogue in the New World, at what is today known as *Joden savanne*, Jew savanna.

Hindustanis, Javanese, and Chinese add to the ranks of peoples brought to Suriname to work the plantations as contract laborers after slavery was outlawed in 1863. These indentured servants managed to maintain their ethnic identities in the New World, and their descendants live in harmony today in Suriname. In the capital city of Paramaribo, Hindustani women wear white lace shawls and sell pungent curries from wooden stalls on the streets; Javanese boys entertain themselves with Indonesian shadow puppets; old Chinese men with wispy Ho Chi Minh beards play mah-jongg in the shade of giant tamarind trees; Maroons carve wooden paddles for a voyage upriver; and Dutch engineers inspect the condition of the dikes built at the end of Keizerstraat Street, where the synagogue and the mosque sit side by side.

As exciting as I found the diversity of Suriname's capital, I was eager to get out into the jungle and to learn from the Maroons. On the face of it, they were not an obvious people with whom to begin my ethnobotanical research. The basic premise of ethnobotany is that the longer tribal peoples have used local plants to meet their needs, the greater their knowledge will be of those plants' secrets. Thus, the indigenous peoples of Africa and Asia—who have inhabited two of the world's three major tropical regions for close to a million years—should have extraordinarily detailed knowledge of the local flora. By comparison, the Maroons, relative newcomers to South America—the third major tropical region—should know less, having lived in Suriname for not quite four centuries.

The reality, however, is that many indigenous groups in Africa and Asia seem to have only limited expertise when it comes to recognizing the useful properties of plants. The most sophisticated "native botanists" known to scientists today are found among the South American Indians. So why didn't I begin my research with the Surinamese Indians instead of the Maroons? Because my interest in African-American ethnobotany had been piqued by the results of a study conducted in Jamaica in the late 1950s that revealed that blacks in Jamaica—who, like the Maroons of Suriname, are descendants of African slaves—were using a tea brewed from the rosy periwinkle as a remedy for "blood problems." Laboratory analysis later found the plant to be an effective treatment not for diabetes, but for childhood leukemia and Hodgkin's disease. If such powerful compounds were being used as medicines by the Jamaicans, I wanted to know what potent curatives might be awaiting discovery in the Amazonian rain forest, which was far richer in plant life than

Jamaica. Furthermore, the Maroons all spoke Sranan Tongo, which I had already begun to learn from Mittermeier. The Maroon territory in the interior could be reached by boat, whereas the lands inhabited by the Indians were accessible only by chartering a small cargo plane. Since renting a plane cost over ten times the price of hiring a boat, my decision to work with the Maroons was at least as much driven by financial considerations as it was by scientific ones.

During World War II, Suriname served as a major source of aluminum ore for the Allied war effort. To get the ore out of the country, Americans built an airstrip that could handle heavy cargo planes. Constructed on the flat terrain of the savanna belt, where soil drainage is much better than in the mangroves to the north or the rain forests to the south, this airstrip is known today as the Pengel International Airport and serves as the major point of entry to Suriname. It is located some thirty miles south of the capital city of Paramaribo. Despite its impressive name, the airport only has a single gate and receives on average about one flight a day.

The heat of the tropical night enveloped me as I walked off the plane in December 1979. Tree frogs croaked and chirped from the forest that surrounded the airstrip on three sides. The diesel exhaust of the jet engine mixed with the scent of tropical jasmine that wafted out of the jungle. Ahead lay the little airport terminal filled with people waiting for returning friends and relatives. I was alone, and felt it.

Inside, the terminal hummed with life in many colors. Beefy, sun-burned Dutch businessmen awaited colleagues from Holland; turbaned Hindustanis greeted family members from Trinidad; black baggage handlers—the urban blacks called Creoles—sweated and strained as they unloaded heavy suitcases and crates. An errant bat swooped into the light, then beat a hasty retreat. A three-foot-long emerald-green iguana sat motionless in a corner on the concrete floor, impassively watching the commotion.

I passed through customs in a daze, trying to absorb the exotic sights, sounds, and smells. Following the instructions Russ Mittermeier had given me—he had helped me set up the trip—I grabbed my suitcase and backpack and jumped on one of the local Volkswagen buses that provide public transportation. The buses are mobile works of art; mine had a yellow roof and white sides, one of which was nearly covered with a gigantic mural of reggae king Bob Marley, his eyes reverently closed as he strummed his guitar and inhaled the intoxicating smoke of an enormous joint hanging from his lips. The bus driver jumped into his seat, turned the key, and pushed the gas pedal to the floor. He switched on the radio and reggae blasted from the speakers at such an ear-splitting volume that my insides began to vibrate in time to the music.

The air was heavy with humidity and thick with the sickly sweet scent of frangipani blossoms. The headlights of the bus illuminated a Technicolor botanical paradise blooming along the roadside: cone-shaped purple petreas; fuzzy red acalyphas that hung like pendants from their stems; buttery yellow cassias; climbing purple bougainvilleas; twining white morning glory vines; orange and black heliconias; and the ubiquitous fiery-hued ixoras. No less impressive was the tropical cornucopia of breadfruit, mangoes, bananas, Brazil nuts, cassava, malacca apples, limes, oranges, coconuts, papayas, and pineapples.

As we roared toward the city, I noticed how the buildings along the highway reflect Suriname's multiethnic society. Huge Dutch warehouses dwarf Maroon palm-thatch huts, and rickety wooden shacks squat next to modern bungalows set high atop pilings. By far the most arresting structures are the Hindu temples. As the bus roared around the bends in the highway, its headlights struck the windows of the huge white buildings, illuminating the carefully carved and vividly painted deities inside.

After a forty-minute ride, we reached the outskirts of the city. Midnight had come and gone; the streetlights had been turned off, and a few mangy stray dogs were the only signs of life. A brackish breeze off the Suriname River provided some relief from the heat and humidity as the bus dropped me off in front of a small rooming house.

I managed to get a few hours of sleep, then headed by taxi to the Forest Service headquarters, where I had an early morning appointment with the director of the Nature Protection Division, an old friend of Russ Mittermeier's. The division's headquarters were housed in a dilapidated white wooden building on the riverbank. Behind the building and across the river was the wreck of a German ship, lying on its side in the water. When the Germans invaded Holland in 1940, the ship had been docked in the Paramaribo harbor. In order to prevent the

Allies from commandeering the boat, the crew scuttled it on the spot. The Surinamese, being an easygoing people, simply left it there, reasoning that the river was wide enough to accommodate it without impeding other traffic. Forty years later, trees grow out of its rusted remains, proof of the local vegetation's robust nature.

Inside the frigid, air-conditioned office sat the director. He was a burly Dutchman, a holdover from the days when Suriname was a colony of the Netherlands and known as Dutch Guiana. He had red hair, a sun-scorched face, and a handshake that could crush walnuts. As I was to find out, he personified all that the Surinamese love and hate about the Dutch: he was honest, thrifty, reliable, blunt, and stubborn as a mule.

"Come in," he said. "Please sit down."

We sat in silence as he pecked out a form on an ancient Smith-Corona typewriter. Then he ripped the sheet out of the machine and, putting it on the desk in front of me, announced, "Welcome to Suriname. Please sign here." He pointed to the bottom of the page and handed me a pen.

Intimidated, I signed the paper without reading it. I only noticed the heading—*Application to Conduct Research in the Republic of Suriname.*

"Now," he began, "Mittermeier notified me of your interest in collecting medicinal plants used by the Maroons. I'm glad you're here. I have already made arrangements for your trip to the interior, but I need to ask you a favor. The son of one of my best workers is very ill. The doctors believe he may have sickle-cell anemia, but they aren't certain. In any case, they can't do anything more for him and recommend sending him to a medicine man in the interior. I know this is not how your doctors function in the States, but such an occurrence is not unusual here in Suriname. In return for this favor, I have arranged for you to have the best guide in Suriname—Fritz von Troon!"

His question as to whether I would be willing to do this favor was clearly rhetorical. He knew there was no way I would turn down free transportation into the interior and an experienced guide, just as I knew that my trip allowed him to justify the use of Forest Service boats to get the son of a colleague to a bush doctor. I accepted the terms readily. He phoned his secretary and asked her to send in von Troon.

With a name like Fritz von Troon, I was expecting a blond Dutchman with a pageboy haircut, short pants, and wooden shoes. The door opened and a large black man entered. He was six feet tall and moved with a grace that belied his extremely muscular build. His hair was short and he wore a mustache and huge muttonchop sideburns. As we shook hands, the guide asked, "How do you do?"

A Maroon who spoke English! I was ecstatic.

"Fine, thank you, and how are you?"

"How do you do?" he repeated.

I asked, "Do you speak English?"

"How do you do?" he replied.

The director told us we could use Forest Service field equipment, saving me the expense of hammocks, mosquito nets, machetes, cooking pots, eating utensils, and flashlights. The plan called for taking a truck south past the end of the paved highway, then traveling another seven miles on a dirt road to where we could catch a motorized canoe going upriver into Maroon country. There we would find the medicine man, and the sick boy could be treated while Fritz and I lived in the village and collected plants. The truck was scheduled to leave Paramaribo at eleven o'clock that morning. We had only two hours to prepare.

Fritz and I left the office and caught a taxi to the waterfront market. As we approached, we could see little wooden fishing boats bobbing in the water; they had arrived at sunup to unload their early morning catch. Inside the market's main building—little more than a giant aluminum hangar—the last of the fish were being sold. People of all shapes, sizes, and colors had jammed inside to buy and sell a seemingly endless variety of goods. Besides the catch of the day, merchants hawked dried food such as salted fish and dried shrimp, and canned goods such as tuna, sardines, and baked beans. There were also lanterns, hammocks, cassette tapes, wooden canoe paddles, clothes, parrots, folding chairs, chain saws, tools, appliances, baseball caps, and old issues of *Sports Illustrated* magazine. We were among the last of the shoppers; the market would close by midday, when it was too hot to transact business.

I trailed behind Fritz, openly gawking as we walked from stall to stall and Fritz haggled his way to acceptable prices. We bought huge bags of rice, bottles of palm oil, packets of dried shrimp, and cans of sardines and tuna. I soon learned that basic jungle etiquette dictates that one never shows up in a village expecting to eat what everybody else is eating. Forest peoples often live in a feast or near-famine situation and a visitor can't simply appear and expect to be fed. Some forest tribes are almost painfully hospitable and will offer so much food that they may go hungry themselves that day. A good rule of thumb is to always carry in enough rations to feed yourself and a few others as well.

The Forest Service truck was waiting when we arrived back at my guest house. Fritz had loaded the field supplies that morning; we stowed my gear and the food we'd just bought; then Fritz climbed in up front with the driver and I jumped in the back. We headed south and soon entered the savanna belt. Savannas are tropical or subtropical grasslands dotted with scattered clumps of small trees and shrubs. Most savannas owe their origin either to shallow soil conditions or to a climate cycle where prolonged periods of rainfall are followed by equally long periods of withering drought. The grasses and trees that grow here have adapted to the harsh environment. In the savannas of Suriname, the most common tree is the savanna cashew, a short, gnarled, grayish tree with thick green leaves. This resilient species not only survives the abrupt seasonal changes of the grasslands, but has adapted to withstand the fires that periodically sweep through this type of ecosystem. Many are natural fires, touched off by lightning, while others are intentionally set by Indian hunters: the tender grasses that regenerate after these conflagrations attract game animals, including deer and giant anteaters, from the forests to the south. But what suits the Indian hunters also suits the ecological status quo. The burnings keep nonfire-adapted plant species from spreading onto the savanna and destroying the grassland ecosystem.

Temperatures can reach ninety degrees Fahrenheit in December, and without a rain forest canopy overhead to absorb the direct sunlight, the heat beat down on us as we drove slowly over the dirt road. High above, a lone black vulture soared on the thermals that rose off the savanna. The horizon shimmered in the distance.

We had been traveling about four hours when we approached a series of small creeks; soon several palm-thatched huts appeared. These dwellings, I was able to understand from Fritz, had been built by Maroons, none of whom seemed to be around. We pulled up in front of one hut with a corrugated aluminum roof; the driver honked the horn. A tall black man wearing the brown khaki uniform of the Forest Service came out, holding the hand of his ten-year-old son. The boy wore a pair of shorts and a cotton shawl draped over his shoulders. Fritz helped the boy climb into the truck cabin—something the child did with great difficulty—then got into the back with me. The man threw his gear into the truck and joined his son up front.

Fritz spoke a very broken English but indicated that I must learn *Sranan tongo,* the local pidgin of Suriname. Based on Dutch, English, Portuguese, Amerindian, and even Yiddish, *Sranan tongo* provides Suriname's many different ethnic groups with a common language, much the same as Swahili does in East Africa. Although Dutch remains the official native tongue, *Sranan tongo* is spoken throughout the country, while Dutch is restricted to the coast.

After little more than an hour, I could see a green shimmering mirage in the distance: tropical rain forest. A slate-gray river the width of a football field marked the boundary between the end of the savanna and the beginning of the forest. We pulled up to the edge of the water and were soon met by two Maroons in a motorized canoe about thirty feet long and three feet wide. Both the bow and the stern were painted in bright blues, reds, yellows, and white. The boatmen had ebony skin, and each wore only a pair of long pants. Their sculpted torsos were mute evidence to the fact that these were men who canoed, hunted, and farmed for a living. The Maroons gave me a warm smile and greeted Fritz like a long-lost brother, then loaded the boat quickly and efficiently.

When the loading was finished, the man who had driven the truck beckoned me over. He was a short, stocky Creole from Paramaribo who, up until this point, had displayed no sign of friendliness, much less the ability to speak English. "I heard this is the first time you have been to Suriname," he said. "Let me give you some advice. The Maroons are crafty thieves who cannot be trusted. They will steal your underwear without taking your pants off!" He gave me a thin smile, then turned to the truck and began tinkering with the engine.

Many years later, I told Fritz about the advice the truck driver gave me that day. Unsurprised, he smiled and said the Creoles often look down on the Maroons, but that the Maroons hold the urban blacks in even greater contempt. "Why?" I asked.

"Because in the old days, when the white man raised his whip, my ancestors took freedom. The ancestors of the Creoles took the lash!"

Verdant rain forest lined both banks of the river. Most of the large trees, such as the reddish-barked sweet bean or the flat-crowned *Parkia*—known locally as *kwatta kama,* or "spider monkey bed," because the creatures are said to sleep in the tree's broad, flat crown—rose to a height of 80 to 90 feet and formed a solid ceiling of green. Some isolated giants, including the white-barked silk cotton tree, whose fibers were once used to stuff life vests, exceeded 150 feet. All were tangled with vines, lianas, orchids, and mosses that wove the trees into emerald walls flanking a broad, watery boulevard leading to the land of the Maroons.

Rivers are the natural roads into the rain forest. The first European explorers to visit the jungles of South America, Africa, and Asia traveled along the watercourses and saw the forest as I was now seeing it—a riot of vegetation growing down to the river's edge. In fact, the word *jungle* is derived from *jangala,* a Sanskrit word meaning "impenetrable." As I had discovered in the interior of the forest in French Guiana the year before, however, this impenetrability was an illusion.

The river was an obstacle course of rocks, logs, and rapids, but our guides were superb. So sophisticated is their knowledge of the river that the Maroons have twenty-three words to describe different types of rapids. In the fifteen years I have traveled through the rain forests I have never found anyone—Indian, Creole, or campesino—who knew and navigated the rivers better than the Maroons of Suriname.

Evening was coming and the heat began to subside. The nocturnal forest, like a slumbering giant, slowly came to life. Locusts called, frogs chirped, and a few mosquitoes circled our heads when we passed close to the riverbanks. Blue and yellow macaws flew from one shore to the other. Tiny squirrel monkeys chattered angrily in the trees lining the river, as if protesting our intrusion. From deeper within the forest came the booming roars of the red howler monkeys, an unearthly din that one explorer imaginatively likened to the sound of a jaguar making love to a dragon.

After an hour on the river, Fritz volunteered that he knew where we could get fresh meat and called ahead to the fellow in the bow to beach the boat to starboard after we had rounded the next bend. We landed in a small cove surrounded by brownish red boulders flecked with mosses; leading up from the river was a little trail into the jungle. Fritz motioned for me to follow. The others remained with the boat, passing around a bottle of rum.

We hiked about half a mile to a small clearing; in the center was a modest lean-to with a palm-thatched roof. Slung from the spindly wooden poles supporting the structure was a cotton hammock and in it sat an ancient-looking Indian carving wooden arrowheads. At his feet sat his wife, peeling yams. Neither had heard us coming, and they froze when we came into view. The only movement in the whole scene was the thick gray smoke that rose from their cooking fire. On the ground were two clay cooking pots, several long bamboo arrows, a purple snake-wood hunting bow, and what appeared to be a half-woven basket. It was as if we had stumbled into a museum tableau portraying a typical scene in a South American jungle village 2,000 years ago. The Indian's faded red gym shorts and his wife's blue calico dress were the only reminders that the Industrial Revolution had occurred.

Fritz asked the couple if they had any smoked meat to trade; they said they didn't and we headed back to the boat. Fritz later explained that even though this was Maroon country, a handful of Indians maintained seasonal hunting camps in the area. They come to hunt deer and peccary—a forest pig—and then butcher and smoke the meat there. After stocking up on enough provisions to last a few weeks, they return to their villages in the north.

As we tramped back to the canoe, I soaked in the sights and sounds of the forest. Although a childhood of Saturday morning Tarzan movies had prepared me for a forest where snakes hang from every limb and monkeys swing from branch to branch, I learned in French Guiana that the most obvious representatives of forest fauna are insects and birds. A troop of army ants patrolled to our left, while a variety of brown millipedes and green beetles shared our path. Many of the trunks of the larger trees were encrusted with termite nests. Overhead, a large toco toucan flew past, uttering its harsh cry. So astonishing was the size of the bird's yellow-orange bill that its black body seemed almost an afterthought. And from a distance we could hear the peculiar three-note call of the screaming piha bird—a kind of whistling *wee-WEE-o* that is the most pervasive sound in the South American jungle.

When we arrived back at the river, the Maroons hurried us into the canoe so we could reach our campsite before dark. The boy, whose name was Petrus, looked very sick. The whites of his eyes were yellowish and he shivered beneath his cotton shawl. He hadn't spoken a word throughout the journey.

An hour later we beached the canoe at a small island on which stood two empty wooden huts. As the sun was beginning to set, we hung our hammocks and mosquito netting—Fritz taught me how to do this critical job correctly—and one of the boatmen built a fire and cooked several pots of boiled rice. As the night grew cooler, we sat around the glowing logs for light, heat, and companionship. The Maroons took turns telling stories and, even though I could understand only a few words, their musical voices and amiable expressions made me feel as if I were among old friends.

The next morning we were on our way before the sun rose. The river and the weather were cool and gray; it did not feel at all tropical. Once it began to warm a bit, the forest birds stirred. We passed a colorful little red-capped cardinal collecting twigs for a nest from the branches of a fallen tree. A yellow and brown sun bittern, spearing frogs with its long, sharp, orange beak at the river's edge, watched us cruise by. Fritz saw me recording the names of the birds in my journal and indicated that he had something to show me upriver.

By midday, the sun blazed down on us and the forest creatures drowsed in the heat. Caspar, the fellow in charge of the motor, steered us over to a small sandy beach on the starboard side; it was time for lunch.

While most of my companions occupied themselves with preparing a fire to boil rice, Fritz strapped on a machete and silently beckoned me to follow him on a path that led into the jungle. We walked wordlessly along the forest trail; I kept my eyes on the ground in front of me, alert for poisonous snakes. Unsheathing the machete he carried on his belt, Fritz walked over to a tall tree whose black bark was perforated by a series of small holes. After cutting away a slice of the bark, he shaved off several yellow pieces of wood and handed them to me. He said that the tree was called *bergibita*—"mountain bitters"—and tried to explain what it was used for. Seeing that I couldn't understand his verbal description, Fritz staged an elaborate pantomime—he clutched his belly in pain, sliced wood from the tree, feigned putting it into a pot of water and stirring up a tea, then drank the imaginary brew and rubbed his belly contentedly. As I scribbled this information into my notebook, Fritz grinned and beckoned me into the forest off the trail.

Up to this point, all our hiking had been on a clearly defined path and there had been little need for machetes. Now we were entering what in Suriname is called liana forest, where exceptionally poor soils prevent the development of a rain forest canopy. Abundant sunlight penetrated to the forest floor, and a tangle of lianas—woody vines that literally seem to tie the forest together—impeded our progress. Fritz was a surgeon with his machete—a quick *snicker-snack*, and the lianas were sliced aside. We hiked until we came to an area filled with large, moss-covered, yellowish brown granite boulders. Fritz motioned for me to be as silent as possible and we crept around the huge rocks to a small clearing.

In front of us unfolded a scene out of a bird lover's dream—the mating dance of the cock-of-the-rock. The males of this species, which is native to the Guianas and northern Brazil, are a luminescent orange. Atop their heads is an extraordinary crest that looks as if it came right off the helmet of a Roman soldier. These birds build mud nests on ledges in caves near forest streams. The intrepid Prussian explorer Robert Schomburgk, who with his brother Richard demarcated the boundary between Brazil and Guyana (then British Guiana) in the mid-1800s, was probably the first European to witness the mating dance of this species. In a report to the Geographical Society of London, he wrote:

We hit upon a flock of those glorious birds, the Cock-of-the-Rock. . . . I had the opportunity of being present at the birds' dance which indeed the Indians had often talked to me about, but which I had always considered to be a fable. We heard at some distance off, the chirping notes that are so peculiar to the [Cock-of-the-Rock], and two of my guides nodded to me to sneak cautiously with them in to the spot that at some distance from the path formed the gathering-place of the dancers. It was from four to five feet in diameter, cleared of every blade of grass, and the ground at the same time was smooth as if human hands had levelled it. It was on this spot that we saw one of the birds dancing and hopping around while the others apparently constituted the wondering spectators. He now spread out his wings, threw his head in the air or spread his tail like a peacock: he then strutted around and scratched the ground up, all accompanied with a hopping gait, until exhausted he uttered a peculiar note, and another bird took his place. In this way three of them one after another stepped onto the stage, and withdrew one after the other with the proudest self-consciousness back again amongst the others who had settled on some low bushes that surrounded the dancing ground. We counted ten males and two females, until all of a sudden the crackling noise of a piece of wood, that my foot had inadvertently stepped on, scared them—and bang flew the whole ballet-troupe away.

Pleased at the sense of wonder I displayed at the scene before us, Fritz smiled and indicated that it was time to return. We headed back down the freshly cut path through the liana forest to the edge of the stream, where we picked up our original trail and hiked down to the river. By the time we met up with the other Maroons, it was too late to push on and we decided to spend the night at the island campsite. The fragrant air, the chirping frogs, the embracing jungle, and the memories of the cock-of-the-rock gave me a sense of satisfaction and exhilaration I had seldom known. That night there was a full moon. A *buta buta* bird—a type of nightjar—sang in the trees near the edge of the river. According to Fritz, the bird's song professed his happiness at seeing the full moon.

Two days later we reached our destination. Maroon villages are typically built at the river's edge and community life extends out into the water. This village was no exception. Young boys in small dugout canoes fished the river with bamboo poles. Little girls at the water's edge played with wooden dolls. Women sat on a sandy beach, washing both clothes and children with care and thoroughness. Men paddled out from the village toward the hunting grounds upriver, with only their dogs for company.

After we landed, Petrus was helped ashore by his father; the other occupants of the boat melted into the village to greet family and friends. Fritz and I unloaded our provisions, piled them high on the riverbank, and then set off to find the village chieftain.

A main path pointed the way to the village; several narrower paths led out to hunting trails and gardens. The village was a wonderful collection of about a hundred small wooden houses, the facades of which were gaily painted with decorative patterns in red, blue, yellow, and white. The doors were sometimes further embellished with elaborate wood carvings. A few houses had roofs of corrugated aluminum; most, however, were of palm thatch.

As we walked through the village, we watched men clad in white breechcloths use machetes and hunting knives to cut canoe paddles from the yellowish brown wood of the paddle-wood tree. They wielded the big knives with dexterity, piling wood chips deep around their feet as they talked and laughed. To finish the paddles, they carved intricate geometric designs into the blades, some to encourage good luck, others for beauty alone.

While the men carved, the women did the tasks reserved for their gender in this culture. Most were spinning cotton into thread, while one teenage girl pounded rice with a huge mortar and pestle to remove the husks. When the women—who wore only patchwork breechcloths—saw us approach, they quickly tied brightly colored lengths of cloth over their bare breasts.

Near the center of the village, we passed an ancestor shrine—a low, flat altar on which stood a simple human figurine carved from wood. On either side of the shrine, sticks had been planted in the ground, and from them hung multicolored cotton cloths. In front of the altar were several old bottles, which held the sacred libations (usually rum) used during religious ceremonies. The village had several such shrines, each consecrated to an ancestor held in particularly high esteem. Each venerated forebear has a specialty: at one shrine, villagers ask the ancestor's help in finding someone lost in the forest; at another, the ancestor is entreated to help heal a broken bone. Each shrine is erected by, and therefore belongs to, one subgroup of the village, such as the men or women of a particular family. The need to consult and pray at the shrines of others fosters interdependence among the members of the village.

At the edge of the settlement we found the chief's hut. To announce our arrival, Fritz paused about six feet from the entrance and called out, "Krock, krock, krock!"—a verbal knock, as there was no door. A sleepy old fellow of about sixty looked out and, seeing there was out-of-town company, quickly gathered the symbols of his authority—a brown visored naval hat and a walking stick. He came out of the hut, and he and Fritz exchanged musical call-and-response greetings. Then Fritz briefly explained the reasons for our visit. The chief immediately sent his grandson to inform the rest of the village that the official welcoming party was to be assembled. Several minutes later, he was joined by his two subchiefs (the *captains*) and his four subsubchiefs (the *bashas*). These two groups stood behind the chief as we presented him with half a dozen bottles of rum and several plugs of a highly aromatic black tobacco, traditional gifts of welcome in a Maroon village. The chief parceled out these gifts to his subordinates, keeping the lion's share for himself. Then the captains and bashas began a brief dance, taking a few simple steps back and forth and chanting "*Danki, danki, baccra!*" ("Thanks, white man!"). At the end of the performance, the chief formally granted us permission to live and work in his village and assigned us a hut for the duration of our visit.

The day begins early in the jungle; you have to accomplish as much as possible before the incapacitating midday heat descends. By the time I awoke at daybreak, Fritz was already cooking breakfast—a boiled purple yam, which the Maroons grow in their gardens, washed down with a cup of the instant coffee we had purchased in Paramaribo. As we headed into the jungle after the morning meal, I marveled at how clean and orderly the village was. The ground is swept at least once a day, and most of the village is kept clear of vegetation. The only exceptions are the fruit trees planted by the villagers to provide them with oranges, bananas, coconuts, and the luscious guanabana, whose sweet, moist, white flesh tastes like a cross between vanilla ice cream and egg custard.

The forest nudged the edge of the village. Fritz and I hiked into the jungle and were immediately enveloped by the green cocoon. We had stepped only a few yards from the settlement and we were already a part of the forest primeval. As I tried to learn Fritz's language and his plants, I could sense something special about the way he and the other Maroons related to their surroundings. During my stay with the Creoles of French Guiana, I felt that they feared the forest and regarded it as a foe that had to be conquered if they were to wrest a living from it. Fritz and his fellow tribespeople had a more mystical relationship with the jungle; it was not only their home, but, in the case of their ancestors, their salvation as well, a haven from the torturous confines of slavery. The Maroons believed certain trees had magical powers. The giant silk cotton, for example, was thought to shelter protective forest spirits and thus could never be cut down. And it was taboo to urinate under other trees, such as the letterwood. The Maroons regarded these sacred species—and indeed the entire forest—with respect and reverence.

One of the first lessons I learned while working with Fritz was that you cannot rush forest people to make them conform to your "civilized" pace; everything in the jungle happens in its own time. Fritz wanted to begin by teaching me the vernacular names of some of the common plants. We approached a huge tree, a member of the legume family with thick buttress roots and reddish bark; in various places on the tree, fist-sized chunks of the bark had been removed. "This," said Fritz, "we call *agrobigi*. The bark is brewed into a tea and drunk to treat fevers."

I was a bit suspicious because the name *agrobigi* is very simplistic, meaning "it grows big." Scientific literature is rife with tales of native peoples giving researchers the wrong names and of researchers recording the right names incorrectly. For example, an early publication on Surinamese flora listed the common name of one plant as *kakabrokoe*, which roughly translated means "shit in your pants." What is uncertain is whether the species was used to treat constipation or whether the Maroon guide fancied himself a clever practical joker. Conversely, in a well-known instance involving Dutch botanists who were exploring the plants of the coastal plain with local Arawak Indians as guides, the botanists were either overzealous in their note taking or completely baffled by the local language. Published accounts detailing that area's flora list a long Arawak name for one of the species. When translated into English, it means "I don't know this one so I'll have to ask my uncle"!

After walking for several hours and looking at a number of plants, we decided to stop for lunch. I was carrying a daypack into which Fritz had put two pieces of smoked fish he had been given in the village. As I sat down, I brushed my arm against a large liana; I immediately felt a burning sensation. This was the same "fire liana" I had bumped into in French Guiana. Seeing my discomfort, Fritz disappeared from the trail into the jungle. He came back holding a small herb with bright green leaves. He carefully broke off three leaves and rolled them together between his palms, making a cylindrical shape. He folded the cylinder twice, placed it in his palm, crushed the leaves into a thick green paste with his fist, and rubbed it on my burn. By the time we had finished eating, the pain and the redness had disappeared.

Fritz proved to be a jungle druggist par excellence, pointing out healing plants almost every step of the way. We collected the triangular-leaved *mispel* herb, eaten to treat gonorrhea; the fetid wood of the *jarakopi* tree, brewed into a tea to relieve fevers; and the green, heart-shaped leaves of a delicate little herb called *konsaka wiwiri*, which is literally used from head to toe as a treatment for both headache and athlete's foot. Fritz also pointed out the *mokomoko*, a shrub with leaves shaped like arrowheads, which is found only at the edge of the river. The sap of the *mokomoko* is dripped into cuts and other wounds to stanch blood flow. Fritz warned that this is a painful remedy because the plant fluid burns when applied.

But one plant stood out from all the others in terms of healing properties. It was a small green herb growing at the edge of the trail; the plant's unremarkable appearance gave no indication of its curative potential. Pulling the herb up by the roots, Fritz explained that you take a tea of the leaves twice a day—*"te joe habe toomsi soekroe na broedoe"*—when you have too much sugar in the blood. It took a minute for me to realize that the malady Fritz was describing was diabetes. I asked him to explain how tribal peoples living deep in the rain forest were able to diagnose excessive sugar in the bloodstream.

"Simple," he replied. "You taste the urine."

I eagerly collected the plant, and we headed back with several cotton bags full of specimens.

Once in the village, we put the samples in my plant press and stacked them over kerosene burners to dry. Since many herbarium specimens lose their active chemicals, laboratory analyses on voucher specimens in the past have sometimes led scientists to conclude mistakenly that various species are chemically inert. Field botany is becoming more sophisticated, however; new technology will soon allow botanists to analyze specimens of medicinal plants in portable field laboratories or to collect the specimens and freeze them in liquid nitrogen for transport to the city for further testing.

That night Fritz went down to the river to get some drinking water and came back to the hut smacking his lips. One of the Maroons had gone hunting the night before and brought back some meat that his wife had just finished making into stew. She had generously filled a bowl and had given it to Fritz on his way back from the river. As he carefully divided the stew into two equal portions, he told me the meat was from an animal called a paca. It was, quite simply, the best meat I have ever eaten, red like beef but with a slightly sweet aftertaste like the finest pork. After having spent a week eating nothing but rice, yams, fruit, dried soup, and salted fish, the fresh meat was a welcome treat and I greedily devoured it. The next day, while we were out in the forest collecting plants, we saw a hunter returning to the village with a shotgun in one hand and a two-foot-long tailless rat in the other. "What do you call that creature?" I asked Fritz in revulsion.

"Oh," he said, "that's a paca."

After dinner that evening, we strolled through the village to visit Petrus and to find out when we would take him upriver to the healer. Moonlight flooded the village and reflected off the white sandy ground, creating an almost ghostly glow. We heard the *bonki-deef*, a tropical thrush, as it plaintively sang *SEE-suh-SEE-suh*—a plea for rain, according to Fritz. Most of the villagers were inside their houses, but some sat outside around small fires, chatting and sometimes singing together.

Petrus lay in a hammock slung in front of a relative's house. His father sat on a low wooden bench before him, maintaining a vigil over his ailing son. The boy looked even worse than he had when we arrived. There was more yellow in the whites of his eyes and his cheeks were sunken and hollow. The father said that he felt it was better to delay the journey a few more days, so Petrus would be well rested.

Consequently, Fritz and I spent the next three days wandering the forest, returning to the village as the sun set to press our plants and devour a quick meal before retiring to our hammocks. One day Fritz pointed out a tree that was well over a hundred feet tall, a true jungle giant, with several small buttress roots. Unholstering his machete, Fritz made a quick horizontal chop in the bark and a copious white latex poured out and down the trunk.

"That," he said, "used to be money."

He smiled at the perplexed look on my face. "This is what we call balata," he said. "When I was a boy, we would make cuts like this in the bark and collect the latex in calabashes. We would let it dry out and then take it downriver to trade for city goods like shotguns or flashlights. For some reason, people from the city stopped wanting it and we don't collect it to trade anymore."

The change in demand Fritz referred to was the trend among industrialized societies to move away from natural products and replace them with synthetics. Balata latex was long used for coating underwater utility cables, golf balls, and machine belts. It is particularly well suited for the manufacture of the latter because, unlike natural rubber, balata is inelastic and does not stretch.

Balata was at one time such an important commodity that it was the third most valuable export of British Guiana. It is still collected in small amounts and used to make covers for high-quality golf balls, but in other applications the latex has been largely replaced by synthetics.

The Central American chicle tree is from the same family as balata and has an even more colorful history. At least as far back as the Aztec empire, people have chewed the latex of the chicle tree. Aztec prostitutes were said to loudly snap their chewing gum to advertise their trade. The commercialization of chewing gum in the United States got its start with General Santa Anna, the Mexican hero of the Alamo. By the 1860s, the general was in exile, living on Staten Island and plotting his return to his native country. To relieve his tension, he chewed chicle. When at last he left Staten Island for Mexico, he left his chicle behind with his host, Thomas Adams, an amateur inventor. Adams initially tried to vulcanize the chicle to produce waterproof shoes. This venture failed when hot weather caused the soles of his new galoshes to stick to the pavement. Adams's next brainstorm was to market chicle to the dental community as a denture adhesive. When this effort failed, Adams flattened the chicle with his wife's rolling pin, added sugar, cut it into little pieces, and put it in a Brooklyn candy store for sale. The results were immediately snapped up, leading to the birth of the multimillion-dollar chewing gum industry.

As was the case with balata, chicle has mostly been replaced with synthetic materials. In our determination to prove that we can reduce our reliance on nature by developing artificial replacements for natural substances, we have subsequently reduced the economic value of the forest. The harvesting of chicle and balata, when done correctly, can provide a steady income to forest inhabitants over a long period of time and without damage to the forest environment. Fortunately, enough demand for chicle persists that a portion of the rain forests of Mexico, Guatemala, and Belize are still protected and managed for this product.

An ironic parallel to the balata and chicle examples is that of gutta-percha, an Asian species from the same family. In the early part of this century, latex from this species was also used to cover underwater cables and golf balls, and to make splints, telephone receivers, waterproofing, and adhesives. As early as 1867, dentists began using the latex as a filling for root canals. Because gutta-percha is not prone to shrinkage, does not encourage bacterial growth, does not irritate surrounding tissue, and is impervious to moisture, it proved to be an ideal compound for this purpose. But in the 1960s, dentists anxious to move away from such old-fashioned natural compounds started to substitute synthetics for the Asian latex. Ten years later, many of these synthetics started to degrade and had to be replaced, a costly, painful, and altogether unpleasant process. Meanwhile, root canals that had been filled with gutta-percha remained intact. As a result, dentists have now resumed using gutta-percha.

Gutta-percha is not the only rain forest plant product that has played a role in modern dentistry. A short while after Fritz showed me the balata, he led me to another huge tree, well over a hundred feet tall, with a distinctive brownish gray bark. Earlier visitors had punctured the bark and from these orifices the tree oozed a thick, yellowish resin that smelled a bit like turpentine. Fritz explained that his people painted the resin on wounds to accelerate healing.

The exudates of the trees of this family are known as copal, a term derived from the Aztec word *copalli*, which means "resin." The healing properties of copal were known and used by South American Indians for hundreds, if not thousands, of years; copal's use was documented by European explorers as early as the fifteenth century. Copal is sold widely in Brazil—where it is known as *Copaiba*—and is considered an effective remedy for colds and other respiratory trouble. Copal was once used in photography to emphasize halftones and shadows, and has been employed medicinally in the United States as a disinfectant, diuretic, laxative, and mild stimulant. This resin is widely used today to scent soaps and cosmetics and in the manufacture of high-quality artists' paints. It also plays a key role in modern dentistry. When a dentist drills a tooth to fill a cavity, he exposes elongated channels known as dentinal tubules, which will generate a toothache unless properly treated. After these tubules have been exposed, the doctor coats them with a copal preparation that prevents further problems.

Perhaps even more astonishing than the fact that a good many of us are walking around with rain forest tree resins in our mouths is the possibility that copal trees may one day serve as gas pumps. Experiments in the late 1970s by Dr. Melvin Calvin, a Nobel Prize–winning biologist, demonstrated that a single tree can produce up to ten gallons of copal oil each year. This oil, rich in hydrocarbons, can be poured directly into diesel engines, which run cleanly and smoothly on the jungle fuel. Although test results are promising, for now the yield from the copal trees is too small for the sale of the oil to be commercially feasible.

Next Fritz led me to a towering *rediloksi* tree with bumpy gray bark. He slit the bark with his machete and this time the resin that leaked out was a rust color. Fritz scouted around a bit until he found a large stump that he claimed was the remains of another *rediloksi* tree. Using the point of his machete, he dug into the ground at the base of the roots until he unearthed a dirt-covered clump about the size of a plum. Wiping the dirt off against his leg, he handed me his find; it appeared to be a fossilized lump of the rust-colored resin. Asking me for my matches, he lit one corner of the resin ball and it burst into a clear blue flame, immediately filling the air around us with the most delightful scent of pine.

"We use this for two purposes," said Fritz. "If we are out hunting and it has been raining, we use this to ignite a fire. It will start to burn much quicker than wet wood. We also crush it and drink the powder with warm water to cure diarrhea."

Diarrhea is a common problem in the humid tropics, so I asked what else the Maroons use to treat it. Professor Schultes had taught me that an answer about the use of one plant can sometimes lead to information on other plants as well.

"Well," said Fritz, "there is something over here that we sometimes value for diarrhea, but it is better for fevers."

He walked over to a thin tree with gray-white bark and small cherry-red flowers. "Taste this," he said, shaving off a thin sliver of the bark with his blade. I followed his instructions and in so doing tasted a piece of Surinamese history.

During the colonial period, a famous black medicine man named Kwasi was one of the most renowned physicians of his day. There is said to have existed a law in Suriname that held that if a slave escaped from the colony and made his way to Holland, he would automatically become a free man. Kwasi made this journey, and not only did he earn his freedom, he became a well-known healer—aided no doubt by the herbs he brought from Suriname. His most potent concoction was a tea made from an exceedingly bitter wood; it was used to treat fevers and intestinal parasites. In the course of his travels Kwasi met the prominent Swedish taxonomist Linnaeus, who named this plant *Quassia amara*, Latin for "Kwasi's bitters." Fritz explained that the tea is still used by his people to treat illnesses: they carve a cup from the bitter wood, pour rum into the cup, and set it aside for half an hour, during which the liquor absorbs the medicinal compounds from the wood. Then the patient drinks the rum.

Because of its introduction to the Western scientific establishment by Kwasi over two hundred years ago, this species has a long history of use in Western medicine. Extracts of the wood were valued as a tonic, an appetite stimulant, and in the treatment of dyspepsia. It was once thought to be effective as an antimalarial agent, but recent tests have proved otherwise. *Quassia* is still employed in the treatment of human threadworm and is sometimes used as an insecticide, since it is a very potent killer of aphids.

The next resin-producing tree I was introduced to that day was not as well understood as Kwasi's, but full of promise. When slashed with a machete, the bark of the *pritjari*, a small tree with a brownish yellow trunk covered with spines, slowly exuded a clear, sticky resin. Fritz explained that his people soak the bark of the *pritjari* in hot water and wash their sores with the liquid to accelerate healing. Although little is known of the chemistry of this tree, a related species from the Amazon provides us with pilocarpine. This drug, which helps improve drainage from the eye, is used by ophthalmologists to reduce intraocular pressure caused by glaucoma.

Back in the village later that night, we were still putting our specimens into the plant press when a female voice called "krock, krock, krock!" just outside our door. In came the chief's daughter, a beautiful girl of about thirteen. Around her waist she wore a simple cotton cloth of red and white stripes. Her back and shoulders were ramrod straight; she carried herself like royalty. On the girl's belly were cicatrizations, tiny ritual scars forming a triangle on either side of her navel. These markings are considered an important aspect of a Maroon woman's beauty and the height of eroticism by the men of the tribe. The practice is often carried out at the end of a menstrual period, since freshly cut cicatrizations are considered particularly seductive.

On the girl's right shoulder sat a pet capuchin monkey busily chewing a piece of banana. In her right hand she carried a pot of stew made from rice and *sopropo*, a bitter relative of the cucumber that is prized by the Maroons.

"My father sent this over," she said, placing the pot on a tree stump we used as a chair. "He says that Petrus is a bit better and tomorrow you will take him to see the medicine man. My father says be careful. The medicine man is bewitched."

Fritz and I picked up Petrus the next morning; his father had been discouraged from attending the ceremony and remained in the village. When Fritz explained that the healing ritual might be too upsetting for the boy's father to witness, I began to wonder just what was in store.

The medicine man's camp was a two-hour paddle upriver. When we arrived, he was standing on the riverbank as if expecting us. About six-foot-two and powerfully built, he wore only a white cotton breechcloth around his waist. His beard was flecked with gray and he had bracelets of small black seeds around both wrists. As we beached the canoe, he mouthed a series of incantations.

When he spoke with Fritz, it became apparent why he was considered bewitched: he appeared to have suffered a stroke that left his face partially paralyzed. While half of his face was engaged in an animated discussion, the other side was frozen solid. All in all, he projected an aura of mystery and malevolence.

The sun was setting and we hurried up the riverbank into the shaman's hut. A dove cooed mournfully from the forest behind the dwelling.

Petrus had trouble walking, so the medicine man tossed the boy across his shoulder like a small sack of potatoes and carried him inside.

It was a one-room hut with wooden walls and a palm-thatched roof. A yellowed Dutch calendar with a picture of a white windmill set amid a field of white tulips was tacked to one wall, adding a note of incongruity. A small fire burned in the middle of the dwelling; the only other light came from an old kerosene lantern hanging from a hook in one of the walls. Around the fire were several ornately carved wooden benches called *bangis,* and it was on these that we sat and stared into the fire as darkness fell. The medicine man opened a bottle of rum and passed it around, instructing us all to drink deeply. As I turned the bottle up, he asked Fritz to explain what he knew of the boy's ailment. Then the medicine man abruptly stood and walked behind Petrus, who remained seated on his bench in front of the fire. The healer waved his hands in strange patterns just above and behind the boy's head, all the while moaning incantations in a low voice.

After a few minutes of this, he started to massage the child's neck while alternately shrieking and laughing hysterically. The hair stood up on the back of my neck, but Petrus remained huddled on his bench, showing no emotion. The medicine man then ran out into the jungle behind the hut and we could hear him talking to himself while he collected a series of plants. When he returned a few minutes later, he threw a pile of herbs on the fire, instructing the boy to inhale the fragrant smoke. Other plants were dropped into a bucket, to which he added rum, all the while instructing us to continue drinking from the bottle he had given us. Then suddenly the shaman grabbed both Fritz and me by the wrists and pulled us outside. As we stood not knowing what to do next, he began pounding a nail into a tree with a large rock and chanting the same phrase over and over—"Make this boy better"—alternating it with other phrases I couldn't translate. Once the nail was halfway in, he handed me the stone and told me to finish the job. Fritz was instructed to chant the incantations along with him. After I completed the task, the medicine man beckoned us back into the hut. After stirring the bucket containing the medicinal plants and the rum, he handed it to Petrus and told him to drink it all. Meanwhile, the shaman began singing; as he crooned, he picked up his machete and started swinging it wildly over the boy's head. Then, with one great sideways swoop, he brought the blade to within an inch of my neck, stopped, smiled his lopsided smile, and plunged the blade into an empty wooden bench. The handle of the machete quivered from the force of the blow. My heart began to beat again.

The ceremony ended shortly thereafter. We were told to leave the boy and return for him the next evening. Pale moonlight showed us the way and we could hear the shaman chanting in the distance as Fritz and I—drunk on rum and exhausted by the healer's frenzied ritual— began unsteadily to paddle home.

The next day, we again headed upriver to pick up Petrus, this time accompanied by the boy's father. As we came in sight of the shaman's clearing, we could see him sitting on a giant boulder at the river's edge. He did not respond to our shouted greetings, just crouched on his rock, mumbling to himself and absentmindedly scratching his beard. More importantly, though, at the sound of our approach Petrus came trotting down to the riverbank, smiling and laughing when he saw his father. The change in him was nothing short of extraordinary. His eyes no longer had their yellowish pall and although he moved a bit unsteadily, he seemed much more vibrant and alive than the previous day. He jumped in the canoe and hugged his father as we pushed off into the river.

On the way back down the river, I was too stunned by the boy's recovery to say much. But once we arrived in the village, I peppered Fritz with questions. "What plants did he use? What were the dosages? Do you know those chants?"

Fritz gave me a wry smile. "Listen, I know a lot of healing plants, but I am not a medicine man. Last night I, too, was participating in the ceremony, not trying to identify the species he was using. If you want to find that out, you have to come back here and live with him."

I contemplated this possibility. I had been more than a little frightened by the healer's ceremony; looking at that shaman was like staring into a roaring fire at close range—the light compels you to look, but the heat the fire generates makes you retreat to a safe distance. I had witnessed shamanism in all its glory and I was intrigued, but within this man seemed to bubble a caldron of uncontrolled forces. I wanted to work with and learn from people as potent as the Maroon medicine man, but who had harnessed their powers and weren't likely to swing machetes at my neck.

Fritz spoke again. "Look," he said, pointing to an emerald-green dragonfly perched on the leaf of a nearby ginger plant. "We call this insect *grasbarki*. There are many different species here, but we call all by the same name. But the Indians have a different name for each one; the same is true for plants. The Maroons are smart, but in the bush, the Indians are smarter. *Na boesi, ingi sabe ala sani*—in the jungle, the Indian knows everything. When you come back to learn more about plants, you must go deeper into the forest to learn from the Indians."

A year later, I followed his advice.

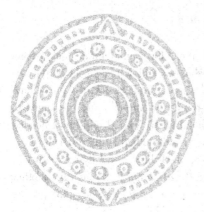

## CHAPTER 4

# Under the Double Rainbow

*Na boesi, ingi sabe ala sani.*
("In the jungle, the Indian knows everything.")    —Surinamese proverb

● ● ● ● ● ● ● ● ● ● ● ● ● ● ● ● ● ● ●

When I arrived in Paramaribo, the capital of Suriname, in December 1982, the country teetered on the brink of a full-scale civil war. The dusty, red-brown streets were empty of people during the day, and the nights were filled with gunshots, the rumble of armored vehicles, and the screams of people being pulled from their houses.

The politics of the situation were obscure—the leftist junta had moved to preempt a coup by the rightist opposition, but no one really knew the details. Rumors spread quickly: depending on who you talked to, the city was being invaded by Cuban mercenaries or was awaiting attack from American, French, or Dutch forces.

The turmoil made it difficult to get into the jungle—borders were closed and there was a curfew on—but I knew that once I reached the country's interior, the green distances would insulate me. To the Maroons of the forest, whom I had visited on my last trip, the killings in the city would be barely a rumor; and in the even more remote Indian lands to which I was headed now, there would not be even a whisper.

In a western suburb of the city I found a small airstrip, a jumping-off point for the interior. This wasn't the type of operation where you purchase a ticket in advance, so I hung around a dilapidated hangar waiting for a plane. I had almost given up hope when a battered white single-engine Cessna landed, bouncing in the ruts of the poorly paved runway. I rushed over to talk with the pilot, a glistening black Creole in white dungarees and T-shirt, who was unloading cages of reptiles and screeching birds. The weather was hot and steamy, a typical Suriname sauna, and he was hustling to get the animals into the shade of a ramshackle shed at the edge of the airstrip. When I told him I needed a ride into the interior, he shot me a gold-toothed smile. "If you've got the money, I'll make the space." The next day he was flying south to a remote Tirió Indian village near the Brazilian border to pick up another load of toucans, parrots, and iguanas for export to zoos and private collectors in Europe. I arranged to meet him at the airstrip the next morning.

There was little I could do that evening to prepare for the trip. I couldn't buy food. No supplies were coming into the city and all the stores were closed up tight. I was heading into the rain forest for eight weeks with my plant press, my machete, a few cans of sardines, and a little dried soup. I spent a sleepless night.

My anxiety only began to recede when the plane lifted up, buzzing and bucking. It passed over rice fields and cattle pastures, leaving behind the rattling trucks and strutting soldiers thronging the city. The houses, fields, and roads soon gave way to pristine rain forest. To the pilot, who flew over it every day, the forest was probably just a jumble of trees and the Tirió village a routine stop in a typical workday. But I was seeing the immensity of the forest for the first time, a mossy carpet stretching out to the horizon, sparkling here and there as sunlight flashed on a hidden stream or pond. Rivers, their waters boiling with white rapids, snaked through the forest on their way north to the sea. Their presence was marked in the canopy by the incandescent yellow flowers of the greenheart trees and by the majestic spreading crowns of the giant kapok trees, which lined the riverbanks at regular intervals.

We flew low enough to see animals. A flock of fiery-hued scarlet macaws scattered like bright red leaves across the green canopy; a troop of red-brown howler monkeys yawned and slept in the top of a black-barked *Swartzia* tree.

Ahead, poking up through the trees like the monumental ruin of a lost civilization, was the Tafelberg—the Table Mountain—part of a chain of mountains that stretches in an arc from Colombia to Suriname. Some of the mountains are so remote and their escarpments so steep that they have never been scaled. Their visual impact and mystery inspired Sir Arthur Conan Doyle, creator of the fictional detective Sherlock Holmes, to use them as a setting in his 1900 novel *The Lost World*. In the book, dinosaurs and ancient plants thrive atop a giant Mesozoic table mountain rising out of the Amazonian forests. Even though evidence of dinosaurs was never found atop the mountains—known as *tepuis*—that inspired Doyle, the isolation of these peaks has made them home to species of bizarre plants and animals found nowhere else in the world.

Professor Schultes is the only person known to have climbed several of the Colombian *tepuis*. In 1988, he described the fabled peaks and some of the myths that surround them:

Remnants of a once continuous highland that stretched from the Guianas across southern Venezuela and nearly to the Andes in Colombia, the isolated quartzitic mountains of eastern Colombia are sentinels of a mysterious past.

The Cerro de la Campana (Bell Mountain) is one of the westernmost vestiges of these hills and is so strikingly awesome that it is wrapped in legend in the Indian mind. All Indians believe that fierce thunderstorms and torrents can be caused by beating upon a thinly eroded slab near the summit. When struck with another stone, it sends forth a bell-like tone. Caves near the base of La Campana have Indian paintings and scratchings of animals on some of the walls, remains probably of the now nearly extinct but formerly numerous and warlike Karijonas who once dwelt in the basin of the upper Apaporis.

The farther south we flew, the less well known was the landscape. According to the pilot, one river beneath us had yet to be named. As we approached the foothills of the Kayser Mountains, enveloped in clouds, the pilot banked the plane and dropped altitude. "Look," he said. We disappeared into a cloud, surrounded for a moment only by vapor, and then broke once more into the light. "There it is," said the pilot. "The Devil's Egg."

It sat on the edge of a mountain, perfectly balanced, seemingly glued in place: an enormous gray-white boulder whose size dwarfed our little plane. It was beautiful, bizarre, unsettling. An oblate remnant of ancient base rock that nature had eroded over time, it seemed to emphasize our inconsequentiality, an awe-inspiring sight in a place that few had seen—or ever would. Here nature did strange and glorious things for her own amusement.

Three hours after leaving the capital city, we passed over several disturbed patches of forest, signs of human presence. The forest gave way to a large clearing, choked with a cluster of thatched huts. As our plane circled overhead, Indians emerged from the huts and when we landed on the crude red dirt airstrip cut between the village and the jungle, they were there to greet us.

The male Indians, dressed alike in red breechcloths and white beaded belts, surrounded the plane and stared at me through the window; the few women, curious but timid, hung in the background, watching as I unloaded my belongings. Several bold little boys rubbed the hair on my arms, a sight they had rarely seen before. The pilot soon had stowed his cargo of birds and reptiles and was ready to go and began to taxi for takeoff. Suddenly he cut the engine and beckoned me over. "My friend," he said, "let me give you some advice—stay away from the women. If you do not, the men will come after you, and all of their arrows have poison tips. Have a good trip, and I will see you in two months."

I watched him go, then gathered up my things to carry into the village, where I hoped to meet the tribal chieftain. As I bent down to lift my backpack, the heaviest piece of equipment, one of the onlookers, a young man of about eighteen, picked it up and tossed it over his shoulder with a dexterous flick of his wrist. He was small and wiry and stood about five-foot-two. Like the other Indians who watched me so intently, he had painted his bronze skin dark blue with the fruit of the *meh-nu* tree. Suspended from a white cotton string around his neck was a charm, a slightly curved, yellowish white jaguar tooth, about three inches long. He introduced himself in fluent Surinamese: "I am called Koita." Then, with my backpack slung over his right shoulder, he strode down the path from the airstrip into the village. Hurriedly gathering up my remaining supplies, I fell in behind him.

The village was called Kwamalasamoetoe, or "Bamboo Sand," for the bamboo trees that lined the nearby riverbanks. It was perched on a bluff, like a sentinel keeping watch over the green-brown Sipaliwini River. The Tirió tribe numbers about a thousand members, and a typical village is home to only ten to thirty people. Kwamala, as the Indians call it, is an exception to that rule, having a population of about three hundred. This is not uncommon in regions visited by missionaries. When the evangelists target a particular area, they try to concentrate the Indians into "supervillages" of several hundred to make it easier and more efficient to convert them.

More than a hundred palm-thatched houses of all different types and sizes dotted the village. Some dwellings were little more than lean-tos, just big enough for a single hammock, while others were great conical communal houses that could sleep twenty or more people. Some homes squatted on the orange-brown sandy dirt like hollow haystacks; others sat six feet off the ground on stilts, like spindly-legged water birds. Some huts had walls and roofs; others had only roofs to catch the rain, and any passerby could look in to see the daily goings-on.

"I did not know that the Tiriós constructed so many different types of dwellings," I commented to Koita.

"They don't," he replied. "The big houses are built by the Waiwais, and the stilt houses belong to the Apalai Indians. There are many different tribes here and each has its own preferred style."

I had stumbled onto an ethnobotanical gold mine—a village inhabited by six different tribes whose presence in Suriname was unreported in the anthropological literature. In this one place alone I might learn six times as much as I could staying with a single tribe. A species used for medicinal purposes by several different tribes, even if it was used for different purposes, would more than likely contain an active compound. I was anxious to begin collecting, but first I had to obtain the permission and support of the village chief.

Heading toward the chief's hut, I was pleased to see that like the Indians who greeted me at the airstrip, almost all of the villagers, male and female, wore only a *kamisa*—a breechcloth woven of native cotton and dyed red by soaking it in a solution made from the crushed seed coat of the *u-shuh* fruit. The fact that most of the three hundred Indians in the village wore traditional dress indicated that much of their culture—including their ethnobotanical knowledge—should still be intact.

The village was alive with the sounds of children laughing and screaming. Packs of young boys fired little arrows from miniature bows at the ubiquitous yellow-green *Ameiva* lizards that constantly prowled the grounds in search of ants and other terrestrial insects. Forest cultures depend on hunting skills for survival, and practice begins at a young age. As we walked through the village, we saw men sitting in cotton hammocks carving wooden arrowheads or carefully checking and rechecking their arrows, making sure that the all but suffocating humidity had not warped the shafts of their weapons.

"What do you hunt?" I asked Koita.

"A little of everything," he replied, "but mostly monkeys, peccaries, and some birds."

"How often do you hunt?"

"When we are hungry."

"What does that mean? How often do you go?"

"In a day, I can kill enough meat to feed my family for three days. When that's gone, I hunt again."

Although only eighteen years old, Koita had a wife and two children. I later found out that among the Tiriós, boys generally marry at age fifteen, girls at age fourteen. Usually, the girl's mother offers her daughter to a prospective bridegroom; if he agrees, the boy must pay a price for his bride, such as helping his prospective father-in-law clear a new garden patch or expand the old one. Occasionally, the boy asks for a girl's hand in marriage. I learned of one instance in which a boy of fourteen asked the parents of a ten-year-old girl for permission to marry; although the request met with approval, the marriage was delayed until the girl's first menstruation, three years later.

I noticed a difference in the reactions of the men and women we passed. The men were curious and friendly; many waved or smiled. The women, on the other hand, either retreated into their huts or looked at the ground when I offered a greeting. I was still pondering their shyness as we strolled around the back of one of the larger circular houses, where I almost bumped into a young woman carrying several brown calabashes of water up from the river. She was beautiful. Flawless light brown skin covered a slightly muscular frame. Thick, lustrous black hair blanketed her soft brown shoulders, and short, straight bangs fringed her face. On either side of her aquiline nose was painted a single elegant red stripe of *u-shuh* berry extract. Standing there with her calabashes, in her red cotton breechcloth and dark red cotton wrappings around her knees, with palm-fiber bracelets circling her elbows and wrists, she would have been the essence of Amazon Indian womanhood but for one thing: a white T-shirt that read JESUS IS LOVE.

American missionaries had first come to southwest Suriname in the early 1970s. They entered the country with "Christianized" Waiwai guides from southern Guyana, who explained to the local Tirió Indians the many alleged benefits—material and spiritual—of the white man's religion. At the time of their first contact with the missionaries, the Tiriós were suffering from diseases that had been introduced to their villages by explorers, Maroons, and other Indians, and possibly even by the evangelists themselves. Tirió ethnomedicine had been ineffective against these strange illnesses. The missionaries, however, provided remedies that worked, thereby "proving" to the tribal elders the superiority of Western culture over the indigenous tradition. While the Tiriós did not completely abandon their native ways in the wake of the evangelists' visits, the role of the shaman, who served as the village medicine man, was weakened. Medicine men no longer found apprentices eager to learn the secrets of the healing plants and, as the old men died, the secrets were buried with them.

In days past, boys—and, very rarely, girls—at about the age of fourteen would express a desire to be the shaman's apprentice. The healer would then paint secret symbols that look like lightning bolts on the boy's body, and instruct him to think carefully about his decision for one month. If the boy was still interested, he would work with the shaman to learn about illnesses, medicinal plants, healing rituals, and sacred songs.

Koita led me to a large rectangular hut at the edge of the river. The palm-thatched roof was supported by eight yellowed pillars, which were nothing more than the debarked trunks of white cedar trees. A slight breeze blew in off the river as my young guide barked a few commands at several small boys who had been watching us. They ran off and soon returned carrying six crudely carved low wooden benches.

Koita placed four of the benches end to end in a straight line. The fifth he positioned six feet in front of this line. In between and a bit to the side he placed the sixth bench. "This," he said, pointing to the last one, "is mine."

Before I could ask for any further explanation, one of the boys who watched us from outside the hut came forward and handed me a well-thumbed book bound in blue leather. The writing was foreign to me, but the pictures of bearded prophets were not. Koita confirmed my suspicion. "That is the Bible in Tirió. The missionaries did that two years after they first came here."

As he spoke, a light rain began to fall even though the sun continued to shine. Hearing a commotion behind me, I turned to view an extraordinary sight. The tribal chief and his three subchiefs entered the hut. Unlike Koita, they were not wearing traditional clothing. Instead, each wore long pants and a cotton shirt with a button-down collar. Adding to his air of Western urbanity, the chief had abandoned the characteristic Tirió hairstyle—bangs in the front and shoulder-length tresses in the back—for a short haircut, parted on the left and combed to the right. It glistened as if slicked down with a commercial pomade; I later learned this hair tonic was oil extracted from a *maripa* palm fruit.

The chief was perhaps fifty years old, stood about five-foot-three, and was somewhat portly, unusual for a forest Indian. His skin was a beautiful copper brown and his high cheekbones were typically Amerindian. His face showed no emotion as he silently looked me over before sitting on one of the four aligned benches. The subchiefs followed suit and Koita indicated that it was now appropriate for us to sit down. He took the bench off to the side and I sat on the one that faced the tribal leaders. With a nod of his head, the chief signaled it was time to begin the palaver.

Speaking in Surinamese, I explained that I had come to learn from the Indians. Perhaps not all of their dealings with white men had been pleasant ones, I said, but I had not come to pursue their women or teach them my religion. On the contrary, I was there to learn about the medicinal plants that the Indians knew and used. To me, the forest was a strange and complicated place—a place that the Indians understood much better than the white man ever could. I concluded by saying that I had come as a guest who wanted to stay and learn and that I hoped this would meet with their approval.

The chief spoke with his assistants in Tirió and then looked at me for a few moments as if he were both evaluating me and choosing his words carefully. He seemed a trifle perplexed—undoubtedly most of the whites he had dealt with in the past had regarded Indians at best as equals and more often as inferiors. Yet here was a foreigner who wanted to learn from him.

The chief leaned forward and addressed me in Tirió. Koita translated.

"You say you come to learn but this is difficult to believe. Why does the white man—the *pananakiri*—want to learn from us? Are not his medicines better? When the missionaries were here and I almost died of malaria, our medicine did not work. The missionaries gave me bitter white pills, and that cured me!"

At this point I broke in.

"Those pills are called quinine. Where does the chief think quinine comes from?"

"The missionaries brought those pills from America."

"Yes, those pills are made in my country. But they were made from a tree that grows to the west of here in a country called Peru. The Indian taught this tree to the white man. Quinine is an Indian medicine!"

The chief again conferred privately with his subchiefs. Then he looked me in the eyes and continued.

"So why should we teach you about our medicines? Though the missionaries have left here, once a month they send a plane with the white man's medicine, which is stronger than ours. Why should we teach you about our plants?"

His tone was a combination of cynicism, curiosity, and genuine bewilderment. I groped for an answer.

"Remember that the chief is a Christian," hissed Koita under his breath.

"The chief is a Christian," I began, clutching at straws. How could I convince him? I stumbled a bit before coming up with an answer. "The chief is a Christian," I repeated, "a man who reads the Bible. I, however, am a Jew, a member of the same tribe as Abraham, Moses, Jesus, Saul, and David." Remembering the drawings in his Bible, I stroked my beard for emphasis and continued. "Thousands of years ago, Saul and David wrote down the psalms of the Bible, which you probably sing in church. If my ancestors had not written down these psalms, no one would know how to sing them today. The songs would be dead.

"Just like Saul and David," I continued, "I want to write a book. I want to write about the plants your shamans use to cure illnesses. I want to help your wisdom live. Please help me to write this wisdom so that in a thousand years your grandchildren and my grandchildren will still know the traditions of your ancestors."

The chief mulled this over a bit, then told Koita that I could stay in an empty hut at the edge of the village. He would tell me of his decision after further discussions with his tribesmen.

Koita led me to a hut near the airstrip and helped me hang my hammock and mosquito net. By the time we finished the task, the sun was beginning to set. He left, promising to come back at sunrise to show me around the village. For the first time since I had arrived, I was alone.

Famished, I dug one of the precious cans of sardines out of the backpack and opened it with my machete. When I tried to unscrew the lid on my canteen, I discovered that it had cracked and all the water had leaked out. With my flashlight in one hand and my canteen in the other, I headed off through the village to get some water at the river.

The sun had set, and the Indians had all retired to their huts. Looking through the thatch, I could see their muscled bodies silhouetted against the cooking fires inside. Each hut had two or three small, mangy hunting dogs tied up nearby. The Tiriós are noted for their hunting dogs, which are deliberately underfed to keep them edgy and aggressive. As I passed each hut, the dogs rose and bristled; I kept a healthy distance from their bared teeth.

I filled my canteen and started back. It was a moonless night, and many of the dwellings looked alike in the darkness. Soon I was completely lost, heading first in one direction, then in another. The dogs were excited now, and snarled and lunged as I passed; soon they were howling in unison. Two Indians came out to investigate the commotion, but when I tried to explain myself, they couldn't understand and went back into their huts.

In a panic now, sweating with fear of the dogs, the Indians, and the night, I ducked into what looked to be a vacant hut. There was no fire, so I thought I was alone. But I heard a sound and pointed my flashlight at the other side of the hut. There a pregnant woman lay in a hammock, staring at me in fright and blinded by my flashlight. Recalling the pilot's admonition that morning, I tried desperately to calm her. I begged her to be quiet, but she didn't understand a word of Surinamese and began to sob. Frozen with fear myself, I was too exhausted even to decide whether to run back into the night or to wait for the arrival of this woman's angry husband.

Just then, someone crawled into the hut. "My friend, are you lost?" asked Koita. I let out a whoop of relief and hugged him tightly. I was still shaking as he showed me the way back to my hut. In the soothing embrace of my hammock I fell into a deep, dreamless sleep.

I was awakened by the intense cold. During the day, the temperature in the village had been in the nineties; overnight it had dropped at least fifty degrees. Morning mist cloaked the village. Walking down to the river, which was embarrassingly close to my hut, I bathed and then sat on the riverbank to collect my thoughts. Gazing upstream to where the Sipaliwini originates in the Tumuc-Humac Mountains that mark the border with Brazil, I saw wispy clouds covering the forest and shrouding the trees that line the river. I felt as if I were looking at the forest primeval, unbroken and unchanged since time began.

Koita interrupted my reverie. He had already spoken with the tribal chief, who informed him that I was welcome to live in their village and learn their plants. Later that day, the chief would tell this to the shamans.

Breaking into a broad grin, I again thanked Koita for rescuing me the night before. Enthused by the chief's assent, and feeling certain that Koita had done some lobbying on my behalf, I unsheathed the hunting knife attached to my belt and handed it to him. "This is for you."

The mixture of surprise and delight that registered on his face told me that he had not assisted me with the hope of gaining a reward. As he balanced the weight of the knife in his right hand and tested the sharpness of the blade against his left thumb, I said, "I have only one question. When do we start?" Koita looked up from his knife and smiled. "If you really want to learn about medicinal plants, you'll have to ask the medicine men, the *piai*," he replied. "But I know a few useful plants, so we can go into the forest and look around if you would like."

We returned to my hut and I grabbed my canteen and strapped on my machete. Before we even left the village it was apparent that Koita knew a bit more than he had let on. He showed me a small tree with large, palmate leaves (leaves shaped like a hand), which was growing behind the chief's hut. Holding one of the dark green leaves, he announced, "This is *ku-deh-deh*. We drip the sap of the crushed plant into aching eyes."

This is the point at which a field researcher should have some familiarity with the local flora. If your guide tells you a plant is used for medicine and you know it's from a family thought to be chemically inert—meaning that it would have no significant effect on the human body—you should be suspicious. Chances are your guide is either mistaken or intentionally misleading you. Of course, it could be that your guide is right and conventional science is wrong, so you need to keep an open mind as well.

The first plant that Koita showed me, *ku-deh-deh*, was a member of the fig family. Typically found in the Amazon in areas where the original forest has been altered or destroyed, it is widely used by South American Indians for several purposes, including the treatment of bleeding gums in Colombia and heart problems in Brazil. Alkaloids—nitrogenous compounds that are important components in many medicines—are known to occur in these plants; Koita's pointing this out as a useful species indicated to me that we were off to a good start.

Our next stop was a cashew tree at the edge of the village. Although now planted throughout the tropics, cashews are native to the Amazon. The green cashew "nut" (which is actually the fruit) dangles from the end of a swollen stem that resembles an elongated pear. The nut contains an extremely toxic oil and must be cleaned and well roasted before it can safely be consumed. That the cashew can be so poisonous is hardly surprising; it belongs to the same family as poison ivy and poison oak, both of which contain irritating oils in their tissues.

According to Koita, the local Indians use the green nut to kill botfly larvae, a common problem in lowland Amazonia. A botfly deposits its larva under the skin and the larva hatch and consume living flesh. By slicing the nut in half and rubbing the cut side over the affected area, the toxic compounds kill the larvae, which can then be pulled out of the skin.

After passing the cashew tree, we turned onto a narrow path leading directly into the jungle. We spent the entire day hiking, exploring, and collecting plants. Koita knew the names—if not the uses—of many plants, and when asked a species he did not know, he would apologize and say we would have to ask a shaman. Although his knowledge proved not nearly as extensive as that of the shamans with whom I would later work, we still made several intriguing finds. At the side of the trail, Koita pointed out a short bush with thick leaves of the deepest green. The color of the leaves contrasted sharply with the ruby-red berries growing at its base. Koita plucked two of the thin, waxy leaves, balled them up, and crushed them in his right hand. Then he opened his fist for me to smell the contents. The mashed leaves gave off an appealing gingerlike aroma.

As I knelt down to examine the plant, Koita explained, "This we call *ko-noy-uh*. We drink a tea of the leaves as a treatment for colds and sore throats."

This use fascinated me. I recognized the plant as a member of the ginger family and I knew that the ancient Chinese used ginger prepared in the same manner for the same purpose. Schultes always taught his students to be on the lookout for closely related plants used for similar purposes by disparate peoples. Such a pattern, he advised, usually indicated a biochemical reason for the particular usage. In this case, the ginger family is rich in essential oils, which accounts for the aromatic nature of the plants. Taking teas brewed from these plants can relieve some of the symptoms of coughs and colds, as discovered by the Chinese, the Tiriós, and other groups throughout the tropics.

A few yards farther down the trail, Koita stopped in front of a slender six-foot tree with whitish brown bark and ovate leaves. Borrowing my machete, he cut a diagonal slit in the bark with a quick, sharp, downward stroke. Almost immediately, a brilliant orange sap oozed out and turned bright red as it dripped down the trunk of the tree. The color of the sap identified the tree as a species of the St. Johnswort family, a group best known for such delicious tropical fruits as the juicy, tart-sweet mangosteen in Asia; the sweet, soft-fleshed mammee apple in the Caribbean; and the slightly acidic bacury in Brazil. Other species of this family serve a variety of purposes throughout Amazonia: The sap of the *maniballi* tree is valued as a pitch for making torches in Colombia, while the resin of the buckwax tree is used to caulk boats, attach feathers to arrows, and as a form of currency among tribes who were otherwise outside of the monetary economy.

"What do you do with the sap?" I asked as we watched it slowly seep from the wounded tree. Dipping his right index finger into the ooze and testing its thickness by rubbing it between his thumb and forefinger, Koita replied, "We rub it on skin infections."

Western medicine cannot cure deep fungal infections of the skin. A slight case of athlete's foot can be successfully treated with several different products on the market, but a serious case can only be suppressed, not cured. The hot, humid climate of the rain forest creates a rich breeding ground for these types of infections, but no one in the village seemed to suffer any skin problems. (Granted, I was not examining everyone I met for dermatoses, but the fact that most wore only a breechcloth made it difficult to disguise a serious skin infection.) According to the great French ethnobotanist Pierre Grenand, in the nineteenth century some of this latex was exported from the Amazon to France as a treatment for skin ailments. Preliminary results of recent laboratory testing indicate it is effective in treating fungal infections.

We had collected about ten different medicinal species when Koita suggested we head back to the village while there was still sunlight. We returned along a trail that crossed a small creek and wound its way around a hundred-foot-tall tree with thick buttress roots and smooth brown bark. Koita walked around the tree, studied the ground, then dropped to one knee to gather up several large nuts with thick brown woody shells. "These probably just fell," he observed, "otherwise the agoutis would already have eaten them. These are called *sho* and they are the best food in the forest!"

Again borrowing my machete—an almost indispensable tool in the forest, but not every Indian has one of his own—Koita cracked the hard fibrous shell. Inside was a nut that somewhat resembled a Brazil nut, covered with a tasty oil. The flavor was a revelation: very creamy and slightly sweet, leaving a lingering dairy taste reminiscent of rich ice cream.

More than a hundred years earlier, while traveling up the Essequibo River in neighboring Guyana, Prussian naturalist and explorer Richard

Schomburgk also noted the dairylike flavor of these nuts, known in that country as *sawari:*

> While taking our black coffee in the morning, our host asked us to wait a while because, although not possessing goats or cows, he knew where to get some milk. He soon returned with a basketful of beautiful ripe *Sawari* nuts . . . [he] broke the kernels out of their shells, pounded them in a vessel, and poured the expressed fatty white juice into the dark brown liquid which now bore comparison with the morning coffee of Europeans mixed with the fattest of cream. The sensible fellow did not teach us the little piece of magic in vain because this vegetable milk has often colored our coffee since, and made it tasty.

That evening, comfortable in the cocoon of my hammock, I reviewed the lessons of the day. I could not help but be struck by the balance in which the Indians lived with the forest and how adept they were in extracting a living from it. Jungle trees do not bear fruit all year round, nor do edible animals hide behind every bush. Through necessity the Indians have mastered their environment in a way that permits them to live off of it without destroying it. For the peoples of the forest, hunting involves making a bow and arrow from local plants and learning the tracks, the haunts, diet, and calls of preferred species. Some tribes are known to relish creatures as unappetizing to Western palates as rats, storks, armadillos, lizards, toucans, parrots, and hummingbirds. The Yukpa Indians of western Venezuela eat more than twenty species of insects. Some are staples in their diet, but most are eaten as snacks when Indians encounter them in the forest.

The next morning, I was awakened by the sound of footsteps outside my hut. Koita had brought a visitor. The man was short—about five feet tall—but very muscular. His cheekbones were exceptionally high, framing his flattened nose. A jutting lower jaw and prominent eyebrow ridges gave him a slightly Neanderthal appearance. Not that he seemed dull or unintelligent; rather, he looked like a man who lived not only by his wits but by his physical prowess as well.

Koita introduced him as one of the most powerful shamans in the village, and he did emanate a certain power—a strange mixture of the physical and the metaphysical that was almost tactile. There was a certain dignity and a condescension in his bearing, as if he would show me something of his healing plants only to demonstrate the superiority of his knowledge. Such was my introduction to the healer who would later appear in my telling dream—the Jaguar Shaman, as I came to call him.

Traditionally, the most powerful men in the Tirió tribe were the chiefs and the shamans. The chief served as the ultimate decision maker while the shaman, or *piai*, healed the sick and maintained contact with the spirit world—responsibilities that usually overlapped. Illness was generally regarded as the work of malevolent spirits (sometimes sent by rival shamans), and the medicine man contacted the spirit world to diagnose an affliction and to determine what special plants might be needed to treat it. The typical Amazonian shaman thus served not only as physician but also as priest, pharmacist, psychiatrist, and even psychopomp—one who conducts souls to the afterworld. Today, the Tirió chief maintains his position of power; however, the shaman is no longer held in such regard, due mainly to the influence of outsiders.

The Jaguar Shaman was a master healer. He led the way into the forest, singing songs that Koita described as chants used in healing ceremonies. In the jungle, we paused at herbs, bushes, and trees unknown to Koita as having medicinal uses yet comprising important components of the shaman's pharmacopoeia.

As we came to an old rotting log that lay across the trail, the Jaguar Shaman paused. He pointed to a flat, ivory-colored fungus that grew on the decomposing bark. "*Go-lo-be,*" he said.

"What is it used for?" asked Koita in Tirió.

"*Pana epi,*" he replied. "Ear medicine."

The shaman peeled several pieces of the fungus off the bark and held them in his palm. Making a fist, he squeezed out several drops of a clear, odorless liquid. He indicated that this sap, dripped into aching ears, would provide relief after three days of treatment.

Earaches are a common affliction in the humid environs of the rain forest, and many are fungal in origin. Since most antibiotics are derived from fungi, the aboriginal use of any fungus for medicinal purposes merits special attention. It is difficult for us to comprehend how radically our lives have been changed since the first antibiotic—penicillin—was discovered in 1928. Prior to that, even a slight cut while shaving could lead to blood poisoning and then to almost certain death.

Next we stopped at a large liana, a woody vine that curved and twisted its way skyward through the bushes and small trees at the edge of the trail. The medicine man found a brown bean-shaped pod that had fallen from the vine. Breaking it open, he showed me the fruits, whose spherical shape and peculiar markings resembled little eyeballs. And sure enough, the Tirió name for the plant, *tah-mo-ko ah-nu*, meant "howler monkey eye."

The medicine man indicated that he valued the sap of the liana's stem as a cure for children's fevers. *Tah-mo-ko ah-nu* is closely related to two other species from the legume family, which is rich in alkaloids. These species play important roles in modern medicine. Physostigmine, originally extracted from a species used as a poison in West Africa, has been used by Western physicians since the 1950s to treat glaucoma, myasthenia gravis, and postpartum heartburn. And extracts of another species provides L-dopa, an amino acid in use since the late 1960s to treat Parkinson's disease. In the body, L-dopa is converted to dopamine, which facilitates nerve transmission in the brain.

In our highly specialized industrial society, we tend to think of plants either as foods or medicines or commercial products; the categories seldom overlap: we eat wheat, we take digitalis (which comes from the foxglove plant), and we use rubber. To the Indian, such artificial boundaries do not exist. The Jaguar Shaman taught me how to use the sap of the rubber tree to kill botfly larvae, how to use the exudate of the cotton plant to treat burns, and how to use the sap of edible palms to stanch the bleeding of severe cuts.

Palms exemplify this principle of multiusefulness better than any other group of plants in the Amazon rain forest. Though used and venerated as important symbols in Judaism, Christianity, Hinduism, Buddhism, and Islam all over the world, palms provide the native South American with food, fibers, musical instruments, fuels, oils, waxes, weapons, medicines, and even toys. And the thatched huts in the village were woven from the leaves of the *mah-rah-re-uh*, *wah-pu*, and *ku-mu* palms. The late Harold Moore, the foremost twentieth-century authority on palms, commented on the paramount role these plants play in the indigenous cultures of the Neotropics—South America, the West Indies, and tropical North America:

> The importance of man as a biotic factor in the tropical ecosystem has been argued. . . . However, to whatever extent man has been involved in the tropical ecosystem, palms have certainly been a major factor in making possible their involvement and even today, despite the advent of the corrugated tin roof and the rifle, they are of primary importance to many primitive Indian cultures.

Alfred Russel Wallace, who lived in the Brazilian Amazon from 1849 to 1852 and shares credit with Charles Darwin as originator of the theory of evolution, gave a detailed account of the uses of palms in Indian culture:

> Suppose then we visit an Indian cottage on the banks of the Rio Negro, a great tributary of the river Amazon in South America. The main supports of the building are trunks of some forest tree of heavy and durable wood, but the light rafters overhead are formed by the straight cylindrical and uniform stems of the *Jará* palm. The roof is thatched with large triangular leaves, neatly arranged in regular alternate rows, and bound to the rafters with *sipós* or forest creepers; the leaves are those of the *Caraná* palm. The door of the house is a framework of thin hard strips of wood neatly thatched over; it is made of the split stems of the *Pashiúba* palm. In one corner stands a heavy harpoon for catching the cow-fish; it is formed of the black wood of the *Pashiúba barriguda*. By its side is a blowpipe ten or twelve feet long, and a little quiver full of small poisoned arrows hang up near it . . . it is from the stem and spines of two species of Palms that they are made. His great bassoon-like musical instruments are made of palm stems; the cloth in which he wraps his most valued feather ornaments is a fibrous palm spathe, and the rude chest in which he keeps these treasures is woven from palm leaves. His hammock, his bow-string and his fishing-line are from the *Tucúm* [palm]. The comb which he wears on his head is ingeniously constructed of the hard bark of a palm, and he makes fish hooks of the spines, or uses them to

puncture on his skin the peculiar markings of his tribe. His children are eating the agreeable red and yellow fruit of the *Pupunha* or peach palm, and from that of the *Assaí* [palm] he has prepared a favourite drink, which he offers you to taste. That carefully suspended gourd contains oil, which he has extracted from the fruit of another species; and that long, elastic, plaited cylinder used for squeezing dry the mandioca pulp to make his bread, is made of the bark of one of the singular climbing palms, which alone can resist for a considerable time the action of the poisonous juice. In each of these cases a species is selected better adapted than the rest for the peculiar purpose to which it is applied, and often having several different uses which no other plant can serve as well, so that some little idea may be formed of how important to the South American Indian must be these noble trees, which supply so many daily wants, giving him his house, his food, and his weapons.

The Tiriós are no less sophisticated in the use of palms than the Indians Wallace described over a century ago. The Jaguar Shaman pointed out that in addition to employing the sap of the *kumu* palm to stanch bleeding, the Indians eat the fruit. According to Dr. Michael Balick, a leading modern authority on Amazonian palms, the nutritional content of this fruit compares favorably with that of human breast milk.

Several of the plants we collected that first day were used by the Jaguar Shaman for the "black arts," and Koita knew as little about these secrets as I did. The *piai* indicated that by blowing on the stem of the *kurunyeh* bush he could paralyze the fingers of a rival shaman. And by chanting and waving the branches of the *wah-kah-pu* tree over someone with a stomachache, he claimed, he could cure the condition. Then, as if retreating from the occult, the shaman taught me simple uses of the plants. By rubbing together dead stems of the *ah-de-gah-nah-mah* bush, a wild relative of the chocolate tree that dries well and burns easily, he could start a fire. The stem of a huge *sho* tree yielded a substance containing a saponin, a sudsing compound like that found in many commercial detergents and that could be used as a soap. The bark of the *ayaeya* vine was used to stun fish, as I was to see on a fishing expedition a few weeks later.

After a week of intensive collecting, the old shaman still had not run out of plants to show me. He knew how to treat heart problems, bed wetting, burns, malaria, malaise, rashes, impotence, and gonorrhea. Using the bark of the towering *po-no* tree, a first cousin of the Brazil nut, he taught me how to make straps for a backpack. He produced a barking bird call by cutting the leaf of a small palm and rubbing the stem back and forth across the blade of his knife. Two minutes later, a red-throated caracara hawk flew overhead above the canopy, its piercing caws answering the shaman's call. The old medicine man summoned the hawk down through the canopy, where it perched in a tree above us, cocked its head to one side, and looked down at us quizzically as the medicine man continued to make the bird call. The Jaguar Shaman was proud of his command of the natural world, both plants and animals.

As we hiked through a swamp, the path became more overgrown. I swung my machete to clear the trail, inadvertently hitting a wasp nest that exploded into a cloud of angry insects. Though we ran, I was badly stung, and the stings were excruciating, like hot needles under the skin.

The medicine man walked over to a small green bush not ten feet away. With his machete, he scraped off a small portion of the bark, crushed it in his fist, and rubbed it on my wasp stings. In less than three minutes, the burning pain had disappeared, and in another five minutes, the swelling had gone down. Twenty-four hours later there was no inflammation, no secondary infection, and virtually no sign that I had ever been stung.

When I returned to the United States, I found that the plant—a member of the violet family and known as *ku-run-yeh* by the Tiriós—had not previously been reported as an effective treatment for insect stings. While collecting plants in the jungles of southern Panama nine years later, I was again badly stung by several angry bees. Relieved to find a related species of *ku-run-yeh* nearby, I rubbed it on the stings. It proved equally effective. Such topical analgesics merit our attention. Over two thousand years ago, Asians were using willow bark to relieve pain. The ancient Greeks and at least fifteen North American Indian tribes employed parts of the willow tree for similar purposes. Chemical research on those species began in the early nineteenth century and led to the development of the most commonly used drug in the industrialized world—acetylsalicylic acid (from *Salix,* the Latin name for willow), better known to us as aspirin.

Aspirin's utility exceeds that of a mere painkiller; it also reduces fever and swelling and, when taken in small, daily doses, has been shown to reduce the risk of heart attacks and strokes. Acetylsalicylic acid acts by inhibiting the body's production of prostaglandins, chemicals that play an important role in blood clotting, blood vessel dilation, constriction of the bronchial muscle, and inhibition of gastric secretions and uterine contractions.

Other potential uses for this botanical wonder drug have recently presented themselves to laboratory researchers. It has been found that some malignant tumor cells protect themselves against attack from anticancer immune cells by forming a protective layer of prostaglandins. Modern science may one day develop a way to use aspirin to break through, or at least weaken, this barrier.

Although it seems unlikely that the painkilling bark used by the Jaguar Shaman to treat my wasp stings might have the commercial potential of aspirin, its effectiveness as an analgesic—proved in the field in Suriname and Panama—may hold promise for the future. New analgesics are always in demand; much as ibuprofen is valued by people allergic to aspirin, a new painkiller may find a niche among people who are sensitive to those analgesics already on the market.

Through the course of our days together, the old shaman maintained a detached air. He never smiled or laughed; his haughty dignity underscored his position as master to mine as apprentice. At the end of the third day, he informed Koita that he would teach me no more. Perhaps he was tired of instructing, or maybe he was merely hungry for meat and needed to hunt; regardless of the reason, I felt a deep regret. That night I dreamed of the jaguar, the most intelligent, mysterious, and powerful creature in the jungle, and a symbol of the shaman throughout lowland tropical America. It was an event that marked a watershed in my experience with both the Indians and the forest. In that one fleeting moment, an instant of pure enlightenment, it became totally clear to me that different people, cultures, and places can have their own realities; that just as one can learn the spoken language of a foreign land, one can absorb its spirit—even if that spirit and its wisdom differ radically from those of one's own culture. In a society where people believe hallucinogenic experiences are caused by deities that inhabit sacred plants and that the reality we live every day is merely a dream, why shouldn't a medicine man who consults with the spirit world be able to turn himself into a mighty jungle beast? When I dreamed of the jaguar, I felt the Indians were communicating in a new language of exchange—beyond the plants that I had learned or the words that Koita had taught me, a language of other realities.

After the Jaguar Shaman went off into the forest alone to hunt, Koita introduced me to Tyaky, another Tirió medicine man. Again I was thankful I had found this village, which was large enough to have several medicine men instead of the single shaman found in most small Indian communities. Although Tyaky was probably seventy years old, he had the build of a professional wrestler and the bearing of a U.S. Marine. He also had an impish sense of humor and never failed to find some aspect of my dress or behavior worthy of great hoots of laughter. One morning I was having trouble with my contact lenses and decided to wear a pair of glasses. Seeing this, Tyaky was overcome by a case of giggles, exclaiming that I looked like a not very bright version of a *koikoi,* a crab-eating raccoon.

I was a constant source of amusement to Tyaky in the forest. Forest Indians have an extraordinary balance and grace that I will never match. To cross a stream, they sometimes fell a small sapling often less than three inches wide, lay it across the stream, and run nimbly across it. I, on the other hand, inch my way across, one foot placed gingerly in front of the other. Once, while crossing one of these bridges, I lost my footing and fell several feet down into a stream. As I checked myself for broken bones, Tyaky guffawed so hard he nearly choked. That was eight years ago. For years afterward, every time I visited the village, Tyaky broke into a big grin, pointed at me, and called, "Look, it is the white-man-who-falls-on-his-ass!"

All in all, the Indians regarded me as a sort of dim-witted relative when we were in the forest. They preferred me to walk between them, where they believed they could protect me from treading on poisonous snakes or blundering into wasp nests. I, too, preferred this arrangement, but for different reasons. By following the medicine man's lead, I let him know I respected his authority and his knowledge of healing plants.

And as I began learning more words in the Tirió language, I was also able to communicate directly with the shaman and depend less on Koita's translations.

Koita, Tyaky, and I spent a week walking through the jungle collecting plants. The shaman showed me the *ay-mah-rah-e-wah* tree, whose bark the Tiriós boil for tea and drink to speed the healing of cuts. He also pointed out the lyrically named *pah-nah-ra-pah-nah*, a vine commonly found at the edge of Tirió gardens. This species has a scarlet stem on which grow rows of lime-green fruits about the size of small blueberries. The Tiriós crush the entire plant and rub it into their hair to kill fleas and lice. This was the first time I had seen this plant, a relative of the North American pokeweed, in use in the Amazon. But I knew that in southern Africa native peoples employ a closely related species to kill bilharzia larvae, which cause the dreaded schistosomiasis. Schistosomiasis, which after malaria is probably humankind's most serious parasite infection, affects tens of millions of people. Recent tests at the University of Texas indicate that *pah-nah-ra-pah-nah* does have antiviral properties, and more tests are under way to see if there are commercial applications for this species.

Even though I had now collected nearly a hundred specimens, I devised ways to find out about other plants. "Here are the names of five plants for fever," I would tell the old shaman. "Do you know more?" Challenged in this way, he would rack his memory for more names, which I furiously scribbled in my notes, creating a wish list of plants to look for in the future. I even involved the inhabitants of the village in my scheme to find out the names of as many healing plants as possible. At the end of the day, rather than bring the plants I had collected back to my hut to identify them and put them in my plant press, I began to sort and press them in the central plaza. It turned into an informal ethnobotanical seminar, with the inhabitants of the village crowding around, showing off what they knew and disagreeing among themselves.

"You use that for rashes? Everybody knows that it's really for sprains!"

"Boil it! That's ridiculous! It should be heated before you use it, but *never* boiled."

"What do you mean for headaches? The *best* headache remedy is the *wyanatude* vine!"

From this I got both contradictions and confirmations, but always leads on new plants or uses.

Late one afternoon, while we were hiking through a hilly patch of forest, Tyaky stopped in front of a tree, patted it fondly, and said, "Here is my old friend Kaloshewuh!" I was momentarily confused; I had met a man named Kaloshewuh in the village, but I couldn't figure out what he had to do with this tree. Tyaky explained that his friend's mother had had a difficult time delivering her baby, and it looked as though either mother or child might die. The midwife prepared a cold water infusion of the bark of the *kah-lo-she-wuh* tree and gave it to the laboring woman to drink. The medicine worked and a healthy baby boy, promptly named Kaloshewuh, slipped out.

I was excited by this story, imagining I could find all sorts of new natural drugs to ease pain during labor or to dilate the cervix. Then I realized that very few sexually oriented medicinal plants had been pointed out to me. I asked Koita about it and he replied, "It is the women who know about these plants." I was filled with curiosity, and in my determination to learn more about this aspect of jungle medicine I seriously breached Tirió etiquette.

That night there was a full moon. After dinner with Koita and his family—my meager rations had given out days before—we sat around the campfire in the middle of the village. This was a special time when the older men retold tribal legends and tales of intertribal wars, and recounted great hunting exploits from their youth. Their complex oratory went far beyond the limits of my fragmentary Tirió, and I waited for a lull in the conversation to ask the chief a question. When the time came, I asked the chief if I could go into the forest with Kykwe's grandmother to collect plants. Kykwe was a friend of Koita's, and his grandmother, an ancient crone who shuffled through Kwamala mumbling to herself, supposedly knew more about medicine than any other woman in the village.

There was a shocked silence, and the chief looked horrified by my request. What had I done? Koita leaned toward me and gently explained that I had asked the chief for permission to engage in sexual relations with the old woman. In a culture where most of the houses have no walls, all illicit couplings take place in the jungle. To proposition someone, you ask them to meet you in the forest. I nearly burst out laughing at the idea that I could not be trusted in the forest with someone's toothless, wrinkled grandmother, who, though charming in her own way, was unlikely to incite the passions of even a lonely ethnobotanist. But this was a serious matter, and I depended on Koita to help explain my ignorance and beg the chief's pardon. It seemed there was no way for me to walk into the forest with any woman from the tribe, and no way for me to learn about their special plants.

Although I have little knowledge of the plants involved, I am convinced that there exists a wealth of ethnobotanical treatments for menstrual problems, birth control, difficult childbirth, and so on, which is simply unavailable to the male ethnobotanist. Take, for example, the famous *piripiri* of the western Amazon. In the 1940s, Nicole Maxwell, a New York socialite, packed her bags and headed to the Amazon. Bored by sophisticated Western society, she had decided to set out for parts unknown in lowland Peru and Colombia. Maxwell, who had no formal training in ethnobotany, lived for many years among tribes like the Witoto and the Bora, carefully collecting as many of their plants as she could. A plant called *piripiri* was used by the women of the tribe as a contraceptive. They brewed it as a tea, and anyone drinking only a few cups reportedly would be infertile for a period of up to three years. But Maxwell was never able to get fresh plant material into the laboratory for testing. It was not until 1986 that *piripiri* was collected and tested, by an American woman named Karen Lowell, who was living with the Shuar Indians (better known as the Jivaros, of head-hunting fame) in the Ecuadorian Amazon. In the course of her research, Lowell was taken into the women's gardens and taught about the plants they cultivated. Most, like cassava and papaya, were grown as food. From some of the plants, like cotton and *u-shuh* berry, the women produced trade goods like hammocks or dyes. A few were medicinal. The famous *piripiri*, which Lowell had heard about but never seen, turned out to be a sedge. Laboratory analysis is currently under way at the University of Illinois, and preliminary test results on rats indicate that *piripiri* does have contraceptive properties.

Late one afternoon, Koita, Tyaky, and I had finished our plant collecting and were hurrying back to the village just ahead of a rapidly approaching storm. We could hear the rain pounding on the forest canopy to the south and periodically an ominous rumbling of thunder echoed through-out the forest. Nothing could stop us as we headed for shelter in the village—nothing, except the fruit of the hogplum tree. About twenty of the bright yellow olive-sized fruits were scattered to the right of the trail and Tyaky quickly began scooping them up. Slicing two leaves off a low-growing *wah-pu* palm, Koita quickly wove a small backpack into which Tyaky piled the hogplums. "These we call *mo-pa*," Koita explained. "They are a favorite food of everything from toucans to tortoises. They must have just fallen because in only a few hours they would all have been eaten or at least carried off."

Having piled all the fruit we found into the backpack, we again set off at a rapid pace, eating the *mo-pa* as we walked. Beneath the thin skin was a yellowish orange pulp that had the consistency of a ripe plum—soft and slightly sticky. Following Koita's example, I popped the whole fruit in my mouth. It was sweet like a banana with a pleasant, tart aftertaste like a mango; the pit was brown, hard, and slightly elongated. From Schultes's classes I knew that hogplum was one of the best-tasting and most widespread species in the Neotropics, found from southern Mexico south to northern Argentina. So highly esteemed is hogplum fruit that the tree often serves as a landmark. In Guatemala there is a town named Ocotenango, which in the Cakchiquel Maya Indian dialect means "place where the hogplum grows."

"Do you ever plant this?" I asked Koita as we hiked back to the village.

"No," he replied. "The tree is common and we always know where to find it in the forest. I have thrown a few seeds into my garden, though, to see if they'll come up."

Here was an agricultural and ethnobotanical screening process in action. The Indians make great use of numerous wild species and some are functional, nutritious, or tasty enough to serve as potential candidates for domestication. Thus some species make the transition from the wild into a stage known as incipient domestication, in which a particular plant may be experimented with in one's garden. Maybe it never sprouts, maybe it grows but does not produce fruit, maybe by the time it produces fruit the tribe has moved on and the garden has been abandoned, yet it is this process of taking a wild species with unknown properties and testing and perhaps even growing it that is at the heart of ethnobotany. Plant study and use is an ongoing process whereby some species go from no use to limited use to a highly specialized use.

Nowhere is this more evident than in the case of cassava, as we saw upon entering the village that afternoon. The skies had just opened up as we arrived and we ducked into Koita's round hut to avoid the downpour. The hut was dark, and the only hint that anyone lived there was the two long, cotton hammocks hung at the far side of the dwelling. Koita's wife and sister-in-law sat on benches made from tree stumps, peeling long brown cassava roots with their knives. The constant *snick*, *snick*, *snick* of their deft slicing beat a steady rhythm in the darkness.

If palms are the most important wild plant used by the Amazonian Indian, then cassava is the most essential cultivated plant. A member of the rubber family, cassava (also known as manioc and yuca) originated in the Amazon, where it was domesticated thousands of years ago. Nutritionally, cassava is almost pure starch and, in terms of starch content, produces millions more calories per acre than corn. Ideally suited to the humid tropics, it is insect resistant and tolerates sun, shade, and both wet and dry spells.

The paramount role played by cassava in Indian culture is reflected in the number of instances it appears in indigenous legends. According to the Tukanoan Indians of the northwest Amazon, the first man and woman reached earth from the Milky Way in a canoe drawn by a sacred anaconda. In the canoe they carried the three plants necessary for life in the rain forest: *yagé*, a hallucinogenic vine that allowed them to communicate with the spirit world; coca, a stimulant that helped them work and hunt without fatigue; and cassava, their staple foodstuff.

The Tupi Indians of Brazil have a different, more poignant explanation for the origin of cassava, or manioc. As the story goes, there was once a mother with no food who watched her starving child die. The grief-stricken woman buried the child under the floor of her hut. That night a wood spirit, or *mani*, visited the hut and transformed the child's body into the roots of a plant. This plant, called *mani oca* ("wood spirit root"), grew up to feed future generations of Indians.

Like the starchy taro in Polynesia and true yams in Africa, manioc has long served as the staple of local forest societies. These root crops have two advantages over species that produce edible fruits above ground. First, the underground food is relatively safe from herbivorous predators. Second, the force of gravity ceases to be a factor in limiting the maximum size of the edible plant part. The root or underground tuber can grow much larger than a fruit that must be supported by a branch. A mulberry bush cannot grow and support a six-pound mulberry, but a cassava plant can and does produce a six-pound cassava root.

Though little known in industrialized countries, cassava is one of the world's most important crops, serving as a staple not only in Amazonia but in tropical Africa as well. The manifold uses that the Amazonian Indians have managed to develop for this plant boggle the mind. Cassava has been used to make various poisons, a spice, beer, baby food, porridge, and bread. It is the latter use which is most common—cassava bread is probably the single most common element in the daily diet of the Amazonian Indian.

What makes this so remarkable is that the most widespread form— bitter cassava—contains poisonous compounds that can be fatal if eaten. Almost all tribes have developed a process—which usually consists of some combination of soaking, boiling, squeezing, and cooking —to remove the toxin. That the Indians have taken a deadly plant, domesticated it, and developed a technology that has turned this poisonous species into something that feeds hundreds of millions of people each day throughout the tropical world demonstrates a botanical ingenuity possessed by few, if any, professional botanists. And Amazonian Indian tribes have cultivated innumerable varieties of cassava. While there is usually no appreciable difference in taste among the varieties, the Indians have diversified the crop as insurance in case of disaster: if a blight were to hit a particular type of cassava, the entire staple crop would not be wiped out.

One common cassava end product, however, never became palatable to me. *Cassiri*, also known as cassava beer, is produced in a singularly unappetizing procedure in which the women of the tribe chew a portion of cassava flour or bread and then spit it into a large vat filled with water. Enzymes in the saliva initiate fermentation and three days later the brew is ready for consumption. *Cassiri* is warm, thick, sour, and has slimy white chunks of cassava floating on the surface. It is said to be insulting to one's host to refuse to drink the beer when it is offered and some foreigners are even said to have managed to become fond of it. Not me!

As we sat in Koita's hut, talking and listening to the rain coming down, I again noticed the jaguar tooth charm he wore around his neck. I asked him how he got it.

Koita fingered the yellow tooth, then replied, "A few weeks before you arrived, I had taken my wife and infant son upriver to the savannas to hunt parrots. I built a lean-to of *wah-pu* palm leaves in a little clearing, then set off alone with my bow and arrow. My son was crying when I left and my wife tried to quiet him by offering him her breast.

"Within minutes of leaving the camp, I heard a jaguar cough nearby and suddenly became afraid that it was homing in on my son's cries. As I ran back to camp as fast as I could, I heard my wife screaming. There she stood, her arms wrapped tightly around the baby, staring at a huge jaguar. His back was arched and he was ready to pounce.

"I fired an arrow deep into its neck, but jaguars are hard to kill. It turned toward me. I shot again and again, and soon the jaguar lay dead at my feet, its blood oozing between my toes. I cut out his canine and made this necklace."

Just then, a visitor ducked in out of the rain. Akoi—the name means "snake"—was lanky and taut, and stood about five-foot-eight, tall for a forest Indian. Instead of the red Tirió breechcloth, he wore a pair of old black cotton pants, and his ears were decorated with colorful round earrings fashioned from red and yellow parrot feathers. Yet Akoi's most remarkable feature was his face: it was like an old Dutch door, the top and bottom two distinct and separate entities. An omnipresent smile revealed a missing front tooth, giving him an amiable, almost silly grin. Yet his deep, dark eyes, with huge pupils that never seemed to shrink, were the eyes of a killer.

Shaking the rainwater out of his hair, he looked at me and said in halting Surinamese: "So I hear you speak Portuguese!"

Surprised at this question, I stammered a reply: "I—I studied it a bit in school, but—" He cut me off.

"Then let's speak Portuguese!"

"Where did you learn Portuguese?"

"I'm not a Tirió, you know," he replied, looking at me with a mixture of haughtiness and bemusement. "I'm a Sikiyana from the Trombetas region of Brazil."

I had read about the Sikiyanas, who were noted for their warlike nature. Richard Schomburgk, the nineteenth-century Prussian naturalist and explorer, had once described the tribe as "the dread and terror of their peaceable neighbors."

"What brings you here, then?" I asked.

"A couple of years ago my village was attacked by Brazilian rubber tappers. They destroyed our gardens and we had to leave to find food. After some initial misgivings, the Tiriós allowed us to move here."

As my Portuguese came back to me, we made small talk about the weather, hunting, and our families, and it seemed like I had found a new friend. As the conversation wound down, he looked at me quizzically for a second, then smiled once again. "Well, a white man, huh? You know, I've killed about twenty of them, but you seem to be an okay sort." With a broad smile and a seemingly friendly pat on the shoulder, he turned and walked out of the hut.

Uncertain as to how to respond, I looked over at Koita, who, unable to understand Portuguese, was sharpening the knife I had given him. "Was he kidding?" I gasped.

"About what?" asked Koita. After I translated the Sikiyana's last comment, Koita nodded gravely and then advised, "Take this fellow seriously. He is a real warrior and has killed many rubber tappers who trespassed on his tribe's lands in Brazil."

A year later, about a month before I returned to the village, Akoi had an argument with his twenty-seven-year-old son-in-law. "You," warned the Sikiyana, "will not live long enough to regret having this argument with me."

Two days later they found his son-in-law dead in his hammock without a mark on him. Missionaries on one of their periodic visits from the capital city took tissue samples back with them for laboratory testing. They found nothing.

The Indians attributed the young man's death to witchcraft, but Schultes taught me that black magic often entails the use of poisonous plants. The difference between a poison and a medicine is often just a question of dosage, something only a sophisticated medicine man would know. The Indians of the northeastern United States, for example, have long recognized the root and rhizome of the mayapple plant as toxic and have used it for a variety of purposes—purgative, emetic, and worm expellant, to name a few. One tribe—the Menominee—sprinkled an infusion of the boiled plant on potato plants to kill potato bugs.

In the 1940s, American physicians began using a resin of the mayapple plant called podophyllin to treat venereal warts. When injected with the resin, the warts—which are generally surgically removed—began to shrink and disappear. In the late 1970s, Bristol-Myers began developing a semisynthetic drug based on mayapple compounds. This drug, called etoposide, has been successfully used to treat testicular cancer and small-cell lung cancer; it apparently works by degrading the DNA of cancer cells. The drug now brings in revenues in excess of $100 million a year.

The Sikiyana shaman was obviously someone from whom there was much to be learned. Unfortunately, not all medicine men are willing to take on an apprentice. Akoi and I did become friends of a sort, but he always cheerfully—and unconvincingly—claimed to know little about the useful properties of plants.

Shortly after my encounter with Akoi, Koita took me to meet the local master craftsman—the man who made the best bows and arrows—so that I might have a set of my own. His hut was located near the edge of the village, and it was unlike any other. The dwelling looked like a palm-thatched version of an Eskimo igloo, albeit with a pointed top.

"I haven't seen any other houses like this," I said.

"That's because there aren't any," replied Koita. "This fellow is an Okomoyana."

"Okomoyana? I've never heard of them. Where do they live?"

"They don't. They *used* to live here. You see, the Okomoyanas were a tribe of warriors, the blood enemies of the Tiriós. When my father was a child, the tribes went to war. The Tiriós won and killed all the Okomoyanas, with the exception of the arrow maker, who was a boy at the time."

I ducked through the doorway to meet the last of this warring tribe.

A small cooking fire provided the only light. On one side of the fire sat an old woman, the arrow maker's Tirió wife. She wore only a red breechcloth and softly hummed to herself as she spun cotton on a wooden spindle. On the other side of the fire the ancient craftsman sat on a low wooden stool. He was carving a hunting bow from the purple wood of the spotted snakewood tree. As a carving tool, he used the lower jaw of a peccary—a rain forest pig. He, too, wore a red breechcloth and at his wrists were bracelets made from the tiny brown seeds of the *sho-ro-sho-ro* bush. His black shoulder-length hair had been dressed with the scented oil of the *tonka* nut and it shone in the firelight. He did not hear us enter.

There exists a belief among many tribes of the Guianas that knowing a person's name gives one a certain power over him or her. At the climax of W. H. Hudson's classic novel *Green Mansions*, the protagonist engages in a wrestling match with the sorcerer who has killed his girlfriend. He whispers the medicine man's name in his enemy's ear, thus demonstrating superior power and winning the match. Among the Tiriós, one acknowledges the wisdom and knowledge of elder men by addressing them either as *Paho* ("Father") or *Tamo* ("Grandfather").

Koita announced our arrival. "*Tamo*," he said softly so as not to startle the old man. "I have brought a guest." The Okomoyana stopped what he was doing and carefully looked me up and down. Then he broke into a toothless smile and came over and patted me on the shoulder. He could not have been friendlier, and I found the visit a sad and moving experience. This wonderful old man was all that remained of a once proud, fierce culture. It was like looking at the last of the dinosaurs, the last of the Madagascan elephant birds, the last of the Carolina parakeets. In a few years he would be no more, and the Okomoyana tribe would have vanished from the earth.

The arrow maker beckoned for us to sit by the fire; his wife handed us short benches made of roughly hewn logs. Reaching into the coals of the cooking fire with a machete, she extracted two roasted yams and presented them to us. Koita sliced them open to reveal a bright purple, beetlike flesh. I remembered reading about the yams in Schultes's class and knew that the Mexican species had yielded diosgenin, a chemical compound used as the basis for the synthesis of some of the first birth control pills. When they cooled enough to taste, I found them to be so wonderfully sweet that I stopped musing about their medicinal uses and greedily devoured both halves.

Since food does not keep well in the tropical climate, Indians eat whatever is on hand, making no distinction between foods served for breakfast, lunch, or dinner. Yams are eaten as a snack during the day, or as a meal. Other dietary staples include manioc bread, palm fruit, boiled meat, and smoked fish.

The old lady had retired to her hammock and resumed spinning cotton. As was the custom, we did not just begin our visit by asking whether the master would be willing to make me a hunting bow. Instead, Koita launched into a long and flowery speech about who I was and what I was doing there. When he had finished, the old Okomoyana still had many questions. Where had I come from? What did people hunt in my country? How old was I? Why didn't I have any children? I liked women, didn't I?

Once the friendly interrogation was completed, Koita asked whether the old man would be willing to make a bow for me; in exchange, he offered my flashlight. The Okomoyana accepted our terms and we stood up to depart. On the way out, his wife handed us two more yams.

A week later, we returned to the arrow maker's hut. The Indians of the region do not have shelves in their houses; they store things by sticking them into the roof thatch like pins in a cushion. As we entered, the old man stood up, pulled a bow out of the thatch, and handed it to me. It was a work of art. Six feet in length, the bow had been carved from the deep purple wood of the spotted snakewood tree. By rubbing it with beeswax, he had given the wood a soft, almost sensuous feel. He had tinted the beeswax with a bit of *u-shuh* berry, so that the purple color of the wood was burnished with a reddish tinge. At both ends of the bow he had attached red, yellow, and orange parrot feathers; they were held in place by the bowstring, which was made from a strong, white, flexible fiber extracted from the tops of wild pineapples. The old craftsman had also wrapped the fiber around the middle of the bow to produce a six-inch band of material that I at first took to be a handgrip. Koita saw me examining this part of the bow and asked if I knew what it was for.

"Isn't this where you hold the bow as you draw the arrow with the other hand?" I asked.

"No. When you are in the forest hunting and the bird is too far away to hit, you rub the arrow against the string and it produces a noise that will cause the bird to fly closer to investigate."

Pleased with my new bow, I was anxious to leave so that Koita could give me a few archery lessons. Before we could depart, however, the old man gestured toward the back of the hut where he indicated he had made a little something extra. Reaching behind his hammock, he pulled out a large wooden club and handed it to me. "This," he said, "is a *siwaraba*, a war club. I haven't made one of these in many years, but I wanted to make you something special in honor of your visit."

About forty inches long and two inches in diameter, the cylindrical stick was made of a very heavy wood, presumably to add to its lethal effectiveness. It, too, was stained red with the *u-shuh* berry extract. As I weighed the club appreciatively in my hand, the old man pointed out a feature I had missed. Six inches from one end of the stick was a raised knot of wood. The club was made to be held at the other end with the knot facing down. "That way," said the old craftsman, "when you hit your opponent's head, his skull collapses like an overripe pumpkin!" He looked at me and smiled sweetly. Apparently he was still an Oko-moyana at heart.

Early the next morning Koita told me I would soon have a chance to use my bow. "In two days," he said, "we will all go fishing. Today we have to go into the forest to get the wood for the fish."

A bit puzzled by this last statement, I nonetheless grabbed my canteen and machete and hurried after him. As we walked through the village, we fell into line behind about thirty other Indians who were heading into the forest en masse. All carried machetes, but none brought their bows and arrows, which struck me as highly unusual. Indians seldom enter the forest without a hunting weapon in case they see something suitable for the cooking pot. One fellow in our group carried only a flute, made from the leg bone of a forest deer, on which he played a lively tune.

We headed into the forest at a pace I had to struggle to maintain. The trail was carpeted by tiny green *Selaginella* herbs interspersed with brown, red, orange, and black leaves in various stages of decomposition. At the edge of the trail grew tiny forest bamboos and behind them flourished wild ipecac bushes with showy red flowers.

On the trunks of some of the trees *Brassavola* orchids bloomed, producing floral clusters that looked like a cascade of white spiders. The image of the rain forest as bursting with flowering orchids is false. Only at higher elevations, where there are cloud forests that are constantly soaked in mists, do orchid species flourish. In the flat, hot lowlands of Amazonia where I was working, orchids are not rare but are certainly not common.

With very few exceptions, orchids are not used by Amazonian Indians for medicinal purposes. In his forty years of studying the healing plants of the northwest Amazon, Schultes found less than ten species of orchids in use versus well over a hundred legumes—even though the orchid family is twice the size of the legume family.

Although most orchid species are found in the tropics, some occur as far north as the Arctic Circle. After its legendary beauty, the most striking characteristic of an orchid is its incredible diversity. Most of us think of orchids as small, green, fleshy-stemmed plants, but some orchids resemble shrubs, while others are vines. They range in height from less than one inch to over ten feet. Orchids grow on the ground, on trees, on rocks, or, in the case of several Australian species, underground.

The ancient Greeks valued orchids as treatments for sexual disorders. Indeed, the name *orchid* is derived from the Greek word for testicle and describes the swollen underground stems common to many European species. The botanist Dioscorides and his students, among others, were devout believers in the Doctrine of Signatures, which holds that if a plant looks like a human organ, it is good for treating ailments of that organ. The shape of the orchid root was proof that it was of value for treating sexual problems. References to the healing properties of orchids abound in the herbal guides and other medical books written in Europe during the Middle Ages.

We derive no modern medicines from the orchid family. Although alkaloids were found in one species during the latter part of the nineteenth century, until recently most plant chemists have considered orchids to be relatively inert chemically. But new research at Harvard University has demonstrated that orchids are much more alkaloid-rich than previously believed. Over 30 percent of the species analyzed were found to contain alkaloids, and many of these compounds were of a unique type, potentially useful for modern medicine.

Of the thirty thousand species that comprise the orchid family, the most important from a commercial standpoint is vanilla. Native to the Neotropics, vanilla was widely used in Central America in pre-

Columbian times. The Aztecs concocted a drink that combined vanilla, chocolate, and chile peppers. Although vanilla is believed to have been sampled by Spanish explorer Hernando Cortez at the court of Montezuma in 1520, it was not described botanically until 1651. The name *vanilla* comes from the Spanish word *vaina*, meaning "little sheath" (because of the shape of the pod), which is itself derived from the Latin term for vagina.

Although there are over ninety species of *Vanilla*, only two are economically important. *Vanilla planifolia* is native to Central America and is the species of choice for plantations in the Old World. *Vanilla pompona* is native to the West Indies and parts of South America—including the northeast Amazon, although the Indians apparently do not have a use for it. Artificial vanilla can be synthesized from wood pulp, but most people prefer the natural product. Today vanilla is used in the manufacture of perfumes, as a spice, and is a key component of the secret recipe for Coca-Cola.

We stopped for water at the edge of a gentle stream and everyone took a drink; tiny brown and silver minnows darted about in the clear, cool water. Crossing the stream, we entered a liana forest similar to the one in which the Maroons had shown me the mating dance of the cock-of-the-rock. Instead of huge forest trees—there were few of those—the most common element in this forest were large lianas, which creeped along the ground. As if forest pythons in search of their next meal, the woody vines snaked up and over large orange, moss-covered boulders. The boulders emitted a sweetish smell of mildew.

The Indians immediately set to work, slicing the lianas into twelve-inch sections. As they cut, the wood released a cucumberlike odor. Within twenty minutes, they had assembled a waist-high mound of *ay-ah-e-yah*—a type of liana that was yellowish in color. Each Indian then cut two large fronds of the *wahpu* palm and wove them together into backpacks; into each of these they loaded about seventy pounds of *ay-ah-e-yah* wood. Next, they cut the long, brown aerial roots of Philodendron plants to use as ropes to secure the wood to the backpack. Finally, they peeled long strips of bark from the *me-de-bo-no* trees, of the Brazil nut family, and wove them into shoulder straps for the packs. One of the older Indians caught my eye. "*Pananakiri! Oheweuh*," he called. "Hey, alien! Come here." In no time, he had fashioned an extra backpack full of the yellow wood. He helped me put it on and we set out for home. The whole operation, from the time we arrived at the site until the time we departed with backpacks full of *ay-ah-e-yah*, took less than an hour.

Back at the village, we unloaded the wood at the edge of the river, then took turns crushing it with wooden clubs. When all that remained was a huge pile of yellow pulp, we loaded it into the dugout canoes. That task complete, we returned to our respective huts, exhausted.

On the next day, the day of the great fishing expedition, wake-up call was before dawn and I headed down to the river still rubbing the sleep from my eyes. Everyone had turned out for the event, including the women, children, and the hunting dogs. With the canoes loaded to the gunwales with yellow liana pulp, bows, arrows, and provisions for the trip, we set off downriver. The day was glorious and there was continuous banter between the canoes, echoed by a squawking flock of mealy parrots overhead. The owner of my canoe pointed out landmarks as if I were on a sightseeing tour. "I once shot a toucan in that tree. See that rock? I once caught two big catfish right in front of it. Right up ahead my brother has his cassava garden. An old jaguar lives nearby!"

We stopped to camp just before sunset. Dinner was *ki-yah-mah*, manioc meal at its most unappetizing, according to my taste. The Indians said that they always traveled with *ki-yah-mah* because it never spoiled. It is dry and gritty, ground to the size of aquarium pebbles and just about as difficult to chew.

Once the sun had set, mosquitoes from a nearby *wapoe* swamp attacked us in waves. Everyone had already slung their hammocks and mosquito nets and climbed in for the night. Unless the mosquito net is tied correctly, so it hangs around the hammock without actually touching it, you are at the mercy of the mosquitoes and/or vampire bats. There was no sign of bats that night, but the ubiquitous mosquitoes swarmed through my poorly tied netting. At one point I was perched in my hammock on all fours and the relentless insects continued to bite my palms and knees. No matter how I tried to resling my mosquito net, I was unable to screen out the pests. That night was one of the very few occasions in the jungle when I wished I was somewhere, anywhere, else.

The division of labor in Indian cultures is clearly defined. The men hunt, clear fields, make gardens, build houses, and craft weapons; the women raise children, tend the gardens, haul water and firewood, and prepare food. Seldom does a man carry water from the river or a woman cut a tree. Each sex has a set of tasks, which complement each other neatly. Nowhere was this mutually beneficial cooperation more evident than in the course of the fishing expedition.

At daybreak on the second day of our expedition, the women were already down at the river, wading into the still-cold gray water with handfuls of the crushed yellow *ay-ah-e-yah* wood. Their powerful brown hands kneaded the pulp just below the surface of the water, releasing a whitish, bubbly substance that first floated to the surface and then began to drift with the current. As the compound made its way downstream, the men grabbed their bows and arrows, jumped into their canoes, and set off with shouts of glee and anticipation.

The compound released from the wood was rotenone, a vasoconstrictor that enters the fishes' gills and closes the capillaries responsible for the intake of oxygen from the surrounding waters. The fish basically suffocate. In the canoes, one man stood up front with bow and arrow at the ready, while another man, seated in the stern, steered and paddled. As the rotenone started to take effect, the surface of the river boiled and churned with fish gasping for air. The poison did not discriminate —baby brown catfish with white whiskers fought for oxygen alongside huge silver-blue, piranhalike *pacu*. Torpedo-shaped *aboikan* fish gnashed their teeth next to the blue-gray *mologoiemah* that floated silently to the water's surface. Some fish were so stupefied they could have been scooped up easily with a net; others lolled on the surface until the approach of an oncoming canoe sent them diving for the river bottom in a futile attempt at escape. Yet each and every fish was shot with a hollow arrow that floated to the surface, dragging the hapless prey with it. Often the Indians would fire three or four arrows in rapid succession—all true to the mark—before stopping to haul in their catch. Their accuracy defied belief. I vividly remember seeing the mere flash of a dorsal fin at the edge of the river an instant before Koita quickly pivoted and fired an arrow. It traveled thirty feet in an almost horizontal shot to hit the fish—just below the water's surface—right behind the eye.

The boats drifted with the river's current and the Indians casually flicked arrows here and there in a kind of tropical ballet. A century ago British explorer Barrington Brown wrote an excellent account of a similar expedition in neighboring Guyana:

> It was a most exciting scene for a time, as the Indians shot arrow after arrow into the bewildered dying fish and hauled them ashore or into the canoe. In about an hour the murderous work was over, and 150 fine *pacu* and *cartabac* were lying dead upon the rocks around the pool, the victims of Indian prowess and poison. During the whole proceedings I stood on the rocks of the upper end of the pool, and had a fine view of the scene, the finest part of which was to see the naked savage, in all his glory, drawing his bow with strength and ease and letting fly his arrow with unerring aim.

So deceptively easy did it all seem that I decided to try my hand at what looked like the jungle equivalent of shooting fish in a barrel. I failed miserably. Standing in a canoe, drawing a bow, aiming at a fish underwater, and shooting an arrow are *all* difficult maneuvers, and trying to accomplish them simultaneously is akin to shooting skeet while riding a motorcycle along a bumpy road. After three unsuccessful attempts to spear a large, unconscious *pacu* drifting my way, I lay down my bow and reached for the fish with my hand. As I did so, an Indian from a neighboring canoe fired an arrow at the same fish. Just as I grabbed for my catch, the arrow passed between my third and fourth fingers, striking the fish in the gills. I looked over at the other canoe, stunned. "Better not to use your hands," said the Indian with a sheepish smile.

You may not see *ay-ah-e-yah* used at your local trout stream, but the substance it yields, rotenone, now serves as one of our most important biodegradable pesticides. Although it has little effect on warm-blooded creatures and limited effects on fish, rotenone is devastating to many insects. First discovered by indigenous peoples, it is now one of the most effective multipurpose pesticides known and has been an ingredient in flying insect sprays, horticultural sprays, flea powders, and animal dips. Used extensively by Allied troops in World War II to ward off mites, lice, and other skin parasites, rotenone first appeared in the international marketplace in the 1930s. Demand for rotenone increased over time until the advent of synthetic chemical pesticides in the 1960s. Recent interest in organic gardening has led to a resurgent demand for rotenone. Rain forest peoples use other toxic plants as well, to poison fish, make curare, even to settle personal quarrels with their enemies. Several of these plants—such as curare, which yields the muscle relaxant d-tubocurarine—have important uses in the outside world. Some species have no uses at this time but may in the future. Only the native peoples can guide us to them.

When we returned to camp late that afternoon, the women had built babracots, barbecue grills of green wood, on which to cook the catch of the day. The fish were gutted and then placed on the grill and a delicious aroma enveloped us. As soon as a fish was done, it would be pulled from the grill by its tail and handed to the nearest hungry person. No effort was made to distribute to each man the exact number of fish he caught; everyone simply gorged themselves until they could eat no more. Many of the Indians, exhausted from their efforts and stuffed to the point of somnolence, retreated to their hammocks after the feast and a few were soon snoring contentedly.

While the men wandered away from the babracots, the women continued to grill the remaining uncooked fish. I asked Koita why they were still cooking.

"They have to," he replied, "otherwise the fish will spoil. The women will grill everything that was caught and that will keep them overnight until we get back to the village tomorrow. There, the fish will be smoked and will keep for weeks and can be distributed to everyone."

Just then there was a commotion. A canoe carrying three Indians had beached at the riverbank. One man, the heavyset, slow-witted, amiable fellow named Kykwe, was slumped forward. The fellows who accompanied him put an arm under each of his armpits and slowly dragged him up the bank to the encampment. Kykwe groaned loudly and began weeping with pain. He had made the mistake of stepping on the creature most feared by the Indians—not the anaconda, the jaguar, or the electric eel, but the stingray.

The stingrays of the Guianas are bottom dwellers who lie partially buried in the mud. When stepped on, they arch their tails forward, driving their saw-edged, poisonous spines into the offending foot. So strong are these animals that they can bury their spines deep into the wooden bottom of a canoe. A serious sting is said to cause convulsions and even death.

British explorer and geologist Barrington Brown described such an encounter with a stingray in 1870:

> My interpreter, William, was unfortunate enough to step upon one, which, being of the colour of the bottom, was not observed. It drove its spine or sting deep into the side of his instep, producing a jagged wound which bled profusely. I immediately put laudanum [tincture of opium] on the wound and gave him a strong dose of ammonia. In a quarter of an hour after he was writhing on the ground in great agony, screaming at times with the pain he felt in the wounded part, in his groin, and under one armpit. His foot and leg were so cold that he got one man to light a fire and support his foot over it, persisting in trying to put it in the flames. I gave him two doses of laudanum, one shortly after the other, without relieving his sufferings in the slightest degree. After three hours of intense pain he became easier, but had returns of it at intervals during the night. For a week he was unable to put his foot to the ground, and the wound did not heal thoroughly for six weeks.

The Indians half-carried, half-dragged Kykwe to a nearby hammock and gently laid him in it. One of the older men trotted down to the river and gathered some of the yellow *ay-ah-e-yah* pulp that had been left behind that morning. He rolled it into a ball, added some water from the river, and crushed it flat between his hands. He then applied this poultice to Kykwe's wound and tied it in place with fibrous strips cut from the bark of a tall *me-de-bo-no* tree. The treatment seemed to provide Kykwe with some degree of relief; one of the women gave him some fish to eat, as much to distract him from his pain as to assuage his hunger. Apparently, almost all of the Indians know basic ethnomedical first aid, such as how to use plants to treat common forest accidents like machete cuts, spider bites, or stingray attacks. But only the shamans possess the more specialized knowledge of healing plants. When he got back to the village, Kykwe went to the Jaguar Shaman, who performed a curing ceremony of special chants, then cleaned the wound and repacked it with fresh *ay-yah-e-yah* wood to kill the pain and *go-lo-be* fungus to fight infection.

By now, my stay in the Tirió village was drawing to a close. The rainy season had started and the plane that would carry me back to the capital city was due to return in a few weeks. But before I left, there was one more aspect of forest life for me to experience. A festival was imminent and the village hummed with excitement as the big day approached. Ten of the men set off on a major hunting expedition to ensure there would be a surfeit of game for the celebration, while the women sewed anklets of tiny brown *sho-ro-sho-ro* seeds to be worn as adornments during the dances.

Most Indian ceremonies revolve around either the harvest or the various rites of passage—puberty for males, first menstruation for females, and marriage, birth, and death. To pay homage to a loved one who has died, for example, the Yanomamos of Brazil and Venezuela wait a year, then grind up the bones of the deceased and mix the powder with fruit pap or juice and drink it. Koita explained the reasons for this Tirió festival. "Cassava is our most important crop, but pineapple is our favorite. This festival celebrates the harvest of *nah-nah*—the pineapple."

Like the cassava plant, pineapple is native to Amazonia and was domesticated many thousands of years ago. By the time the Spaniards arrived, the pineapple had spread throughout lowland South America and was cultivated as far north as Mexico. Columbus first encountered this plant on November 4, 1493, during his second voyage. Peter Martyr, chaplain to Queen Isabella and a historian of the new discoveries, recorded that pineapples were part of the cargo shipped back to Spain during Columbus's exploits. Although King Ferdinand declared it the world's best-tasting fruit, Martyr could not pass an opinion: "I have not tasted it myself, for it was only one which arrived unspoiled, the others having rotted during the long voyage."

Botanically, the pineapple is known as a *synconium*, a specialized type of compound fruit. Flowers appear on the central stalk and then fuse to form the fruit as we know it. Unfortunately, pineapples do not ship particularly well, since they do not ripen much once they are picked. Consequently, the taste of pineapples we buy in our grocery store hardly compares with the vine-ripened version the Indians cultivate. Furthermore, there are many different indigenous varieties to which we do not yet have access. According to Schultes, the Witoto Indians of the Igaraparana River in the Colombian Amazon have twelve different types of pineapples—from one the size of an orange up to a giant eighteen-inch version that he says is the sweetest fruit he has ever eaten.

On the morning of the pineapple festival, I awoke as a bright red hunting dog trotted past the door of my hut. I sat up in my hammock in time to see two other vermillion dogs amble by. Apparently, in preparation for the fete, each dog had been painted with *u-shuh* berry extract. When I went outside, I saw that the women were already at work, tending the cooking fires and heating leftovers from the previous night's dinner. In honor of this special day, three teenage girls were sweeping the central plaza with palm-leaf brooms.

At a prearranged signal from the chief—a wave of his hand—the Indians assembled in the plaza and began singing a Tirió song. After the impromptu concert, the Indians retired to their huts to don their finery. The men girded their waists with fabulous white belts made of thousands of tiny glass beads carefully sewn together. The Indians had acquired the beads in Brazil by trading pet parrots to other Indians, gold miners, or the military. Some augmented these belts with the spotted pelts of jungle cats such as ocelots and margays, mute testimony to their skills as great hunters. Most wore orange and blue beaded armbands into which they stuck elaborate ornaments called *tasha*, made from ebony black spider monkey tails, ivory white harpy eagle down, and scarlet macaw feathers. A few had also put tufts of harpy eagle down into their hair and crowned themselves with red, yellow, and black toucan feathers.

The women were dressed more simply yet no less colorfully. Around their waists they wore red and blue beaded aprons. Long strands of orange and blue glass beads were slung bandolier-style from each shoulder. Around their wrists and ankles they wore bracelets of brown *sho-ro-sho-ro* seeds. When the women all joined hands and danced a backward two-step, the bracelets produced a hissing rattle that kept the beat.

After their dance, the women returned to their huts to collect huge vats of *cassiri*—the dreaded cassava beer. As I dutifully downed calabash after calabash, I recalled an early explorer's classic description of the hideous brew: "an abominable, ill-tasted [sic] and sour kind of fermented beverage!" The drinking of the *cassiri* was followed by the presentation of huge platters of smoked fish and boiled monkey—the spoils of the large hunting expedition. Everyone plunged in with gusto; I stuck with the fish. Dessert was huge helpings of luscious red and yellow pineapples.

When most of the food had been eaten, the chief announced an archery contest and all the men retreated to their huts to get their bows. A large palm spathe was hung as a target and everyone lined up to take a shot. There was much breast beating and promises of bull's-eyes from the younger men, trying to impress the younger women. The contest was won by a most unlikely Robin Hood—a skinny little old man of about sixty, with stooped shoulders and a perpetual squint. He possessed an almost supernatural ability to hit the bull's-eye, and in this village of skilled marksmen, he had no equal.

Koita, meanwhile, had gone off into the forest with several of his compatriots in search of a highly prized treat—wild honey. On one of our jaunts the week before he had evidently spotted a dead tree containing a beehive. After the morning's singing and dancing, he led the others to the site. They cut into the hollow tree and then climbed up inside to collect the honeycomb. When Koita strode into the central plaza carrying the comb on a banana leaf, a cheer went up from the crowd. As Koita shared his sticky prize, I could see that he was still covered from head to toe with the honey that had rained on him when he cut the comb from the tree. The angry bees, fortunately a stingless variety, buzzed around his head.

I sat off to the side, enjoying the spectacle and devouring the ambrosial pineapple until several Indians my age beckoned to me. I strolled over and they half-invited, half-pulled me into a nearby hut. I was startled when two of them started peeling off my clothes. Then I realized what they were doing. They dressed me in a red breechcloth and white beaded belt and invited a woman in to paint my entire body red and blue for the occasion. One fellow disappeared, then returned a few minutes later carrying a huge headdress made from the feathers of the scarlet macaw and the harpy eagle. He put it on my head and they all stood back to admire their handiwork.

As I walked out of the hut, all heads turned, and a howl of laughter swept through the crowd. Even the old Jaguar Shaman, whom I hadn't seen since our time together in the forest, began to giggle.

Later that afternoon, when the festivities were over, I discovered the difference between a vegetable paint and a vegetable dye. When I scrubbed myself with soap, the red stain of the *u-shuh* berry—a vegetable paint—came right off. When I rubbed at the zigzag lines created by the blue *meh-nu* fruit—a vegetable dye—nothing happened. It had bonded with my skin and would wear off only over time. When I landed in the capital city a week later, most of my body was still a dark blue, a sort of corporeal souvenir.

As I stood on the little airstrip at the edge of the village, waiting for the cargo plane that would take me back to the city, an extraordinary double rainbow burst over Kwamala as if to crown this magical place. Koita was heading for the forest, his bow and arrow slung over his shoulder. He stopped to greet me, saying, "I have enjoyed our work together. I look forward to your return."

I replied, "You have been very patient, helpful, and kind. I, too, look forward to working together again." We stood silently for a minute and then he walked on toward the jungle. After a few steps, he turned and came back. Without a word, he took off the jaguar tooth hunting charm he always wore around his neck. He smiled, put the charm around my neck, and disappeared into the jungle without saying a word. Looking down as I flew off an hour later, I thought I caught a glimpse of him as he hiked deeper into the forest.

# CHAPTER 5
# A Recipe for Poison

Some of these nations use bows and arrows, a weapon which is respected for the force and rapidity with which it inflicts wounds. Poisonous herbs are plentiful, of which some tribes make a poison so fatal that an arrow, stained with it, destroys life the moment it draws blood.

—Cristóbal de Acuña, 1641

● ● ● ● ● ● ● ● ● ● ● ● ● ● ● ● ●

To the ethnobotanist, curare represents a sort of Holy Grail. Prepared from jungle plants and smeared by the Indians on the tips of their arrows and blowdarts to give them a deadly effectiveness, this lethal poison embodies all that we seek in the course of our research. Its preparation often shrouded in secrecy and ritual, its complex chemistry still incompletely understood by Western scientists, curare has fired the imaginations of Western explorers for almost five hundred years.

*Curare* is one of the few words in the English language derived from Amazonian Indian dialects. Also called *woorari, wourali, urari,* and various other names, curare is actually a blanket term for all arrow poisons prepared by tribal peoples from tropical plants. Most curares function by interfering with the transmission of electrical impulses from the nerves to the muscles. This causes the muscles—including the diaphragm, which controls breathing—to relax and to eventually stop working. A curare victim can suffocate within just a few minutes. But new types of curares are still being discovered. While working in northern Brazil in the late 1960s, Professor Schultes discovered an arrow poison that, instead of killing its victims outright, apparently stuns them by inducing hallucinations. The animal lies there, presumably tripping to the Amazonian equivalent of "Sgt. Pepper's Lonely Hearts Club Band," while the hunter calmly moves in for the kill.

Though curare is still used by some Indians as a potent weapon in the hunt, physicians in industrialized countries have long used curare to treat a variety of conditions. Initial experiments concentrated on using curare to ease the stiffened muscles caused by polio and to treat such diverse conditions as lockjaw, epilepsy, and chorea, a nervous disorder characterized by irregular and uncontrollable muscle movements. More effective treatments were eventually found for those illnesses, but researchers pinpointed a number of uses for a curare that originated in the western Amazon. An alkaloid known as d-turbocurarine, the active principle in this curare, is extracted from a liana in the moonseed family, then injected into a patient as a muscle relaxant during throat, rectal, and abdominal surgeries. This compound is also used to relax patients receiving shock therapy to lower the incidence of spinal fractures suffered during treatments, and in the diagnosis of myasthenia gravis, a muscular disorder. This alkaloid cannot be synthesized in the laboratory in a form that has all the attributes of the natural product.

Each Amazonian tribe has its own unique recipe for making curare, and ethnobotanists dream of stumbling across a secret arrow-poison plant containing an unknown compound that may prove beneficial to the world at large. Once again we are involved in a race against time: as indigenous peoples come into increasing contact with the outside world, they almost always lay down the bow and arrow and the blowgun in favor of the shotgun, and so their knowledge of how to make the curare is often lost, possibly forever.

My interest in curare led me back to the land of the Tiriós for four weeks in September 1983. My first trip had been devoted to building relationships with the Indians and learning about their medicinal plants; clearly, many more expeditions would be necessary to master the range of the Tiriós' natural pharmacy. But now I set myself an ambitious new goal: to learn how the Tiriós prepared their curare.

To prepare for this journey, I immersed myself in the vivid accounts of the early explorers of South America—men like Sir Walter Raleigh, Alexander von Humboldt, and Charles-Marie de la Condamine—whose matter-of-fact scientific observations are punctuated with tales of madness, cannibalism, and witchcraft. In my research, I stumbled across the works of two forgotten figures who had carried out the first field studies of curare in the Guianas. These intrepid eighteenth-century explorers, American Edward Bancroft and Englishman Charles Waterton, not only made great contributions to ethnobotanical research but rank among the most extraordinary characters produced by Western civilization.

Edward Bancroft, ethnobotanist, physician, philosopher, politician, and spy, lived a life right out of an espionage novel. Born in Westfield, Massachusetts, in 1744, Bancroft went to sea as a boy and likely served as a surgeon's mate on board ship. He may have seen British Guiana first as a sailor. In the 1760s, Bancroft moved to British Guiana and worked as a physician despite his apparent lack of any formal education. Fascinated by the plants, animals, and indigenous peoples of his new home, he published in 1769 a book with the ponderous title *An Essay on the Natural History of Guiana in South America Containing a Description of Many Curious Productions in the Animal and Vegetable Systems of That Country Together with an Account of the Religion, Manners, and Customs of Several Tribes of its Indian Inhabitants Interspersed with a Variety of Literary and Medical Observations in Several Letters from a Gentleman of the Medical Faculty During his Residence in That Country.* In his book, Bancroft gave the recipe for the curare of the Akawaio Indians, and correctly noted that each Indian tribe had its own unique arrow-poison formula.

A year later, in 1770, Bancroft moved to London, where he studied medicine and became a popular physician to the rich and the royal. Bancroft also met and befriended Benjamin Franklin, who was then visiting England. Probably at least in part due to Franklin's influence, Bancroft traveled to the colonies to support the colonies' fight for independence. When Franklin was sent to France by the rebel American government in 1776 to garner support for their cause, Bancroft accompanied him as his personal secretary.

After the war, Bancroft went to England again, and established himself as the leading authority on vegetable dyes, then of paramount importance to the British textile industry. His fame as a chemist was far-reaching and he was made a fellow of the Royal Society, a rare honor for someone born in the colonies and who was such a prominent member of the opposition during the Revolution.

While ethnobotanists remember Edward Bancroft for his contributions to our understanding of curare, history remembers him for his startling secret life. Seventy years after Bancroft's death in 1821, examination of his private papers revealed that during the Revolutionary War, Bancroft acted as a double agent, serving as England's most important spy. While in France with Benjamin Franklin in 1776, he supplied the British government with virtually every detail of Franklin's negotiations and of French troop movements to the colonies. Bancroft wrote his reports in invisible ink and used a hollow tree in the Tuileries as a dead drop. In one particularly remarkable instance, he transmitted a copy of the Treaty of Alliance between France and the United States to the British government just forty-two hours after it was signed.

If Edward Bancroft concealed any activities that might tarnish his reputation as a scientist, British naturalist Charles Waterton did just the opposite. A flamboyant character, apparently without a secretive bone in his body, Waterton's eccentricities constantly threatened to undermine his work as a biologist. Passionate about his calling, at the age of eighty Waterton was still climbing to the tops of tall trees and sitting next to nesting birds to better observe their behavior. He turned his estate in Yorkshire into one of the world's first bird sanctuaries, complete with artificial nesting boxes and wooden decoys to mislead would-be poachers. He was also a tireless crusader against the pollution produced by the Industrial Revolution, and a best-selling author. Waterton's classic 1826 work, *Wanderings in South America,* is still in print and is believed to have inspired many an English schoolboy—including Charles Darwin, Alfred Russel Wallace, Henry Walter Bates, David Livingstone, and Henry Morton Stanley—to devote their careers to tropical forest exploration. His writings range from the ludicrous ("[Indian] women never die in childbed, owing, no doubt to their never wearing stays") to the humorous ("I never saw a sloth take to his heels in such earnest; but the expression will not do, for the sloth has no heels") to the prescient ("No doubt there is many a balsam and many a root yet to be discovered [in these forests], and many a resin, gum and oil yet unnoticed").

A man of many talents, Waterton was also a skilled and innovative taxidermist. Rather than stuffing the animals, as is the usual practice, he soaked the creatures in a highly poisonous solution of bichloride of mercury. This unique method produced completely hollow museum specimens, which were not only well preserved but extremely lifelike. A passionate Catholic who railed against the Church of England, Waterton contorted preserved toads and lizards into caricatures of famous British Protestants; he called the work "The English Reformation Zoologically Demonstrated."

At the age of twenty-three, Waterton was sent by his family to British Guiana to manage a sugar plantation. He spent seven years as a wealthy colonial, then abandoned that life to travel into the uncharted interior. Despite the fact that it was the rainy season, Waterton set out barefoot, accompanied by six Indian guides and a black slave, traveling more than eight hundred miles through unexplored jungles and among previously uncontacted tribes. He eventually crossed into Brazil, an extraordinary trek by any measure. Waterton collected numerous birds and reptiles along the way for his personal taxidermy collection, but his major reason for making this journey was to collect *wourali*, the deadly arrow poison of the Macushi tribe of northern Amazonia.

Waterton claimed to have survived the rigors of Amazonian travel by following two practices: downing purgatives and bleeding himself regularly, which he did throughout his life. He sometimes extracted up to twenty-two ounces of blood at a sitting and once wrote, "If you desire to drink health's purest juices/ shun care and wrath and drain your body's sluices."

If his written accounts are to be believed, the intrepid adventurer survived encounters with some of the most powerful animals in the jungle. He claimed to have once caught a huge black caiman—the flesh-eating crocodilian that can grow more than twenty feet long—by jumping on top of it, twisting its forelegs over its back, and using them as a bridle. To silence critics who might have questioned his veracity, Waterton wrote, "Should it be asked, how I managed to keep my seat, I would answer—I hunted some years with Lord Darlington's fox hounds." He once claimed to have caught a ten-foot boa constrictor by grabbing its tail and then shoving his hat down the snake's throat. Ever the classics scholar, Waterton sat down after finishing his battle and wrote an account of the struggle in Latin hexameters.

Waterton's behavior scandalized the British natural history establishment, who tended to dismiss him as a liar and a fool. His description of the sloth as an animal that spends most of its time hanging upside down was disputed by "professional" scientists who had only seen specimens incorrectly preserved as right-side-up quadrupeds. Waterton understandably held these biologists in contempt, referring to them as "closet-naturalists." (It would be a little easier to sympathize with him if he had not included artist and naturalist John James Audubon in this category.)

As he traveled through the Kanuku Mountains of southwestern Guyana en route to Brazil, Waterton entered the heart of Macushi Indian country. He vividly recalled a visit to one of their huts:

> Their blow-pipes hung from the roof of the hut, carefully suspended by a silk-grass cord; and on taking a nearer view of them, no dust seemed to have collected there, nor had the spider spun the smallest web in them; which showed that they were in constant use. The quivers were close by them, with the jaw-bone of the fish *Pirai* [piranha] tied by a string to their brim, and a small wicker basket of wild cotton, which hung down at the centre; they were nearly full of poisoned arrows.

The explorer not only witnessed the Macushis' laborious preparation of the *wourali* arrow poison, he also obtained enough of the material to later carry out a series of experiments on animals. Waterton sought to understand how curare functioned in the body and to find therapeutic applications. Although he never succeeded in curing any ailments with the arrow poison, his research led to the use of curare in medicine today and when a sample of his Macushi curare was tested in the laboratory in 1983, more than 170 years after his expedition, it still retained its lethal toxicity.

The nineteenth-century French physician-adventurer Jules Crevaux also encountered the mysterious poison. After participating in the Franco-Prussian War, Crevaux moved to French Guiana and began exploring the Tumuc-Humac Mountains that form the border between Brazil and the Guianas. He visited the Brazilian Tiriós living on the Paru River and was astounded by the virulence of the arrow poison they used.

A small monkey playing was hit in the shoulder by one of these [curare-tipped] arrows. He started running for about one minute, then stopped. I saw him make several grimaces before his hands became paralyzed and he fell on his back. Six minutes after the initial wound, he was inert with his muscles unresponsive to the pricks of a needle. Within seven minutes he was nothing more than a cadaver.

Despite this detailed account of the monkey's demise, Crevaux provided a frustratingly incomplete description of the plants used to make the poison. After reading his account, I was more than ever determined to find the curare myself and detail its deadly ingredients.

The small plane back to the land of the Tiriós carried me over the carpet of forest green. The Devil's Egg looked as defiantly unnatural as ever. Three scarlet macaws soared below us in formation. The reflection of the sun in the rivers seemed to race just ahead of the plane like a will-o'-the-wisp, teasing and beckoning but remaining just out of reach. That awe and reverence and a sense of oneness with nature—a feeling never taught in biology classrooms—overwhelmed me once again.

As we flew over Kwamala in preparation for landing, I looked down fondly on the yellowish brown palm-thatched huts on the northern bank of the Sipaliwini River. At the sound of the plane, the Indians poured out of their homes and headed for the airstrip. We made a smooth landing, and the Indians surrounded the plane.

When I opened the door and slid out of my seat, I was greeted by about thirty Indians. I scanned the crowd for Koita, but he was nowhere to be seen. Many of the Indians recognized me and they seemed almost as excited as I was.

"Remember that tree that my father told you about last time, the one used to treat mouth sores?" shouted one fellow, "There's one that I found along a hunting trail and it is full of flowers!"

Another chimed in: "Hey, you know that plant that's good for colds that my grandfather told you about but couldn't find? There's one growing behind my garden!"

I was tempted to pull out my notebook and begin scribbling immediately, but protocol dictated otherwise. First I needed to see the chief and ask his permission to continue my research. One of the subchiefs was at the airstrip; the boss was upriver, he said, working on his manioc plantation. I would have to confine myself to a hut at the edge of the river, he instructed, until they could find somebody to take me to the chief for our talk. A bit taken aback at this version of house arrest, I picked up the supplies that I could carry and made my way to the deserted hut. Several of the Indian boys shouldered the rest of my equipment and followed along behind me, single file.

I hung my hammock and mosquito net in the appointed hut and started to unpack my plant press and notebooks. A familiar voice hailed me from the river, and looking out I saw Koita paddling up in a small dugout canoe. A scruffy white hunting dog stood on the bow of the canoe happily wagging its tail—until it saw me. Then it began growling menacingly. Ignoring both the dog and the subchief's order that I remain in my hut, I ran down to the river and embraced Koita as he stepped ashore.

Wearing his usual costume—a long, red cotton breechcloth over skin painted blue in a wildly impressionistic pattern—Koita was a welcome sight. He immediately handed me one of the enormous pineapples he had picked from his garden. The fruit must have weighed four pounds, so ripe it was more red than yellow. We walked up to my hut, where I cut the pineapple with my machete and shared the slices with my friend. As we ate, Koita plied me with questions about my trip: How long would I stay? What was I looking for? Would I really keep returning each year? Koita mentioned that he was helping his father-in-law cut a new garden and might not be able to work with me every day. No matter, he said; there were several of his friends who were very knowledgeable and reliable, and they would fill in for him when he wasn't around. Just then a four-year-old miniature version of Koita came by and told him that he was expected home for dinner. As he left, Koita promised to return at sunrise to take me upriver to speak with the chief. An hour later, as I was about to open a can of tuna, he reappeared with a plateful of "pepperpot," a specialty of his mother, a Waiwai Indian from Guyana.

A single bite of this fiery stew of red peppers, wild game, and chunks of cassava can just about cauterize the roof of your mouth. I thanked him sincerely and inhaled the delicious aroma. Having learned from experience, I went down to the river and filled my canteen to the brim before I began eating.

The next morning we headed upriver. I let Koita do most of the paddling while I rehearsed my speech to the chief. Every field scientist wants to be accepted by "his" people and I was still a bit shocked at having been confined to quarters after my arrival. I wondered whether this showed some displeasure about my return or some insecurity or indecision on the part of the subchiefs. In any case, my first talk with the chief a year earlier had been a bit testy and this time I wanted to make sure that everything went as smoothly as possible. We traveled about an hour on the river, then turned into a large, sluggish stream fringed by feathery-leaved *wah-pu* palms. Here we paddled only for another ten minutes before the water became too shallow to continue. We tied the canoe to a tree stump and hiked in.

The chief was swinging slowly in a hammock slung under a thatched roof at the edge of his garden. He smiled, waved, and beckoned us to sit on short wooden stools that his wife placed next to him. Koita immediately launched into a long introduction; although I couldn't make out much of what he said—flowery, formal oratory in Tirió was still beyond my ken—it must have been quite eloquent, judging from the older man's pleasant expression. At the end, my friend turned to me for the presents I had brought: red cloth, knives, fish hooks, and salt. He handed them to the headman, who then began his response. He thanked me for the gifts and welcomed me on the occasion of my return to his village. Altogether lacking was the rancor and skepticism the chief had exhibited at our first meeting. After he finished his welcome speech, he dismissed us and shook my hand. Walking back to the canoe, I asked Koita why his attitude had changed so dramatically. Basically, Koita replied, the chief had been pleased that I had worked so hard the last time and had not chased the women. My gut feeling was that the headman regarded me as a harmless oddball.

As we paddled back to the village, my thoughts were interrupted by an earthshaking clap of thunder. The sky parted and sheets of rain pelted us. We made for shore as quickly as possible, pulling up next to a little hut perched high on a bank overlooking a bend in the river. We ran laughing and hollering up the slippery red mud of the riverbank, quieting down only once we were sheltered under the thatched roof. We saw an elderly woman quietly tending a cooking fire nearby. She didn't say anything in the way of welcome, just reached into the ashes with a pointed stick and pulled out two baked yams. As we waited for our yams to cool, we could hear two pairs of feet running toward us to escape the steady downpour. I immediately recognized one of the two men who entered the hut: he was Nahtahlah, one of the paramount shamans of the Tiriós. I had never met him, but he had been pointed out to me during my previous stay as someone with whom I might wish to study. I guess I was enough of an oddity that he knew who I was too, though we had not really been introduced. "*Jako!*" he cried when he saw me. "Brother!"

To be addressed as brother by a shaman is a great honor. I never called any of the medicine men *Jako;* the more respectful *Paho* ("Father") or *Tamo* ("Grandfather") was more appropriate. Now I no longer felt as much the *pananakiri* ("alien") as I did when I first arrived. Nahtahlah was short and compact, and wore his hair like Prince Valiant. Nearly toothless, he nonetheless had a warm and friendly grin. Nahtahlah was famous for his black magic as well as white magic, and it was said that for his enemies his curses were deadly. Unlike the other shamans, he had a lively sense of humor and regaled me constantly with the most outrageously ribald tales, once confiding that the male members of a neighboring tribe have such an overwhelming sex drive that they have intercourse with knotholes when there are no women around.

Before working with Nahtahlah, I wanted to pay my respects to my original mentor and headed for the hut of the Jaguar Shaman. His circular house, situated at the edge of the village, had no walls; its privacy was protected by a thatched roof that came down to within a few feet of the ground. As I bent down to crawl under, I could see the medicine man dozing in his hammock, his powerful body silhouetted against the cooking fire at the far end of the dwelling. He began to stretch and slowly awaken as I walked over to him. "*Tamo,*" I whispered. "Grandfather." He opened his eyes, smiled sleepily, and gently tickled my arm. It was good to be back.

———

Day after day I ventured into the forest with Koita and the Jaguar Shaman in search of healing plants. Much of my time was spent rechecking the results of the year before, recollecting samples and making sure that a certain tree was indeed used for a particular infirmity. Even though I felt the Indians were becoming my friends, Schultes had warned me that forest peoples sometimes exaggerate or mislead an outsider for a variety of reasons. The only way to be sure my notes were accurate was to check and recheck them; if I was being led astray about something, it was unlikely the Indian in question would remember his exact words year after year.

The shaman was a fountain of information on forest ecology. "Here a tapir slept last night," he said, pointing to a cozy corner formed by buttress roots of a large *pono* tree. "This fruit is the favorite of the scarlet macaws," he observed as we passed under a wild fig. When he wanted fibers to weave into a basket, he cut the aerial roots of a wild philodendron hanging down from its perch high in the canopy. If it rained, he sliced the broad leaves off a heliconia plant and we used them as biodegradable umbrellas. One day I mentioned that I was hungry and he disappeared from the trail. A few minutes later he returned, his hands bulging with yellow, grape-sized fruits he called *ah-ku-de am-pe-de*. The name meant "agouti smell," a reference to the similarity of the fruit's acidic aroma to that of the agouti, a small forest rodent. Although the stone was large, it was surrounded by a sweet, slimy pulp that tasted like a lychee with just a hint of orange. Once again, spending endless hours trekking through the bush with my friends, I felt myself falling into the rhythm of the forest.

Although I was eager to learn the plants the Tiriós used to make curare, Professor Schultes had warned me before my trip that it might be rude to ask for the recipe outright. I would have to be subtle, so I waited for the appropriate moment to broach the subject.

As we walked through the forest on one particularly hot and humid afternoon, Koita heard a turkeylike bird called a guan hopping about in the branches above us. In a single fluid motion, he launched an arrow almost straight up. The arrow flew wide of its mark—the only time I ever saw Koita miss a shot—and the bird noisily flew off. As Koita retrieved the arrow from the trail in front of us, I casually mentioned that I would like him to show me the plant used to make the arrow poison. Neither he nor the Jaguar Shaman said a word, so I let the matter rest.

Rounding a bend in the trail, I noticed a tree that was about my height with pale green fruit growing directly out of the tree trunk rather than at the ends of the branches. The fruit was the size of a large avocado, but shaped something like a football; it had ten parallel ribs that ran from one end of the fruit to the other.

Koita twisted a fruit off the tree and broke it open.

"This tree we call *ah-kah-nah-pah-to-do-to-do*," he said, passing me some pulp-covered black seeds from the heart of the fruit. I chewed off the juicy white, sweet-tart flesh and spit out the seeds.

From its peculiar methods of producing fruit, I recognized this species as a distant relative of the chocolate tree. I asked Koita if this species could be crossed with *weh-deh-guh*—the Tirió name for the cacao, or chocolate tree. Although the trees look somewhat alike, he replied, they did not crossbreed as far as he knew.

Plant breeding has typically entailed crossing closely related plants, usually within a species, to add desirable traits to a valuable—usually commercial—species. This might produce a fruit with a higher sugar content, for example, or one that is resistant to pests and disease. With genetic engineering, however, scientists are now able to move particular genes from one plant species to a totally unrelated species. While the chocolate tree and its distant relative do not crossbreed in nature, they may one day be crossed by genetic engineers to enhance the value of commercial chocolate trees in some way.

Potentially more important, however, are the crosses of unrelated species, which emphasizes the need for conservation of plant diversity, particularly in the Amazon. Though most of the plants found in Amazonia are not close relatives of commercial plants, through genetic engineering the species in the Amazon—and in the Congo, Indonesia, and North America—may contribute valuable genes that can be bred into commercial species.

The implications for this type of crossbreeding are far-reaching, and one important benefit of strengthening commercial species would be felt by the people of Amazonia. The staple dish in almost every Latin American country is beans and rice; the poor often subsist on little else. While a fairly healthy meal, they do not provide a complete set of the amino acids needed by the human body; beans only contain the tiniest amount of methionine, one of these essential amino acids. At the University of Hawaii, Dr. Samuel Sun and his colleagues have had some preliminary success in inserting genes from the methionine-rich Brazil nut into other plants; their ultimate goal is to crossbreed methionine-rich legumes. Thus Brazil's rain forests, if they can be brought back from the brink of destruction, may one day feed the country's starving population.

Hearing thunder in the distance, we turned back. As we neared the village, Koita told me to wait. He left the trail and headed off to visit an abandoned garden to see if he could find any trees that were still bearing fruit. Expecting him to return with some unusual jungle treat, I was more than a little surprised when he came back with a handful of oranges.

Oranges are believed to have originated in tropical China and are not a common sight in the more remote corners of Amazonia. Such masters are the Indians at coaxing crops from their poor soil, however, that early explorers who stumbled on isolated tribes were amazed to find the Indians growing nonnative species such as sugarcane and bananas. Novel food plants were routinely traded from tribe to tribe, becoming staples in areas unseen by the outside world.

Oranges were probably introduced to the New World tropics as early as 1493, during Columbus's second voyage. They were first brought to Europe from China by the caravans traveling the Silk Route across central Asia, and from there carried westward with the Muslims during the period of Islamic conquest. Because citrus juice prevents scurvy, sailors during the Age of Exploration planted orange and lime trees on tropical coasts around the world to help ward off the disease during their travels. Lime juice became part of the British sailors' official ration, hence the nickname "limeys." In temperate zones, citrus fruits remained the dessert of choice among royalty and other members of the ruling elite. This led to the construction of orangeries, extravagant glass houses that protected the trees from cold weather and served as status symbols for their owners.

Despite their names, many oranges are not orange in color. The fruits Koita plucked from the jungle trees were bright green, yet as sweet and ripe as any orange I have ever eaten. One of the elements that turns supermarket oranges their brilliant hue is cold air, which causes the breakdown of chlorophyll and the release of an orange pigment called carotene. Some brokers expose their fruit to ethylene gas, which causes green oranges to change color and conform to consumers' expectations of an orange.

The next morning Koita appeared at the door of my hut accompanied by two remarkable friends. Particularly dazzling was Yaloefuh, the most resplendently painted Tirió I had ever seen. He was about five-foot-six, with the strapping build of a weight lifter. His arms, back, and legs fairly rippled, and the sinews were enhanced by the paint he wore on his body. With the dark blue juice of the *meh-nu* fruit, Yaloefuh had drawn a series of parallel designs that began at the tops of his feet, ran up both legs, and ended at his waist. Solid blue lines traced his ankles, followed by serpentine squiggles, more lines, then dots, lines again, then more dots at his waist. His brilliant red breechcloth made a startling contrast to the *meh-nu* blue. Around his bulging right bicep was a thick band of tiny orange beads; around his left, a band of blue. His powerful chest was bare, a visual pause before my eyes absorbed the work of art that was his face and hair.

As was the custom with Tirió men and women, whose bodies are generally hairless and who regard body hair as somewhat repugnant, Yaloefuh had plucked out his eyebrows completely. This softened his countenance and accentuated his large dark eyes. A jagged red line of *u-shuh* berry pigment ran across his forehead and down the center of his wide, flat nose. His shoulder-length black hair glistened from a rubbing with the vanilla-scented oil of the *tonka* bean, and plastered to his head with *tonka* oil were white feathers of the great *piahnah*—the harpy eagle.

Gazing at Yaloefuh with his long hair, smooth face, and high cheekbones, I was reminded of the accounts of Cristóbal de Acuña, a Jesuit priest traveling through Brazil in the 1640s. Acuña had tried to pinpoint the exact location of the female warriors said to have attacked Francisco de Orellana, a Spanish soldier and the first white man to navigate the Amazon. The Indians told Acuña that the tribe lived near the Tumuc-

Humac Mountains. Later, a noted historian studying Acuña's journal concluded that the Tiriós, with their somewhat feminine features, must have been the Amazon supposedly female warriors.

Accompanying Yaloefuh, but nowhere near as elegantly done up, was Kamainja, who would one day prove to be more than Yaloefuh's equal as a friend, confidant, and guide. Kamainja was not a Tirió but a Wai-wai, a tribe found to the west, deep in the rain forests along the Brazil-Guyana border. Born in the jungle in Brazil, he was married to a Tirió and had settled in Kwamala. (Although most marriages take place within tribes, marriages between members of different tribes are not unusual; in those unions, the couple tends to live in the woman's village.) Kamainja stood about five-foot-two, with high cheekbones highlighting an open and particularly handsome face. Not one for dressing up, Kamainja wore only a faded pair of cotton gym shorts. His sole nod to fashion was an old black Timex watch whose hands had long since fallen off.

We decided that Kamainja would come to my hut at sunrise and we would work with old Nahtahlah; that would give the Jaguar Shaman a chance to go hunting. Kamainja was going fishing at the end of the week and Yaloefuh would then take his place as my guide.

The next morning I awoke to the sound of Kamainja's bare feet on the dusty path that led to my hut. He gave a sad, soft whistle, the roosting call of the tinamou fowl. Hearing him, I swung my legs out of the hammock. As I tried to stand, I felt a sharp pain in my left ear; I lost my balance and fell over on the dirt floor. Kamainja rushed in to help me back into my hammock. Despite being six inches shorter and many pounds lighter than I, he handled me as though I were a rag doll. He looked into my eyes and felt my brow with the palm of his right hand. Saying he needed to get help, he trotted off.

My ear continued to throb. I was feverish and dizzy, and could not find a comfortable position in my hammock. As weakness began to wash over me, I felt sad, sick, abandoned, and a long way from home.

I could hear people around me, but could not see them. I wondered, through a muffled fog, if I had come down with malaria or been poisoned or cursed. Days (three, I would later learn) seemed to pass without interruption. Then I sensed someone standing above me, but I couldn't make out his face. The nameless shape spoke in a language I could not understand and then bent over and looked deep into my eyes. A familiar yet frightening face loomed out of the inky blackness: the Jaguar Shaman. I tried to concentrate on his movements. He threw branches and leaves on the fire and a thick, aromatic smoke filled the hut. He loomed in front of me once more and from the waistband of his breechcloth he pulled a short yellow bamboo container whose brownish yellow top was made from the bladder of a paca, the large, tasty, tailless rat. Twisting off the cover, the Jaguar Shaman knocked the contents—several pieces of white fungus—into his open palm. Turning my head to the side, he squeezed sap from the fungus first into one ear and then the other. Finally, he began chanting a slow and soft mournful dirge and washing me with a warm solution; he gave me a tea to drink, and I fell asleep.

When I awoke, I could not tell how much time had passed or even whether the healing ritual had actually occurred. Several little boys were playing outside my hut, noticed me struggling to sit up, and ran off. Soon they were back with Kamainja in tow, who brought me water. When I asked what had happened, he simply said, "You were sick."

I was familiar with the fungus the medicine man had used to treat what must have been an ear infection and I believe that antibiotic compounds in the sap cured the illness. But I could never pry out of him or Kamainja the names of the herbs he had steeped in the warm water or the meaning of the words he had spoken as he bathed me with the infusion. I thought about this experience a lot over the years as I came to know more of the Indians and their way of life. The reality of the Tiriós—and of some other non-Western cultures around the world—is peopled by were-animals, malevolent spirits, and talking plants. In this reality, the cure for my earache could have come from a dream, a healing plant, or a chant. Over the course of my research, there has never been a shortage of incidents, apparitions, dreams, and coincidences impossible to explain through the prism of Western science. The secret of healing does not lie only in the biochemical weaponry of the plants themselves. Healing of serious ailments in indigenous Amazonian societies almost always involves ritual.

As I relaxed in my hammock, my strength slowly returning, Kamainja told me he would soon be heading west to Guyana to participate in a festival held by his tribe. (The Indians think nothing of walking a hundred miles to visit family or special hunting grounds.) He usually made the trip home once a year to see his family and to take part in special ceremonies; occasionally his wife accompanied him, but most of the time she remained in Kwamala with their children. Perhaps we could work together when he returned, he offered, but in the meantime, Yaloefuh would step in as my guide.

As we entered Yaloefuh's hut, we caught him lying in his hammock, checking his face paint in a cracked hand-held mirror he had traded for in Brazil. As the local Beau Brummell, he wouldn't dare venture out of his dwelling until every aspect of his attire was absolutely perfect. Today's choice accessory was a *kuruwehmpo*, a headband made of luminescent yellow, red, and black toucan feathers.

Yaloefuh looked up and saw me admiring his headpiece. With hardly a pause, he took it off and handed it to me, saying, "*E-pah-wah-nah.*" According to Tirió tradition, if you admire something belonging to someone else, it must be given to you as a present—"*e-pah-wah-nah.*" This works fine in a forest culture where virtually everything is made from local plants, but the practice tends to break down when different cultures collide. The contemporary American anthropologist Napoleon Chagnon wrote of being given a banana by a Yanomamo Indian who then appeared in his hut a week later and demanded a shotgun in exchange.

I was touched by Yaloefuh's generosity; he had obviously spent a lot of time crafting the headband, probably weeks. Yet his gift was so genuine, so utterly lacking in some sort of reciprocal demand or expectation, that I took an immediate liking to him. He suggested we try to work with Ijuki, the oldest and most powerful of the Tirió shamans. We strolled over to Ijuki's hut to see if he was willing. Outside his house Kamainja called out "*Tamo!*" and a small, frail, white-haired figure came to the doorway. Few Indians have white hair, but when they do, they look hundreds of years old. Ijuki was about eighty. Kamainja and Yaloefuh explained the situation and asked his assistance, but he demurred, claiming to have a sprained ankle, a headache, a stomachache, a bad heart, dandruff, and several infirmities I had never heard of. His list of ailments did little to convince me of his curative powers and I was discouraged. But Yaloefuh insisted the old man knew a great deal about plants, so I joined the negotiations. "Tell him," I said to Kamainja, "I will give him six fishhooks a day, a bag of salt, and, if things go well, a flashlight at the end of the week." Hearing my offer, Ijuki disappeared into the hut; I thought the deal was off. Just then he reappeared, holding his machete. "*Mmpah!*" he exclaimed. "Let's go!" My two companions erupted in laughter. They explained to him that we would not start out until the morning, and bid him a good night. On my way home I wondered aloud if the old man would be able to keep up with us. Yaloefuh laughed. "*Jako*, that old man moves through the forest so fast he's going to leave you in the dirt!"

We headed east out of the village, leaving the palm-thatched huts behind us as we entered the forest. After a ten-minute walk through the jungle, we entered the *tebitas*, the gardens of the Indians. They had cleared an area about half the size of a football field and planted it with manioc. The plants had reached a uniform height of about six feet and their palmate leaves interlaced to form an almost uninterrupted ceiling of green. Hiking along the trail through the gardens, I could see that the soil was little more than white sand, yet my friends were managing to eke a living from it. As we walked, Yaloefuh explained the basics of Tirió agriculture.

"Before you is not one person's plantation, but the fields of many people. Large tree trunks, which you cannot see from the trail, mark the boundaries between each person's property. Everyone knows more or less where his fields begin and end and if there is any question, disputes are settled by the chief."

Borrowing my machete, Yaloefuh walked off into one of the gardens and came back with a huge pineapple. He divided it into three pieces, one for each of us.

"This is from your garden?" I asked, biting into the tangy fruit.

"No, this belongs to my brother-in-law. Just because you see someone taking something out of a garden does not mean it belongs to him. If you are hungry, you may take what you want, but you must always tell the owner when you get back to the village. You see, everyone helps everyone else. Once a patch of forest has been chosen, we clear the undergrowth and then cut down the trees, usually in June or July. After leaving the trees to dry for two or three months, we burn them, which enriches the soil. A month later, just when the rains begin, the women plant the manioc and the other crops."

"What other crops?" I asked. "All I see is manioc."

Yaloefuh beckoned me off the trail and into the garden, showing me how blind I had been. Throughout the plantation there grew countless banana trees, heavy with ripening fruit. What I had taken to be weeds were chile pepper bushes, although without their fruit they were hard to identify. Papayas, yams, cotton, tobacco, cashews, and squashes dotted the garden. With Yaloefuh's help, I saw that not even all the manioc trees were alike. Nearly twenty varieties grew there—one to make bread, another to make sweet cassava beer, another to make manioc meal, and so on, much like a farmer in the United States who grows one type of corn to feed his animals and sometimes several others to feed his family and to sell as a cash crop.

The gardens contained no plants for medicinal purposes, however. For that, we had to follow the shaman into the forest, into which he had disappeared while we were talking.

We came into what at first looked to be a clearing. Unlike other clearings, however, the canopy above this one was intact, indicating that no trees had been felled. We had entered what in the northwest Amazon is known as "the Devil's Garden," in which no underbrush will grow. It is believed that certain trees release toxic substances called allelochemicals through their roots, which inhibit the ability of other plants to grow in these areas. As I marveled at this strange phenomenon, I saw the old shaman seated on the stump of a *Duroia* tree. He was perfectly still, his eyes were closed, and he hummed softly to himself. Yaloefuh turned to me and whispered, "This is where he comes to work his magic."

The old man opened one eye and, seeing our arrival, stopped humming; he opened his other eye, then stood up and stretched. The stage seemed eerily set for a speech or some act of sorcery. But instead, Ijuki yawned, scratched his crotch, and headed farther down the trail. As we followed, Yaloefuh told me more about him. "He is one of the oldest men in the village, and one of the best hunters. While most of us prefer to hunt with friends, he always goes out alone, accompanied only by his dog. His wife is very young, but all the men are afraid to even look at her. Two friends of mine, convinced that the old man could no longer keep her happy, tried to seduce her. Later, one went hunting and never came back; the other was bewitched and is now impotent. Some fear

Ijuki, but he has never harmed anyone who did not first provoke his wrath."

I pondered this new information as I saw the medicine man raise his machete and slice off the top of a small sapling. Handing me the stem, he pointed to the alternating bands of white and green, and said, "*Eh-ru-ku-ku*"—the name for a poisonous snake of similar coloration. I smiled, thinking that he was pointing out the visual similarity between the tree and the snake, but he persisted, "*Eh-ru-ku-ku, eh-ru-ku-ku epi.*" (*Epi* means "medicine.") I then understood that the plant not only looks like a poisonous serpent, but also provides the medicine—a tea brewed from the plant's stem—for treating its bite. I started taking notes.

I was becoming proficient enough with the Tirió language to ask basic questions—What do you call this tree? Is it medicinal? How do you use it?—but was not yet at the point where I could discuss the finer points of cosmologies, for example. Yaloefuh, Koita, and Kamainja were patient language teachers, although my efforts seemed to alternately amuse and bewilder them. (One time, for instance, I tried to ask Yaloefuh whether he would be sad when I departed but later learned that I had asked him if he would whip me as I left!) I tried not to use interpreters whenever possible, though, so that little of the shamans' wisdom would be lost in the translation of their words.

At the edge of the clearing, Ijuki deftly used his machete to hack off a section of the *ah-mo-de-ah-tuh* liana, the leaves of which smell like bitter almonds. So enticing was the fragrance that I almost tasted it before remembering that this beguiling smell indicates the presence of a deadly poison: cyanide. In the early 1970s, a Brazilian botanist who collected a large quantity of this species for chemical analysis inhaled so much of the fumes that he almost passed out—permanently. Knowing that this was a poisonous species and mindful of the purpose of my quest, I asked the shaman, "Can you use this species to make curare?" He fixed me with a penetrating stare but didn't answer.

We made few collections that day, and I had the distinct impression that the medicine man wanted to get to know me better before he accepted me as a serious student. I reminded myself of the importance of deference and patience.

By late afternoon, it was time to return to the village. I asked that we go by a different trail so that we could see other plants. As we approached the village, Yaloefuh, ever concerned about his appearance, insisted that we pause so he could freshen up. After a short search, he found the black, spiny, flattened fruits of the *wihkapu waku* tree, with which he fastidiously brushed his hair. Then he looked around for the crowning glory: the aromatic green beanlike fruits of the *tonka* tree. He crushed a few in his hands and applied the oil to his hairdo.

The pleasant, vanillalike smell of the *tonka* bean is due to an abundance of coumarins, toxic white crystalline substances that are used in the preparation of soap and perfumes and to make other chemicals. *Tonka* was once used to make synthetic vanilla and to flavor tobacco, but it proved to be toxic in large quantities. A related chemical called dicoumarol, initially isolated from sweet clover, has been used in medicine as an anti–blood clotting agent. Because *tonka* is common in the northeast Amazon and the beans can be collected without damaging the tree, *tonka* bean extracts are an ideal way to use the forest for commercial purposes without destroying the ecosystem.

During our days in the jungle, Ijuki continued to prove obdurate, refusing to respond to my questions about curare. But Yaloefuh and I became fast friends. He made a special effort to point out aspects of Tirió hunting practices that I would have overlooked if I had concentrated only on medicinal plants. He taught me the *binas*, magical plants or minerals that are rubbed on the body or on the bow to ensure success in the hunt. And he demonstrated superb hunting calls that brought animals to gather near him. The ability of the Tiriós to beckon their game animals is nothing short of astounding. The British explorer Everard Im Thurn, who traveled with the Indians of British Guiana in the late nineteenth century, witnessed their skill:

This Indian habit of mimicry was well illustrated on one occasion when two of my Indians started from our camp in two directions to shoot a maam (*Tinamus*), neither knowing that the other was going. Presently one, hearing the cry of a maam some distance on his right, began to imitate it to draw the bird nearer. The other heard a bird cry on his left, and he too began to imitate it. Each mistook the cry of the other for the real bird, and the two continued calling each other and drawing nearer through the thick bush, until they met; each thinking that he was just about to see his bird, found the other had mimicked the cry of the maam only too well. They came back to camp in very bad temper.

Whenever I was naive enough to believe that I had finally begun to truly understand my new surroundings, inevitably some occurrence would teach me otherwise. A child of a materialistic society, I was impressed by the concept of reciprocity and sharing that the Indians called "*e-pah-wah-nah*." But occasionally I was also baffled by it. One night, Yaloefuh was helping me as I recopied the day's abbreviated field notes into my notebook, patiently explaining everything that we had seen in great detail. Night had fallen and the only thing that could be seen of the rest of the village was the faint flickering of cooking fires in the other huts. I lay in my hammock writing, while Yaloefuh sat on a small wooden stool next to the fire. He stood up, stretched, and said, "*E-pah-wah-nah*. Tonight I sleep with you."

I almost fell out of my hammock. Harvard taught no courses on Tirió sexual customs or preferences and I didn't know what to do. Bounding out of my hammock, I told Yaloefuh that it really was time for him to go home and handed him a cooking pot for his wife.

When I later explained what happened to Koita, he enjoyed a good laugh. "*E-pah-wah-nah* isn't just about exchanging gifts," he explained. "It is an expression of friendship and brotherhood. What he was telling you was that you were such a good companion, he wanted to sling his hammock next to yours so you could continue to talk all night. Relax!"

Early each morning when I walked over to Yaloefuh's hut I would inevitably find him lying in his hammock, carefully painting his arms with *meh-nu*, decorating his face with *u-shuh*, or weaving an exquisite headdress from feathers he had collected in the forest. Once, while he worked on his toilette, his wife (who seemed considerably older), nagged him.

"You're going into the jungle to look for plants? Why don't you go into the jungle to look for *meat*? We haven't had any fresh game for over a week. Sometimes I wonder why I chose to be the mother of your children. . . ."

Yaloefuh jumped out of his hammock, grabbed his bow and a handful of arrows, and trotted off, gesturing for me to follow. "Today I have decided that we are going hunting," he said over his shoulder. We passed the old medicine man's house and found Ijuki standing in front, picking his fingernails with the blade of his machete. When he saw Yaloefuh with his weapons, his face broke into a broad grin and he dashed back inside to fetch his armaments.

We set off into the forest at a steady trot, a pace I scrambled to maintain. The Indians clearly relished the idea of a hunt. "What are we going after?" I asked, breathlessly trying to keep up.

"*Ahdeme*—spider monkey," yelled Yaloefuh from somewhere up ahead. The trail wound into the forest and then out again through a small cassava plantation. We splashed through a palm swamp, maneuvered around boulders in a liana forest, and ascended and then descended a steep hill. Only occasionally did I glimpse the two red breechcloths sailing through the forest far ahead of me. By now we had left any semblance of a trail and bushwhacked our way through the jungle. Using my machete to clear the sparse underbrush only slowed me down and I was frightened of being left behind. As I struggled to keep up, I crossed a cold stream with a sharp current. Stepping on an algae-covered rock, I lost my footing and went down, twisting my ankle in the fall. I must have cried out because the two Indians reappeared within moments.

Taking off my shoe, I felt my ankle to see whether anything was broken. The old medicine man knelt down, gingerly took my foot in his hands, and did a detailed examination. Finding that I was okay, he placed my foot in the stream to keep it from swelling and indicated that we would take a short break before continuing. Both men carefully rested their bows and arrows on boulders at the edge of the stream and helped themselves to a drink of the cold water.

Hoping to sit long enough to catch my breath, I asked Yaloefuh to explain the variety of arrows that he carried.

"When we hunt," he began, "we usually carry four or five different arrows. The arrow shafts are all made from the giant cane grass that grows at the edge of our gardens. We make the fletching from the feathers of the big *hoko* [a turkeylike bird, also known as a guan], unless we are hunting something special such as a jaguar. Then we use the feathers of the harpy eagle."

"So then the shafts and feathering are basically always the same?" I asked.

"That's right," he said. "Only the arrowheads are different. The biggest and most important arrows are called *para*." He pulled out an arrow that had a large, razor-sharp lanceolate head made from bamboo. "This we use for large terrestrial animals like tapir and peccary."

"Where is the curare?" I asked.

"We do not use curare when we hunt these animals."

Ijuki held up his arrow.

"See how the arrowhead is perpendicular to the ground when you draw the arrow? That is because the ribs of these animals are also perpendicular to the ground, so these arrows can enter between them. When we went to war with the Okomoyanas, we made our arrows so the heads were parallel to the ground—like the ribs of a man!"

His words were few, but well chosen.

"What about this one here, the arrowhead carved with barbs?" I asked.

"That we call *tuhyehteh*," Yaloefuh replied. "It is primarily for use on large birds like curassows or macaws. If we shoot them with *para*, they can sometimes wiggle free. With these barbs there is no escape," he said with a satisfied smile.

The remaining three arrows looked anything but lethal. One had a flat arrowhead, one had a small bone arrowhead, and the third had only a small slit where an arrowhead should have been. Yaloefuh anticipated my question. "The one with the big tip is *ehyahkurah*, which is used to stun birds like toucans or toucanets when we want just a few feathers to make headdresses. For small terrestrial mammals, we use *ahdeme eyehtuhpuh*, which is the sharpened bone of a spider monkey."

"But what about the other one?" I asked. "It has no arrowhead."

Yaloefuh smiled as if he were trying to be patient with an eager but slightly dim-witted student. From the band of his breechcloth, he untied a small bamboo tube, similar to the one in which the Jaguar Shaman kept his earache-curing fungus. Twisting off the *paca*-skin top, Yaloefuh gently tilted the tube over my open palm and six bamboo arrowheads slowly slid out. Each was encrusted with the reddish brown residue that was the object of my search: curare.

I started to ask why the curare-tipped points were carried separately, but was able to figure that out on my own. For an Indian racing through the forest in hot pursuit of dinner, poisoned arrows in hand, tripping would be a mistake he might not live to repeat. Charles Waterton once wrote of an incident told to him by an Arawak Indian guide that amply illustrated curare's deadly capability.

His companion took a poisoned arrow, and sent it at a [howler] monkey in a tree above him. It was nearly a perpendicular shot. The arrow missed the monkey, and in the descent struck him in the arm, a little above the elbow. He was convinced it was all over with him. "I shall never" said he "bend this bow again." And having said that, he took off his little bamboo poison-box, which hung across his shoulder, and putting it together with his bow and arrows on the ground, he laid himself down close by them, bid his companion farewell, and never spoke more.

Suddenly Ijuki shushed us and cocked an ear in the direction we had been traveling. In the distance I could hear what Koita had impishly called the Tirió dinner bell, the *plop-plop-plop* of falling fruit as unsuspecting animals foraged in the forest canopy. They were moving toward us and we froze, perfectly still. The anticipation of an imminent kill made me fidgety, but I held my ground and waited for the drama to unfold. Just when it seemed as if the animals were going to pass directly overhead, Ijuki popped the cap off his curare tube, planted an arrowhead at the end of the shaft, strung the arrow, and let fly. Remarkably, he completed all these actions in one single fluid motion and the "Hunh!" he exhaled as he released the arrow was the only evidence that he had exerted any energy whatsoever. A capuchin monkey landed a few yards away with the arrow through its heart, dead before it hit the ground.

The rest of the monkey troop screamed and fled. I was flooded with conflicting emotions: the exhilaration of a successful hunt and a primal sense of conquest, compromised by a wave of revulsion at the sight of the dead animal. Capuchin monkeys have very human features and I found myself unable to look at its face.

Ijuki, beaming, borrowed my machete and cut several slender green vines. He used these to tie the animal's limbs together, and then slung the six-pound package over his shoulder for the trip back to the village.

Yaloefuh continued the lesson. "We always use curare when we hunt monkeys," he began. "These animals are very intelligent and they have tails. It is sometimes difficult to get a good shot at them, and even when you do, they wrap their tails around a limb and die in the tree. With curare, even a scratch is fatal and the poison relaxes them so they fall to the forest floor."

We headed home, and I tried to minimize the pressure on my sore ankle as Ijuki told us tales of the great hunts of his youth. Suddenly Yaloefuh stopped and gave a soft whistle. He turned right and slithered through the forest without making a sound, even though he moved through dead leaves at the height of the dry season. He studied the canopy and silently drew an *ehyahkurah* arrow, sending the flat-headed missile soaring skyward. From the forest heights tumbled the most beautiful bird I had ever seen—a paradise tanager, with an emerald-green head, jet-black back, vermillion rump, royal purple breast, and an iridescent bluish green throat. In true Yaloefuh fashion, he plucked a few feathers, then let the stunned bird go. He held the feathers up close to his face and admired them, saying, "These will make a fine headdress." He gently placed the feathers in the curare tube for safekeeping and we moved on. I smiled to myself. In his excitement over the makings of a new headdress, Yaloefuh had completely forgotten his wife's request for fresh meat; he headed home with only the colorful feathers to show for his day in the jungle.

The extraordinary marksmanship of South American Indians is obvious to all who visit them. Even six-year-old Tirió boys can easily hit a small target thirty feet away with their miniature bows and arrows. The great German ethnologist Theodor Koch-Grünberg, who traveled through the northern Amazon in the late nineteenth century, noted that the Indians were consistently accurate at 120 feet. In 1977, while visiting a Jivaro Indian village in Peru, Russ Mittermeier saw an Indian casually fire a blowdart at a tiny hummingbird, hitting it through the left wing. The Indian walked over, picked up the bird, and gently withdrew the dart. He released the hummingbird, which flew off seemingly none the worse for the wear. As he let it go, Mittermeier asked the Indian if that had been just a lucky shot. The Indian smiled, picked up his blowgun, aimed it at the departing bird, and put the blowdart through the right wing. A similar story surfaced several years ago from an American ornithologist collecting birds in the Ecuadorean Amazon. Anxious to help him, the local Indians offered the American several birds they had blowgunned. He politely declined, noting that he was collecting specimens for an important museum in the United States and could not use birds with holes in their skins. The next day, the Indians returned with a bagful of birds they had blowgunned through the eyes.

That evening I went to Yaloefuh's house, where I found him feeding two baby spider monkeys he had caught and given to his daughter as pets. The little monkeys huddled on a rafter in his house, refusing to have anything to do with him until he sat in his hammock, peeled a banana, and placed half on each shoulder. The monkeys chatted excitedly, then climbed down and perched on his shoulders to devour the fruit.

I reclined in a nearby hammock and, in the best Tirió custom, launched into a long-winded discussion of this and that before getting to the point: I wanted to learn about curare. Yaloefuh was silent for a few minutes, carefully considering his response. "Curare is not like the other plants we have taught you," he began. "The Tiriós paid a tremendous price for the knowledge and it is only passed on to those who can appreciate its value.

"When the world began, there was only one man, and he was a Tirió. He had three pets—a howler monkey, a yellow-headed parrot, and a yellow-headed vulture. One day, he returned from hunting to find that someone had made cassava bread; the next day he hid, hoping that the bread maker would return. From his hiding place he watched as his pets changed themselves into men and began to prepare the cassava bread. When he confronted the animal-people, the howler monkey changed into a beautiful woman, and the woman and the Tirió married.

"One day in the forest, a harpy eagle showed the man his talons and said, 'This is my curare.' The eagle then showed the man a liana and said, 'This is your curare,' and taught the man the proper way to make the arrow poison. The man was anxious to try the curare. A troop of howler monkeys was passing overhead, and the man shot first one howler monkey, then another, and another, until there was only one howler monkey left in the forest. 'Please don't shoot me,' the monkey—a female—begged. But the Tirió ignored the monkey's pleas and shot it dead; when it fell to the ground, the monkey turned into the lifeless body of the Tirió's wife."

I was quiet for a moment, letting the impact of the story sink in. I chose my words carefully. "My friend, I did not know the price the Tiriós paid to learn curare. I have come to hear, to listen, and to record. My promise to the chief was to write down all the plants that the Tiriós use and their method of preparation. Teach me this and your children will have a written record from which to learn."

He sat there quietly, deep in thought. "My friend," he said, "I must think about this tonight. Tomorrow I will give you my answer." As I walked back to my hut, the village was bathed in the silvery iridescence of a full moon. Behind me I could hear the monkeys chattering in the rafters of my friend's house.

The next morning I was awakened by Yaloefuh's youngest son, who was carrying one of the spider monkeys. "My father asked me to bring you to the house of the curare master." I assumed this boded well and I pulled on a pair of pants and a clean T-shirt. As we walked across the village, I wondered what the curare master would be like. We stopped in front of the hut of my old friend Tyaky and the boy told me to enter. As soon as I walked in, Tyaky, who was busy making a set of baby rattles out of dried gourds, looked up. "Why, it's the white-man-who-falls-on-his-ass." He chuckled. Then I saw Yaloefuh sitting next to the fire; he pointed to Tyaky and said, "He has agreed to teach you based on the terms of our agreement."

To seal the deal, Tyaky passed around a pot of cassava beer. After we drained it, Tyaky grabbed his machete and the three of us set off for the forest.

As we walked, I romantically assumed we were headed for the deepest, darkest depths of the forest where the secret plants grow. Leaving the main trail, we hiked only as far as an overgrown garden, where Tyaky started to dig into the sandy soil with his machete blade. With a few quick jabs into the dirt, he uncovered the end of a thick root, which he pulled until he held about two feet of liana. He sliced it off, gently scraped away a portion of the bark, and sighed appreciatively as the root exuded a bright red sap.

"Aha!" he exclaimed. "Blood!" This reddish exudate, according to

Yaloefuh, was proof that the specimen was highly toxic. Tyaky collected several other pieces of the thick root, tucked them under his arm, and we then retraced our steps to the village to get the other materials necessary to prepare our poison.

Early explorers were both fascinated by the curare poison and terrified of it. Because they were not permitted to witness its preparation, strange tales circulated regarding the process. José Gumilla, a Spanish Jesuit who lived among the Orinoco tribes of Venezuela in the seventeenth century, wrote of a rumor that only old women are allowed to make the curare and when one dies from the fumes that arise from the cooking pot, she is replaced by another. Similarly, Peter Martyr, court chaplain to Queen Isabella and official historian of the Indies, wrote that old women condemned to death for various crimes were assigned to make the poison; their death was a sign that the curare was ready for use. But the Tiriós did not involve women in the making of curare; quite the opposite. As we hiked back to the village, Tyaky told me the rules governing the preparation of flying death.

"Man makes the poison and women must not see it being prepared. It is said that if children are near when the poison is made, they may sicken and die."

By now we were back at the village and had entered Tyaky's hut. His wife, almost always at home tending the cooking fire, was nowhere to be seen. The old man helped himself to a stalk of tiny yellow bananas and passed them to us. He then rummaged around the back of his hut and came up with an old aluminum pot, a handful of flat bamboo arrowheads, and a monkey-fur brush that he would use to paint the arrowheads with poison. Yaloefuh picked up the pile of curare roots and we walked back into the jungle.

Just past the outskirts of the village, Tyaky borrowed my machete and swiftly hacked down several fronds of the *wapoe* palm. With these leaves and a few saplings he quickly made a simple shelter, large enough for just two people. Next, he wandered off with the pot to get water from a nearby stream while Yaloefuh collected twigs to make a fire.

Tyaky returned with the pot and hung it over the fire, suspended from a stick that Yaloefuh had pounded into the ground next to the flames. With his machete, the old man began to scrape long strips of root bark into the water, which turned a brownish yellow. Once this was done, he handed the machete to Yaloefuh and told him to get the other plants. Although I soon lost sight of him, I could hear him wielding the machete close by. Within a half hour he returned with a handful of herbaceous plants, handing them to Tyaky. One by one, the old man crushed each plant and added it to the pot.

"This," he said "is *ah-lah-ku-pah-ne,* and it causes the victim to bleed from the ears. Next is *ku-neh-beh-beh,* which helps paralyze the victim. Then *poi-fuh,* which causes convulsions, and after that *pom-weh,* from my garden, which causes the poison to burn its way into the blood. Finally, the stems of *tow-tow,* whose oil helps the poison to stick to the arrowhead."

As I watched the age-old ritual, Yaloefuh handed me a stem with leaves. "This," he said, "is from the curare plant. I thought you might want to see what the leaves look like."

From the specimen he handed me, I could finally identify the curare liana as *Strychnos guianensis,* a common jungle climber that was already known to be the main curare component in the arrow poison of several neighboring tribes. It was a bit anticlimactic to find that the plant the Tiriós were using was well-known, but my temporary disappointment was overshadowed by the pleasure of observing the ritual.

Tyaky took a great deal of care alternately lifting and lowering the pot to ensure that the water temperature was controlled. At first he kept the water warm but not hot, then hot but not boiling, then boiling rapidly to condense the poison. As he worked, he told me of a curare he had made that was especially effective for killing spider monkeys (his favorite dish), and of what a great marksman he had been as a young man. He also told me he sometimes added large stinging ants to the brew to make the potion more virulent.

The whole question of admixtures—the components used in addition to the curare plant itself—has caused vigorous scientific debate over the years. Both arrow poisons and hallucinogens tend to have a similar pattern to their recipes, basically an active component plus several admixtures. Many scientists have been quick to dismiss these admixtures as just so much mumbo-jumbo. When the Indians refused to show Prussian naturalist Robert Schomburgk how to prepare the poison in 1837, he decided to attempt it himself. Knowing which plant served as the major component, he collected it, soaked it in water overnight, and boiled it down to the consistency of syrup. He tested the poison on domestic chickens and found it fatal, leading his brother Richard to write, "This was a sure demonstration that the *Strychnos toxifera* alone, without any mixing of the other ingredients, developed the deadly properties and that all the other additions of the Indians did not contribute essentially to its strength."

But Charles Waterton (whom Richard Schomburgk insisted on referring to as the "famous traveller," as if his work was of no scientific merit) concluded otherwise:

Here it might be asked, are all the ingredients . . . necessary, in order to produce the wourali poison? Though our opinions and conjectures may mitigate against the absolute necessity of some of them, still it would be hardly fair to pronounce them added by the hand of superstition, till proof positive can be obtained.

Charles Waterton was correct. Recent laboratory investigations using state-of-the-art technology have demonstrated that some of these admixtures augment and intensify the effects of the arrow poison and/or the hallucinogen. Once again, indigenous peoples in red breechcloths, living deep in the Amazon, had proven to be our equals—actually our betters—in organic chemistry.

Just when I thought my quest for curare had ended—and rather anticlimactically—I found I had not completely unraveled the mystery of the arrow poison. Several nights after Tyaky showed me the secrets of the poison preparation, I was busy reading my field notes by lamplight when I felt a nearby presence. Looking up, I saw the Jaguar Shaman standing silently in front of me. Clenched in his right hand was a small bush I had not seen before.

"Grandfather," I said, "you startled me." The old man did not reply.

"What's that?" I asked.

"Curare," he said, flashing a rare smile. He handed me the plant.

"That is not curare," I said. I thought he was trying to trick me.

"The *pananakiris* have more than one kind of shotgun. Why can't we have more than one kind of curare?"

I examined the plant closely under the light of the lamp. Professor

Schultes had taught me enough about the arrow poisons of the Amazon I knew that this plant, an herblike species of *Strychnos*, had never been recorded as a species of curare. When I looked up to ask the old medicine man more questions, he was gone.

It is both interesting and instructive to learn what happened to Charles Waterton's beloved Macushi Indians, the proud and hospitable blowgun hunters whose curare sparked the interest of the Western scientific establishment and led to its use in modern medicine. In 1981, R. J. Lee, the UNESCO representative to Guyana, retraced the explorer's steps and eventually located the village where Waterton found the curare. He wrote:

> Little of the southern half of Guyana has changed in the last 2,000 years, let alone the 200 since Waterton's birth. Little, that is, except the people. The Amerindian . . . has been Christianized and westernized, bullied and cheated. His culture was ridiculed by early European missionaries and has slowly been abandoned. In the Macushi territory, between Toka village and Pirara, none of the men know how to make arrow poison and few have ever seen a blowpipe. Their diet is still based primarily on the root cassava and some of the women can make up a "bush tea" to cure fever, but they are no longer part of the land. During my stay in Toka village, I was the guest of the village captain. The hut was thatched with a rough dirt floor, mud walls, and little furniture—but they possessed a radio. It was tuned around the clock to the BBC world service.

Ten years after Lee's journey, I was able to travel to Macushi country to recheck his conclusions. The Indians had many of the "blessings" of Western civilization: boom boxes, rap music, sunglasses, bicycles, and Bibles. The missionaries from England and the traders from Brazil had introduced the shotgun over a century ago and the Indians quickly lost the art of making blowguns and preparing curare. When the local economy began to deteriorate in the 1960s, the Indians no longer had access to shotgun shells or spare parts. Their livelihood threatened, they wanted to go back to the traditional ways of hunting, but the old people who knew the secrets had already died off. Today the Macushis hunt with primitive bows and arrows and even with machetes, but without the curare their ancestors discovered and introduced to Western civilization. Yet we have curare in virtually every major hospital in the United States.

There was no guarantee that the Tiriós, like the Macushis, would not one day abandon the old ways for the new. But for now, at least, the recipe for the tribe's curare—and an important part of their heritage—had been preserved through my notes. I felt honored to have been trusted by these gentle people, whom I would always consider friends, and was grateful to the Jaguar Shaman for sharing with me a new and previously unknown arrow-poison plant, a species whose potential, when unlocked in the laboratory, might be as far-reaching as the arrows that carried it.

## CHAPTER 6

# Across the Savannas of the Sipaliwini

There is still a vast amount of field work to be undertaken, not only there, but in Suriname and [French Guiana], and if haste be not made, the information which it is now possible to glean will probably be lost forever. The so-called opening up of the country for the trader, the rancher, the timber getter, the balata and the rubber bleeder . . . may or may not exert a beneficial influence on the welfare of the Creole, the Negro, and the European; but for the aboriginal Indian, it means ruin, degradation, and disappearance. —Walter Roth, 1916

● ● ● ● ● ● ● ● ● ● ● ● ● ● ● ● ● ●

By the end of my second expedition to the land of the Tiriós, I was becoming restless. I had spent a total of twelve weeks in the bush with the Indians and gathered about a hundred plant specimens. No matter which of the old medicine men I worked with, at least half of the plants they pointed out were specimens I had already collected. I was greedy for more knowledge. Then one of the Indians told me of a large village called Palu. One of three Tirió villages in the area—and the only one not in Suriname—Palu is situated at the edge of a savanna across the border in Brazil, about fifty miles from Kwamala. Did they use the same plants as the Kwamala Tiriós, I asked, and for the same purposes? Were they people of the forest or of the savanna? What stage of acculturation were they in? How much contact had they had with the outside? No one quite knew how to answer these questions and countless others that popped into my mind, and I knew then that the only way to satisfy my curiosity was to go there.

Although the Kwamala Indians knew little about ethnobotanical practices in Palu, they told me of life in the village, warning me that I might run into the Brazilian military, who kept a post near the border, and that I might not be as warmly welcomed by the Brazilians as I had been by the Surinamese. Missionaries controlled the village, they said, not the Indians, and peasants who farmed in the surrounding forest were encroaching on the Indians' territory. Their tales only confirmed what I had deduced in more than a decade of studying the South American Indians in Schultes's classroom and in the field: the missionaries were the bad guys. They would move in and forever change the Indians' way of life, all in the name of Christianity. They would wipe out the Indians' native religion, destroy their culture, and extinguish the harmonious balance in which these peoples lived with the surrounding ecosystem. The greedy peasants weren't far behind, plundering the forest and claiming the Indians' land as their own. Little did I know that when I visited Palu I would discover that, like most things in life, the situation wasn't quite so black and white.

Ignoring the cautions of my Indian friends, I made up my mind to travel to Brazil in 1984 to research the Palu Tiriós. I decided to make the trip on foot, wanting to see it as the Indians did. For thousands of years the Sipaliwini savannas have been a crossroads of Amerindian migration: peoples moving east from the Orinoco River in Venezuela, north from the Amazon, and south from the coast had traversed these grasslands. I wanted to follow in their footsteps. Kamainja and Fritz von Troon, my Maroon friend, agreed to help guide me to Palu.

I met up with Fritz in August 1984 in Paramaribo. It had been four years since I had seen him, and as we flew south over an unbroken sea of green, we caught up. I asked about Petrus, the boy whose healing ritual I had witnessed during my research with the Maroons; Fritz confirmed that the boy had fully recovered from his illness and was doing fine.

As we approached the tiny airstrip where we were to rendezvous with Kamainja, about 250 miles from Paramaribo, 40 miles east of Kwamala, and 8 miles from the Brazilian border, the rain forest abruptly gave way to the pale yellow grassland of the savanna. In the distance we could see the gray peaks of the Tumuc-Humac Mountains, marking the border with Brazil.

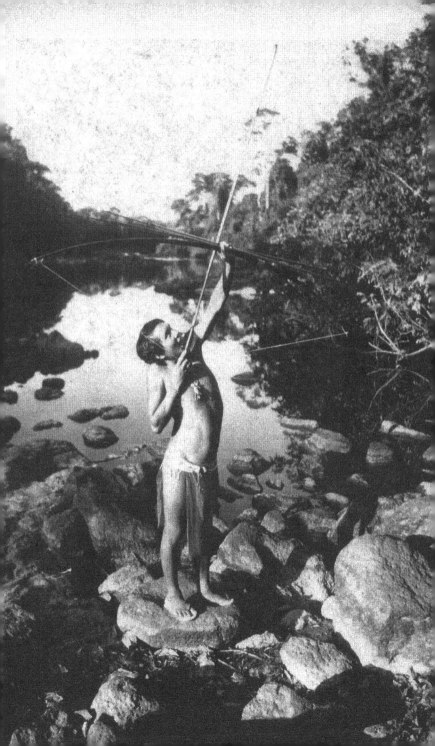

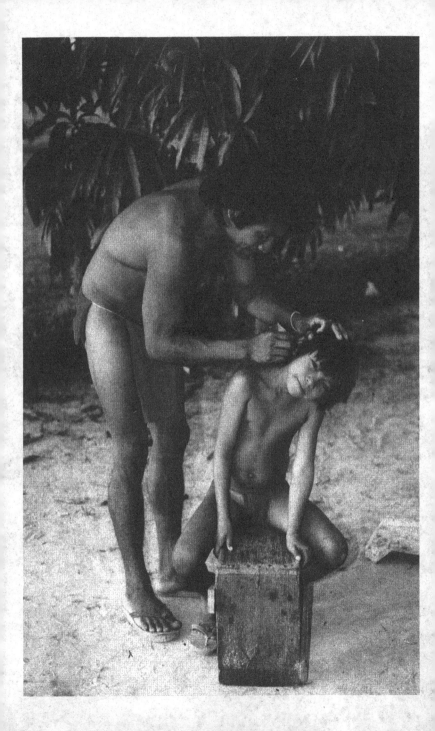

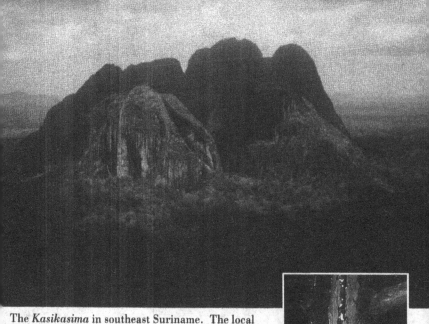

The *Kasikasima* in southeast Suriname. The local
Indians claim that the massif is home to evil spirits and
refuse to climb it. A group of Dutch and Surinamese
explorers tried unsuccessfully to ascend
it several years ago.

RIGHT: *Uh-kuh-pu-ru* of the St. Johnswort family.
The sap of this tree is used by the Tirió Indians to
treat fungal infections of the skin.

*Go-lo-be* fungus, the sap of
which is dripped into ears to
cure earaches.

OPPOSITE: Kamainja on the
Suriname-Brazil border
dripping *Go-lo-be* fungus sap
into an aching ear.

PRECEDING PAGE: Koita,
wearing a necklace with a tooth
from a jaguar he killed.

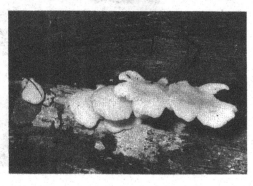

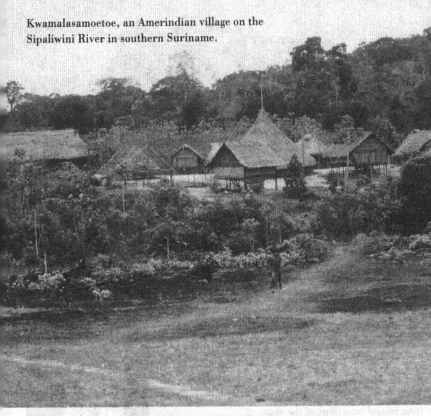

Kwamalasamoetoe, an Amerindian village on the Sipaliwini River in southern Suriname.

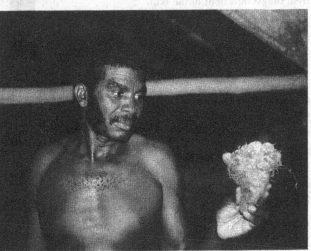

Fritz von Troon with wild yam.

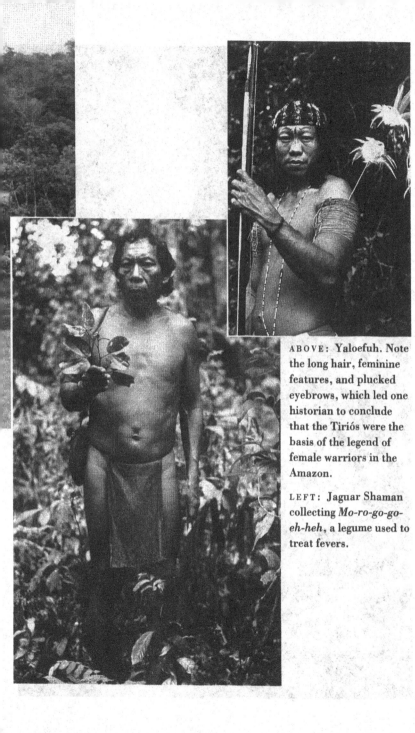

ABOVE: Yaloefuh. Note the long hair, feminine features, and plucked eyebrows, which led one historian to conclude that the Tiriós were the basis of the legend of female warriors in the Amazon.

LEFT: Jaguar Shaman collecting *Mo-ro-go-go-eh-heh*, a legume used to treat fevers.

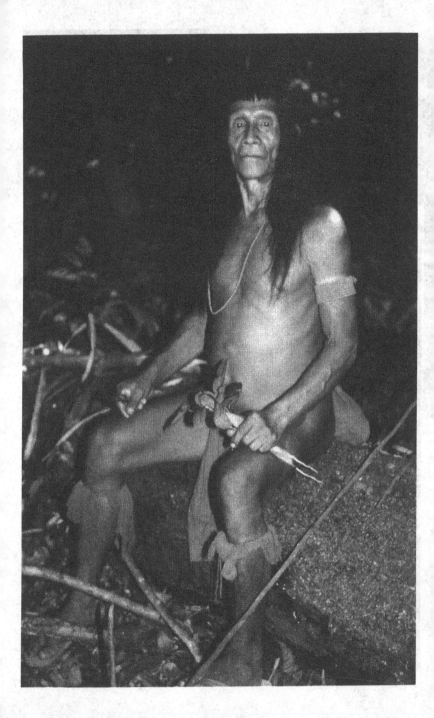

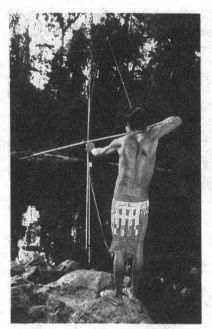

LEFT: Tirió Indian bowfishing after having thrown crushed *Ay-ah-e-yah* stems into the water to stun the fish. This plant is the source of rotenone, an important biodegradable pesticide.

BELOW: Tyaky with arrow poison admixture from the black pepper family. These admixtures, although themselves sometimes chemically inert, often amplify the toxicity of the poison itself.

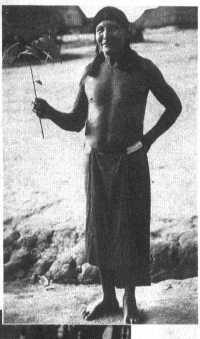

OPPOSITE PAGE: Witch doctor of the Wayana tribe, upper Tapanahony River, southeast Suriname. Some of the plants he is holding are from the frankincense family and are used to treat colds.

BELOW: Tirió women using cassava flour (center) for preparing cassava bread (right) and cassava beer (left).

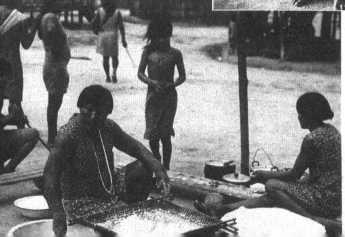

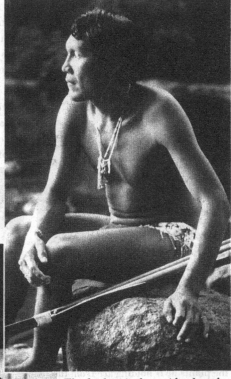

The frighteningly rapid cultural
erosion in the northeast Amazon
is illustrated by the changes in
Koita's dress, seen here in 1982
and 1992.

Nearby squatted three small one-room buildings erected by the government to house workers during construction of the airstrip. Kamainja was on hand to meet us, and he helped carry our gear into the dwellings. Once we were settled, he beckoned us around to the back of the buildings, where we found a palm-thatched hut, in which an old Tirió woman fanned a cooking fire while her daughter sat in the far corner peeling cassava. An elderly man in full traditional garb—breechcloth, simple feather headdress, and face paint—sat on a low wooden bench and bid us welcome as we entered. A younger man sat at his feet, drinking a huge calabash of cassava beer.

After he had finished the beer, the young man reached back and picked up the black and yellow shell of a redfoot tortoise, a common Amazonian species. Tucking it under his left arm, he rubbed the heel of his right hand against the shell's edge. Displeased with the sharp hollow sound the shell gave off, he stopped and picked up a grayish black lump of *mah-tah-ke* resin from the *Symphonia* tree, and used it to rub the lip of the shell. This produced a much clearer sound, and the older man, as if on cue, lifted a bamboo flute to his lips and joined his son for a duet.

That evening the Hindustani who manned the airstrip made us dinner. We feasted on rice and boiled green papaya. Although many Americans consider papaya native to southern California, the fruit actually originated in Andean Colombia. A staple crop in South America, the papaya is prized not only for its sweet flesh, but for the enzymes it produces. One, called papain and extracted from the latex of the unripened fruit, is effective in breaking down proteins; it is the active ingredient in meat tenderizers and in some digestion aids. Since the early 1980s, another papaya enzyme—chymopapain—has been used as an enzymatic cleaner for contact lenses and as a treatment for slipped disks. The enzyme is injected into the center of the problem disk, where it dissolves the soft jelly that fills the disk. This shrinks the disk and relieves pressure on the adjacent nerves. In some cases, injection of the drug into damaged disks has eliminated the need for back surgery.

After the meal, I went back to my little house to prepare for the upcoming trek. Working under the light of a single bare bulb hanging from the ceiling, I folded clothes and put them into my backpack. Then, out of the corner of my eye, I saw a gray blur near the door and felt a sharp burning in my leg. Looking down, I saw a *munu*, or vampire bat, clinging to my ankle. As I yelled and jumped back, the bat's incisors slit my flesh and it lapped at the blood that oozed from the wound. Fritz heard my howl and came running, machete in hand, thinking I had stepped on a poisonous snake. Quickly he pried the bat off my ankle with the blade—the bat had a wingspan of about eight inches—and crushed it flat with the heel of his boot. I watched in shock as blood dripped from my leg onto the concrete floor.

Fritz sat me down in my hammock, bathed the wound with soap and water from my canteen, and bound it with one of my T-shirts. "Tomorrow," he said, "I will find some plants to help it heal. I have done all I can for you now. Perhaps you should get some sleep." He patted me kindly on the shoulder, picked up his machete and the bloody remains of the bat, and headed for the door.

"Fritz!" I cried. "Will I get rabies?"

"Uh, no," he said reassuringly, then asked, "What's rabies?"

I listed the symptoms as best I could remember them—the fevers, the madness, the foaming at the mouth. He recognized the description and said, "No, probably not. Don't worry!" And with that he headed off to his hammock.

I was too agitated to sleep, so I hobbled over to Kamainja's hut for a second opinion.

He was asleep. "Kamainja," I said quietly. He rolled over and stuck his head out from under the mosquito netting. "What is it?" he asked.

I pointed to the blood-soaked T-shirt bandage and explained what had happened. Kamainja sat up and motioned for me to put my foot in his lap. He unwrapped the bandage and had a look at my ankle. The bat's teeth were so sharp and the puncture wound so clean that it took him a minute to find where I had been bitten. "That's the work of a vampire bat, all right," he pronounced, rewrapping the bandage. "Try and get some sleep."

"I'm not going to get rabies, am I?"

"What's rabies?" he asked.

The vampire bat lives entirely on blood, a high-protein diet for which the creature has a specially adapted digestive tract. It pierces the skin of its victim with sharp incisors, and an anticoagulant in the bat's saliva keeps the blood flowing while it drinks its fill. Originally, the vampire bat probably feasted on large forest mammals such as tapirs; when live-stock were introduced to savanna areas, it added those animals to the menu as well. Some vampire bats do carry rabies, and what scared me—besides the attack itself—was that this bat had flown into a lit dwelling to bite me, highly irregular behavior for these nocturnal crea-tures. Fortunately, Fritz and Kamainja were correct in saying I had nothing to worry about, but at the time their reassurances had a rather hollow ring.

The night was long and sleepless. The airstrip lay on the flank of the Tumuc-Humac Mountains and the evenings were cool at the higher elevation. The chill multiplied my discomfort and, despite my fatigue, I was glad to see the sun rise.

While I went down to the river to wash, Fritz headed off to the forest to collect plants. By the time I returned to the house, he was boiling two pots of water: one contained tea bags, the other bubbled with long, thin, waxy leaves that were light green in color. "What kind of leaves are those?" I asked.

"Smell," he said. "They're the leaves of the *masoesa* bush. It is ex-cellent for cleaning wounds."

The boiling pot gave off a pleasant tangy smell and the water turned a light green. I recognized the plant as a member of the ginger family, rich in essential oils. Species of this family are used throughout the tropics, brewed as teas to relieve the symptoms of coughs and colds and swabbed on wounds to accelerate healing. The essential oils may have antibiotic properties but need to be examined in the laboratory; I would collect a specimen for my plant press.

By now it was hard to see any evidence that I had been bitten. There were no marks on my ankle other than a slight bruising at the wound site. As Fritz bathed the wound with a piece of cotton soaked in the medicinal brew, I could feel the cooling effect of the essential oils.

We decided to postpone our trek for a day to let my ankle heal. At loose ends, I went to the thatched hut to visit with Kamainja and the other Indians, who were eating a breakfast of cassava bread with a cassava beer chaser; because of my previous night's trauma, I was able to pass up the meal without seeming impolite. Sitting down in an empty hammock, I asked the older man how far it was to the village in Brazil.

"Seven days," he replied.

"What?" I asked in dismay.

"No, one day," his son corrected him.

"One day?" I repeated.

"Yes, for an Indian," said Kamainja. "For you, three days. You walk like a white man."

"I am a white man," I said. "Three days?"

"No," said another Indian, who had just made the trek. "For you, two days."

"Two days?" I asked hopefully.

"No," said the old man. "For you, seven days."

The argument continued and estimates flowed faster than the cassava beer. Of course, I had checked the distance before setting off on the trip and calculated it to be about eighteen miles as the crow flies. But Indians seldom take the shortest route to a place; trails detour to pass by a fruiting tree that attracts toucans, to avoid a rock shaped like a face that is thought to harbor evil spirits, or to take advantage of a lovely waterfall to bathe in. I had to rely on the Indians who knew the trail to tell me how long the hike would take. Although I trusted Kamainja completely, the mental and physical preparation for a two-day trek and a seven-day trek are different, and I wanted to know how long we would be gone. But I was never able to get a satisfactory answer. Time and distance have a different meaning for the Tiriós, and my Western cultural obsession to know how far and how long went unheeded.

As the sun came up the next morning, Fritz, Kamainja, and I hoisted our packs and prepared to hit the trail. Because he didn't have a passport, Fritz would be going with us only to the border with Brazil.

As we set off, Kamainja asked to borrow a shirt.

"What for?" I asked.

"*Fre-fre ku-deh-tah!*" he replied. "The bugs are bad on the savanna!" This proved to be the understatement of the journey.

Although the airstrip was built on a small savanna, the trail to Brazil began in rain forest. We fell into an easy rhythm, with Kamainja leading the way down the path, me in the middle, and Fritz bringing up the rear. We had been traveling a few hours when Kamainja suddenly froze and, raising his right hand, signaled for us to stop as well. Leaning his head back, he sniffed the air and said one work—*pingo*—meaning "white-lipped peccary." The collared peccary is the Amazon's most common; it ranges from northwestern Argentina to the deserts of the American Southwest, where it is known as the javelina. It is a relatively docile animal who usually flees at the sight of humans. The white-lipped peccary is an entirely different beast. Weighing in at well over a hundred pounds, this piglike animal may travel in herds of up to two hundred. Found only in the rain forest, it has earned a reputation for orneriness. Confronted by humans, white-lips will click their teeth menacingly and then charge.

The herd we approached must have been intent on feeding, because the animals didn't pay us any attention; eventually we heard their barrel-chested grunts as they moved off in another direction. We soon came upon the remains of their feast: *mu-ru-mu-ru* palm nuts, which the peccaries crushed with their huge teeth. Kamainja also pointed out where they had used their tusks to dig up the ground in search of jungle roots and tubers.

We soon came to the edge of a cold, swift stream flowing through a bed of black rock, where an Indian had built a thatched hut as a way-station for travelers. I stopped to fill my canteen and heard Fritz and Kamainja talking quietly. We had been traveling about three hours, and Fritz was beginning to worry that we were approaching the border. He was clearly reluctant to turn back, but I didn't want all three of us to end up rotting in a Brazilian jail because we had entered the country illegally. I thanked him for his help and he headed back toward the airstrip.

Soon after crossing the stream, the trail began a slow but steady incline. Stepping over a log, Kamainja whooped with joy and scooped up a redfoot tortoise that had taken shelter under the fallen tree. Its shell, an elongated dome about a foot in length, had large yellow spots scattered over a dull black background. It blended perfectly with the dead leaves that littered the forest floor.

Kamainja carried the tortoise over to a fig tree with large buttress roots. He handed me the turtle for safekeeping while he used my machete to cut several short poles from a dead limb at the edge of the trail. He then placed the turtle gently on the ground between the buttresses and drove the poles into the ground in front of the animal to form a natural holding pen.

"What's that for?" I asked.

"A feast!" he replied. Kamainja was a man of few words.

I was witnessing a practice as old as humankind—preserving food in the most basic form possible. In the humid tropics, one way to keep the next week's meal from spoiling is to keep the animal alive. Pre-Colombian turtle pens have been found throughout the Neotropics and Kamainja was carrying on his ancestors' tradition.

We finally reached the top of the hill and looked down on a magnificent sight. Before us were the Sipaliwini savannas, the four-foot-high pale yellow grass stretching as far as the eye could see. The only trees were a few scattered *sabana-kasjoes*—savanna cashews—whose dark green leaves provided a stark contrast to the buttery savanna grasses. In the distance, the pinkish gray Tumuc-Humac Range rose from the savanna floor against a clear blue sky. Both Kamainja and I stood silently savoring the beauty of the scene.

"*Mmpah*," he said. "Let's go."

We eased our way into the high grass; it was difficult to see where we were putting our feet. Indians tend to walk by putting one foot directly in front of the other and the trail through the tall blades was less than six inches wide. As I tried to follow Kamainja along the path, I quickly learned why he had donned a shirt.

The bugs descended on us in droves, invading our noses, our ears, our hair, our eyes. They were tiny flies—you could hardly see them, much less swat them away—and their bites on our skin were like pinpricks, not particularly painful, but maddening and relentless.

The heat beat down on us as well. Many people believe the tropical forest is humid and stifling, but the canopy shades you and the inside of the rain forest is surprisingly cool. On the savanna, however, there is no umbrella of trees and the equatorial sun is merciless.

The mud was our third torment. It had recently rained on the savanna and the ground had turned to mush. Many tropical biologists wear boots, but I find them hot, heavy, and slow to dry, and long ago gave them up for running shoes. Now I wished for my boots as I sank into the ooze, which sometimes literally sucked the shoes off my feet.

We moved along like one huge inchworm. Barefoot Kamainja carried on at a brisk pace and then stopped and waited while I caught up. The terrain had become more hilly, and the weight of my backpack—with hammock, mosquito netting, a blanket, cooking implements, food, and clothes—seemed to hold me back on each ascent and then push me forward on descent, making my footing even more uncertain. At one point, Kamainja disappeared over the rise of a small hill. When I finally struggled to the top, I looked down to see him calmly seated on a boulder, patiently waiting for me. He looked up and said in a slightly schoolmarmish tone, "Look at you. You're all sweaty!"

He was right. I might have just stepped out of the shower. And the more I sweated, the thirstier I got; I had already emptied my canteen. Kamainja, on the other hand, was not the least bit winded and had refused every offer of water. (Indians don't usually carry water on a trek; they are adept at finding streams and other sources of water.)

I later learned that physiology was on Kamainja's side. Caucasians tend to have a higher basic metabolic rate than South American Indians and therefore have more body heat to dissipate—an adaptation to a colder European climate. Because the rain forest is such a humid environment, sweating is an ineffective way to cool the body—the sweat never evaporates. As a result, the Indians sweat very little.

I ignored Kamainja's assessment of my appearance and wearily asked, "How much farther to the village?"

"Half," replied my Indian friend.

"Half? Halfway?" I asked excitedly. If we were indeed halfway, we would make it in less than two days. This thought gave me new life. "Halfway?" I said. "You're sure?"

"Half," said Kamainja as he stood up.

We set off again. After another hour, my throat was utterly parched and I asked if we could find some water. He pointed east to a grove of magnificent *koi* palms, noting that such a stand is usually found growing at the edge of a stream.

The *koi* is the most widespread, beautiful, and useful of the Amazonian palms. Reaching a height of over sixty feet, it has leaves with narrow stems and large palmate-shaped leaf blades that look something like the end explosion of a Roman candle. The trunk of the tree is smooth, gray, and often cool to the touch. Nineteenth-century German naturalist Alexander von Humboldt described it as the "Tree of Life" and this was no overstatement. From the palm's leaves, the Indians extract a strong and durable fiber they use to weave their hammocks, starch from the pith is used to make bread, and the *koi*'s fruit not only produces an edible oil, but is richer in vitamin A than carrots or spinach and as rich in vitamin C as citrus fruit. In addition, Indians eat the palm heart, make wine from the tree's unopened flowers, produce a corklike material from the leaf stem, and use the wood of the palm in light construction.

Kamainja told me that many forest creatures also rely on this tree. During the rainy season, when a single *koi* may hold over two hundred pounds of fruit, the scarlet macaw and its relatives—the blue-and-yellow, the chestnut-fronted, the red-and-green, and the red-bellied—gather for a feast. The fruit is also eaten by pacas, agoutis, turtles, and tortoises. Both the blue-and-yellow and chestnut-fronted macaws nest in the *koi*'s hollow trunk.

Kamainja found a ripe *eperu*, a *koi* palm fruit, on the ground, probably loosened by feeding parrots. Covered with small, reddish brown scales, the fruit looked like a botanical armadillo. Kamainja showed me how to get at the mesocarp—the edible pulp—by sawing off the scales with my machete. I had to scrape the firm, orange-yellow pulp off the pit with my teeth. Accustomed as I was to finding each new plant I sampled to be a taste treat—with the exception of cassava—I was surprised at the disagreeably oily taste of the *koi* fruit. It may be the "Tree of Life," but to me it tasted like famine food.

I didn't collect any plants along the trail. For one thing, I didn't have a collecting permit for Brazil, so any plants that interested me would have to wait for another expedition. But the main reason for passing up the savanna plants was that I wanted to learn from the Indians who used them. Kamainja used nothing from the savanna, but I was hoping that once we reached Palu, I would learn about these plants or others and find out new uses for plants I was already familiar with.

After two more hours of trekking, a small island of rain forest appeared on the horizon. It was close to five o'clock and we needed to find a campsite. The trail led directly into the trees, and there was a small hut at the edge of a little stream that cut through the forest glade. The gurgling of the stream, the sound of the wind blowing through the canopy, and the cool shade were a soothing respite from the broiling savanna. Kamainja unshouldered his pack and said, "Here we will camp."

By the time we slung our hammocks, the sun had begun to set. I was anxious to bathe and relax, but Kamainja beckoned me into the forest, saying he had something to show me. We walked over to a large, brownish orange boulder spotted with green mosses. Kamainja pointed to something small sitting motionless on the rock. Once my eyes adjusted to the darkness, I saw a tiny frog that glowed like a forest jewel. His body was a glossy jet-black with iridescent blue splotches. I had heard about this particular species from Russ Mittermeier and knew it was found only in the forest islands of the Sipaliwini savanna. This tiny amphibian was one of the famous poison-arrow frogs, whose name is derived from a species that is native to the jungles of western Colombia. These frogs secrete poisons that are rubbed on the blowdarts of the local Chocó Indians; scientists studying poison frogs have found that one frog contains enough toxins to kill a hundred people. Although only a few species are known to be used for arrow poison, many, if not all, members of this family secrete poisonous compounds. Russ Mittermeier was one of the first biologists to collect the blue frogs of the Sipaliwini, and he made the mistake of scratching some cuts on his legs after handling the creatures. So painful was the result that he spent the better part of an afternoon sitting in a forest stream, scrubbing the cuts with a laundry brush to get the poison out.

Among the scientists now studying poison frogs are Dr. J. W. Daly of the National Institutes of Health in Bethesda, Maryland; and Dr. C. W. Myers of the American Museum of Natural History in New York City. They have discovered in one type of poison frog a new alkaloid that, according to their initial research, works more effectively as a painkiller than morphine.

We went back to the hut and climbed into our hammocks, exhausted, without even bothering to eat dinner. I counted the hours until we would reach Palu. In the early afternoon, Kamainja had said we were halfway there and after that we had walked for another three hours. By my estimation, we were approaching the three-quarter mark and should reach our destination before midday. I decided to recheck my calculations.

"Kamainja," I said.

"Yes?"

"We're almost there, aren't we?"

"Half," he said, and turned over to go to sleep. Within a matter of minutes he was snoring.

Although I never got a straight answer out of Kamainja about what "half" meant to the Indians when they were talking about a trek, I came to the conclusion that, for the Indians, anytime between the starting point of a journey and the destination is "half."

We woke up early and breakfasted on cassava bread. Kamainja wanted to leave as soon as possible, claiming the bugs were less bothersome in the morning. I filled my canteen in the little stream and we were off.

The cool of the morning was a welcome change from the scorching heat of the previous day. Kamainja maintained a brisk pace and I did my best to keep up, figuring that continually lagging behind and playing catch-up was as tiring psychologically as it was physically. We trudged on, not stopping to rest. As we crossed a stream lined by *koi* palms, we spooked what is known as a laughing falcon; it gave a strange cackle as it flew off with a squirming green snake in its talons. High overhead soared a group of king vultures, circling carrion we never saw.

I concentrated on breathing slowly, putting one foot in front of the other, and avoiding any thought of physical discomfort. By the time the sun had risen overhead, however, sweat was pouring into my eyes.

A forest island lay dead ahead and I focused on that as a goal. By this point the heat coming off the savanna was enough to make the distant trees shimmer, but the forest was no mirage. The shade, the cool temperature, and the stream that greeted us felt like paradise.

We dropped our packs and were preparing to jump in when I sounded a note of caution. "*Spari wakin, awah?*" I asked. "There aren't stingrays here, are there?"

Kamainja smiled and shook his head no. We peeled off our clothes and plunged in. The water was cold, coffee-colored, and surprisingly deep. A large log had been felled over the stream to serve as a bridge and since I was unable to touch bottom, I held on to it and lowered myself into the water, relishing the cool current washing over me.

Kamainja had already scrambled out of the water, pulled on his clothes, and was checking our backpacks to ensure they were securely fastened. As I climbed out and began to dress, Kamainja stared into the water under the log from which I had been hanging. His face was ashen.

"What are you looking at?" I asked.

"*Ah-de-me-nah*," he replied. "*Ah-de-me-nah-e-muh*."

Some believe that the first words one should learn in a new language are those of greeting or of thanks. I, however, believe that in the tropical forest one should first master the local names of all potentially unpleasant organisms.

I knew that *e-muh* is a suffix in Tirió that means "big." *Ah-de-me-nah* is the word for "electric eel." I looked down into the water. From under the log floated a brownish gray electric eel that was about four feet long and looked as big around as my thigh. Alexander von Humboldt once had the misfortune to step on one of these creatures—which are found only in South America—and received a jolt that for the better part of a day caused him "a violent pain in the knees and in almost every joint." Although the strength of the shock depends on the size of the electric eel, the maximum jolt is delivered when the eel's head and tail are touching different points of its victim's body. Kamainja smiled at me sweetly, shrugged, and, shouldering his backpack, headed off in the direction of Brazil.

The savanna was monotonous; we saw few animals and none that was unusual. Birds offered the only real distractions. Inside the rain forest, you hear birds all the time but seldom get a good look at them. On the savanna, they are constant companions. Reddish-feathered savanna hawks, perched in the leafless *sabana-kasjoe* trees, scanned the grasslands for their next meal. Flocks of noisy sun parakeets—respendent with their fluorescent yellow bodies tinged with orange, and their black, blue, and green wings—flew overhead scouting for palm fruits. Countless small green parrots, too fast and too far away to identify, flitted over the open savanna.

We were about halfway through our second day of trekking, and the edge of the horizon shimmered in the midday heat. I thought my eyes were playing tricks when I picked up two tiny figures moving in our direction. Half an hour later I could make out the shapes of a man and a woman.

They turned out to be two Tiriós heading north to visit family in

Suriname. The man carried a twelve-gauge shotgun in his right hand and a machete in his left. His wife labored under the weight of a large backpack woven of *wapoe* palm leaves; through the leaves I could see hammocks, mosquito netting, a cooking pot, shotgun shells, a machete, cassava bread, a live redfoot tortoise, a bunch of green bananas, and an assortment of other goods. The fellow took one look at me, wrinkled his brow, and asked Kamainja, "What are you doing with this *pananakiri?*" He obviously assumed I couldn't understand his language.

"He is my friend," Kamainja replied. "We are going to the village."

"Are you crazy?" asked the other Indian. "Don't you know you will get in trouble? The village is full of Brazilian soldiers right now!" The Indian shook his head, then motioned for his wife to follow as he began walking. Behind them, a scraggly hunting dog bounded through the tall grass. It stopped when it saw me, gave a perfunctory growl, then loped after its master.

Kamainja didn't move and stared pensively at the ground. Then he turned to me and said, "We have to turn back."

"Why?"

"Didn't you understand what he said? There are soldiers there. We will both get in trouble."

There was no way I could turn back. We had to be getting close to the village and I just couldn't face coming this far and then going home empty-handed. Also, the thought of retracing our steps through the savanna was more than I could bear. I tried to reassure him. "Kamainja, we aren't doing anything wrong. You know that you have the right to go back and forth; you've done it many times. I have my passport and I speak Portuguese, so I can explain everything to the soldiers. Don't worry!"

Kamainja was silent again, then said, "You go on alone. I am going back."

At this I almost lost my temper. I caught myself, but when I spoke, I let a glint of my anger show through. "Listen, Kamainja, we're friends, and I asked you to bring me here. You agreed. I'm not an Indian; if you abandon me, I will die out here. You promised to lead me to the village, so lead me to the village. You gave me your word, now I will give you mine. If there is any problem when we arrive, I'll swear that you have nothing to do with me. I'll say that I'm a botanist who got lost on the Suriname side of the border and I ran into you on your way here and followed you. I give you my word. *E-pah-wah-nah!*"

At the mention of this last word, he straightened up, paused a second, then said *"Mmpah! Let's go!"* and we were once again on our way. Looking back nine years later and reflecting on the historically bloody relationship between Native Americans and local armies—be they in South America, Central America, or North America—I realize I probably should have backed down. But I was tired, inexperienced, and impatient, and given the heat of the savanna, I was in no mood to evaluate things in a historical or cultural context.

Like many of the Indians, Kamainja was an excellent linguist, speaking not only several related languages—his native tongue (Waiwai), his wife's language (Tirió), and the languages of neighboring tribes (Kaxuyana, Sikiyana, and some Wayana)—but also Sranan Tongo (the local trading language) and a bit of Dutch (the national language of Suriname). Although born in Brazil, Kamainja did not speak Portuguese, a source of embarrassment for him. For some reason, he seemed to have a mental block that made him unable to remember the words. On the rare occasions when we talked as we crossed the great grassland, our conversation usually went something like this:

"Teach me Portuguese!" Kamainja would say.

"Okay. *Chegamos* means 'We arrive.' "

*"Chegamos."*

*"Bom dia* means 'Good day.' "

"Wait. How do you say 'We arrive' again?"

As we approached the end of the second day, I became convinced we would never reach the village; I also worried that Kamainja would change his mind and turn back. We came to a slow-moving stream and Kamainja took off his pack and his shirt and waded in to cool off. I couldn't be bothered with stripping off my clothes; I just dropped my pack and plopped myself down in the water. As I lay there, hoping the stream was too shallow for electric eels, Kamainja looked over at me and cheerily said, *"Chegamos!"*

"What?" I asked.

*"Chegamos!"* he said, getting out and putting on his pack. I looked

up to see two little Indian boys standing on the other edge of the stream, their faces painted bright red with the dye of the *u-shuh* berry. Kamainja was right. We had arrived.

We followed the boys down a winding path that led into the jungle at the edge of the savanna. After a short walk in the forest, we stood at the entrance to Palu.

We met two Tirió women in faded blue calico dresses at the end of the path. When they saw Kamainja, who walked ahead of me, they broke into broad grins and welcomed him back. As I emerged from the forest, still dripping wet from my dip in the stream, they simply stared, speechless.

"*Como vai?*" I asked in Portuguese. "How are you?"

"*Muito bem,*" they replied in unison. "Okay."

I decided to shift gears and offer the traditional Tirió greeting. "*Kudeh manan?*" I asked. "How are you?" At this the women's eyes widened and they ran off giggling. Kamainja explained that it was strange enough for them to see a white man arrive in their village on foot, but when I greeted them in their own language, it was simply too much to bear.

Palu sat on the lovely west bank of the upper reaches of the Paru River, bordered on the south and east by rain forest, while the savanna stretched to the north and west as far as the eye could see. The village itself, though, was something of a shock, especially when compared with Kwamalasamoetoe. Although there were some traditional palm-thatched huts, most of the houses were built of wood and designed in a simple boxlike style that reminded me of urban housing projects. In the middle of the village stood three large white concrete buildings: a church, a dining hall, and the missionaries' house.

The most unsettling sight to me, though, was the Indians. All wore secondhand Western-style clothes, and it seemed that just the act of putting on the shabby clothes had sucked the vitality out of them—they appeared slow, solemn, and downcast. The comparison with my friends in Suriname could not have been more striking: in traditional loincloths, the Indians were the lords of the jungle, but in their hand-me-downs, they looked like the urban poor.

A century before, Prussian explorer Richard Schomburgk noticed a similar loss of joie de vivre among Indians recently converted by missionaries in British Guiana.

One could tell at once the new inmates who only recently had been received in the Institution by the deep melancholy which was inwardly awakened by these scenes and stamped a definite mark upon their faces. The remembrance of their forests, of their free unfettered life, the recollection of the playing grounds for their childish sports had chased away every smile, every sign of life from their boyish features.

Kamainja told me that we had to meet the padre to announce our arrival. Despite what the Kwamala Indians had said about the village, that struck me as odd.

"Don't we have to talk to the chief first?" I asked.

"Here, you begin with the padre," he explained.

I was prepared to loathe this odious creature who seemed to be despoiling Indian culture; I envisioned an obese potentate wearing a black cassock, draped in gold chains, and waited on by Indian servants. I was surprised to find an engaging sixty-year-old Bavarian named Padre Haas, who stood about five-foot-two, was dressed in jeans and a cotton work shirt, and kept a slow-burning pipe clenched between his tobacco-stained teeth.

Spry and hardworking, the padre was a carpenter by trade and we found him in a little woodworking shop he had set up to teach Indians a marketable skill. He had spent many years living among the Brazilian Tiriós, trying to prepare them for contact with the outside world. Although I continue to abhor many of the ideals he personified, I found him to be a kind and thoughtful man.

When we entered, he spoke briefly with Kamainja in fluent Tirió and then greeted me warmly in Portuguese. He said he knew we must be tired and hungry after our long journey and suggested that we wash up and join him for dinner. Turning to Kamainja, he told him that we could stay in the room at the back of the church and to take our belongings and put them there.

I felt as if my friend was being treated as a porter, so I made a point of picking up my own backpack. As we walked through the village toward the small white church, we could see that many of the Indians suffered from severe skin ailments. Kamainja suggested that this was due to the clothes the Indians chose to wear. If you wear a loincloth in a hot and humid environment and jump in the river several times a day to wash, you stay cool and clean. This is not true, however, if you are wearing long pants and a long-sleeved shirt.

Our little room was located behind the altar and we entered through a door at the back of the church. The room was completely barren except for several hooks in the wall, from which we hung our hammocks. After settling in, I sat on the floor and gingerly removed my shoes from my aching feet. I was greeted by an ugly sight: two of my toenails were cracked and had turned black. I also felt a strange itch under the big toenail on my right foot and mentioned it to Kamainja. He looked at the toe and said one word: "*Sika.*" Reaching over to his backpack, he pulled out his machete and, before I could protest, he sliced into the flesh under the nail. He squeezed my toe and a bloody egg case came oozing out. The *sika* is a flea that devours human flesh, and it had laid its eggs under my toenail. As I watched Kamainja perform this hideous operation, I thought of one of Professor Schultes's favorite sayings: "Ah, the joys of fieldwork!"

Wrapping my brutalized toes in bandages, I eased on clean socks and dry shoes and hobbled over to the dining hall with Kamainja. Many of the Indians had built cooking fires outside their huts and they waved to us halfheartedly. At the door to the dining hall, we were greeted by the cook, a rotund, shabbily dressed Brazilian who presumably worked for the church.

Behind him were two screen doors. As he opened one for me, he signaled Kamainja to go through the other. I entered a dining room about thirty feet long and painted a dull white; its only decorations were a large crucifix and a calendar featuring a photo of Rio de Janeiro. Two long wooden tables filled the room and several Brazilian workers were already seated, waiting to be served.

Turning around, I saw Kamainja's face staring at me through a hole in the wall. My friend had been sent to eat with the help in the kitchen. Kamainja, who had looked out for me, who had waited patiently for me as I plodded along on the savanna trail, who had ministered to my injured feet, was being treated like a servant. I clenched my fists and dug my nails deeply into the palms of my hands. It was all I could do to keep my mouth shut, but I knew that as a guest of the village I had to submit to their rules.

The screen door slammed behind me and I felt the padre's hand on my shoulder. "I have an announcement to make," he said to the diners. "We have a special guest, an American who will be staying with us for several days. Let us bow our heads in prayer and thank God for his safe arrival."

Everyone bowed their heads and prayed silently. The padre motioned me to a seat at his left and yelled for the cook to bring in the food. Dinner was *feijoada,* a red bean and rice stew, the Brazilian national dish. I was so hungry that I had eaten half my meal before I realized that everyone else was in the middle of another prayer. Sheepishly, I put down my fork, bowed my head, and tried to look properly devout.

Once dinner was well under way, everyone plied me with questions about who I was, where I came from, and what I was doing there. Clearly, they all regarded me as an oddball—why else would anyone want to walk across the wretched savannas, much less study Indians? Turning the tables, I asked them what they were doing in Palu. All were Brazilian laborers from the town of Belém at the mouth of the Amazon. They had been recruited by the church to work in the village, doing odd jobs like carpentry and simple construction to make life as comfortable as possible for the missionaries. My distinct impression was that the steady work and steady pay, rather than a religious commitment, brought and kept these men here.

As we finished the stew and the cook passed around an old Tabasco jar filled with wooden toothpicks, the screen door opened and four Brazilian soldiers walked in. They said hello to the padre and seated themselves at the far end of the table. I was apprehensive after all I'd heard about the military presence in the village and tried to look as inconspicuous as possible. Several minutes later, I finished my coffee and excused myself from the room.

Kamainja was seated on a stump, waiting for me. With him was an Indian about forty-five years old, dressed in a pair of faded blue gym shorts. They spoke in a language I did not understand.

"This is my friend Shafee," said Kamainja. "He is from the Kaxuyana tribe."

Speaking Portuguese, the Indian introduced himself and told me that he had been hearing all about our journey. "Kamainja says you walk just like a white man," he said.

"I *am* a white man," I said.

Both convulsed with laughter, though I'm not sure why.

I heard the screen door slam behind me and turned around to see a Brazilian sergeant looking me over. "Perhaps we should have a little discussion," he said.

"Yes, sir," I replied. I looked back around, but the Indians had faded into the village.

"Follow me. We will use the padre's office." We walked to a nearby schoolhouse that had been built along the same architectural lines as the church and dining hall.

The padre was evidently a scholarly man. The study was dominated by a massive mahogany desk and a matching high-backed chair. The walls were covered with bookshelves that held works in Portuguese, Spanish, German, Italian, French, and English. The sergeant seated himself behind the desk.

He stared at me for a moment, then said, "Passport!"

I pulled my passport out of my pocket and handed it to him. He examined it slowly and then turned to the page with my picture. He held it up, pointed to the photo, and asked, "Can you prove that this is you?"

How would a philosopher respond to this question? I wondered as I opened my wallet, extracted my driver's license, and handed it to him. After examining the two pictures, he returned both documents and asked what I was doing in Brazil. I explained that I was carrying out research on the medical botany of the Suriname Tiriós. I emphasized that my purpose in crossing the border was to get a brief look at Tiriós of Brazil for comparative purposes and that I had no plans to collect or study any Brazilian plants.

This seemed to satisfy him. He reached across the desk and shook my hand. "*Bemvindo ao Brasil*," he said. "Welcome to Brazil." Despite my weary state, we struck up a lively conversation about Brazilian and American politics and the role of the military in both societies. He was an interesting, educated man. Then he asked warily, "You're not going to steal our useful plants and take them to the States, are you?"

"No," I replied, "I am not going to do any collecting."

"Good. I thought you might be like that bandit Wickham, who stole the rubber tree from the Amazon. Brazil, with all her wonderful plants, would be a rich country if that Englishman had not robbed us of our latex."

The rubber tree, native to the Amazon, was first discovered and used by the local Indians. Not only did they eat the seeds, but they dipped their feet in the latex and dried them over the fire, thus creating the first custom-made sneakers.

All major industrial attempts to use the latex failed until Charles Goodyear discovered the vulcanization process in Boston in 1839. As a result of this discovery demand for rubber rose astronomically—from thirty-one tons in 1827 to twenty-six hundred tons in 1857. Amazonia was supplying the rubber for most of the world's car tires by the turn of the century, and soon rubber was running a close second to coffee as Brazil's main source of currency.

The sergeant had such strong feelings about plant theft because in 1876 an enterprising British botanist by the name of Henry Wickham managed to shift the rubber industry away from Brazil. To do this, he first chartered a British cargo ship that had already unloaded in Manaus, Brazil—the center of the country's rubber boom. Rather than return to the United Kingdom empty, Wickham had the ship stop downriver in Santarém, where he had Indians load the ship with baskets with ripe fruit from the rubber trees. This fruit was officially cleared for export to England. Less than three thousand of the seventy thousand rubber tree seeds Wickham had thus spirited out of Brazil germinated, but the young trees grown from these seeds were distributed among British plantations throughout Southeast Asia, where most of the world's rubber is produced today.

I felt honor-bound to point out to the sergeant that Brazil herself had once benefited from similarly duplicitous behavior.

"Where does coffee come from?" I asked.

"Why, Brazil, *senhor*. You know that."

"Well, most of the world's coffee is produced in Brazil," I admitted. "But it does not come from here. Coffee is native to Ethiopia, in Africa. The history of crop plants is one of movement from their centers of origin."

Though we soon shook hands and parted company amiably, he seemed unimpressed by my line of argument and I suspect I did little to reassure him that I was just a scientist casually passing through. By bringing up the story of coffee, I had only intended to illustrate how the rise of plant-based industries has historically had little to do with the country in which the crop plants originated.

The word *coffee* is said to be derived from Kaffa, the province in southeastern Ethiopia where the plant originated. According to popular legend, the stimulating properties of coffee were first observed in A.D. 850 by a goatherd named Kaldi, who was tending his flock by the shores of the Red Sea. Noticing that his animals romped about energetically after eating the red berries (the "beans") of the coffee bush, Kaldi tried the fruit himself. He liked the feeling of exhilaration the berries gave him and shared his discovery with the monks in the local monastery.

The use of coffee spread rapidly throughout Ethiopia, primarily as a foodstuff. People chewed the leaves and ate the fruit—which has a high protein content—to pep them up and to blunt their hunger pangs. Warriors and hunters carried with them filling, if not particularly appealing, snacks made from balls of fat studded with coffee berries.

The Arabs began importing coffee perhaps as long as a thousand years ago and are generally credited with the invention of the brewing process. Although conservative priests declared it an intoxicating beverage and coffee consumption was prohibited by the Koran, coffeehouses sprouted up all over Mecca and the drink spread throughout the Islamic world. The port of Mocha on the Red Sea was the center of a bustling coffee trade.

The plant reached Europe by way of a Dutch trader, who in 1616 stole a single coffee plant from the Middle East and brought it to Holland. From there, seedlings were taken to Dutch colonies in the East Indies. Meanwhile, coffee was introduced in one country after another in Europe, and the popularity of the drink increased dramatically. London's first coffeehouse opened for business in 1652. In less than a century there were thousands of coffeehouses in England and these served as centers of political, religious, and business life. The famous insurance firm Lloyd's of London began as Lloyd's Coffee House, catering to sailors and ship captains.

Coffeehouses also appeared across the Atlantic in the colonies. According to one account, plans for the American Revolution were first laid out in the Green Dragon Coffee House in Boston. But it was only after the famed Boston Tea Party that coffee became more popular than tea in North America.

One of the most dramatic stories about the spread of coffee across the world involved a single coffee bush sent by the mayor of Amsterdam to France's Louis XV in the early eighteenth century. This treasured gift was planted in the Jardin des Plantes in Paris, in the royal hothouse of the king. In 1723 (some accounts say 1720), a French naval officer named Gabriel Mathieu de Clieu, who was assigned to the island of Martinique but was visiting France, filched a seedling from this bush and set sail with his ill-gotten gains. The voyage to Martinique was not an easy one and water ran low, forcing de Clieu, he later wrote, to share his own scanty ration of water with the plant. His sturdy little seedling survived and spawned a sizable coffee plantation industry on the island.

From Martinique, plants were sent south to French Guiana; they were the first coffee bushes to arrive on the South American mainland. A Brazilian soldier visiting French Guiana struck up a relationship with the governor's wife and received as a farewell present a coffee plant hidden in a floral bouquet. This surreptitious gift became the basis for the Brazilian coffee industry, today the world's largest. As I tried to make clear to the sergeant I met in Palu, Brazil received its first coffee plants in much the same manner that England got its rubber trees.

The next morning was gray and overcast as Kamainja and I made our way down to the river. To the north, above the distant mountain peaks, dark cumulus clouds were gathering. As we bathed in the river, a light rain speckled the surface of the water.

After we washed up, I asked Kamainja if we could meet the village chief. Without uttering a word, he led me to a conical thatched hut on the northern edge of the village. In front of the hut sat a handsome Tirió man wearing a new pair of denim jeans and a red and blue T-shirt that read RIO DE JANEIRO in large yellow letters. On his wrist he wore a Casio watch, and perched on his head, in his sole nod to tradition, was a splendid headdress of red, yellow, and black toucan feathers.

"*Paho, wenehfuh,*" I said in Tirió. "Sir, I have arrived."

Ignoring my Tirió, he replied in Portuguese. "*Bemvindo. Um prazer,*" he said. "Welcome. A pleasure to meet you." He stood up to shake my hand and beckoned for me to sit on a low wooden bench while he chatted with Kamainja. During the course of the conversation, his two-year-old son peered out from inside the hut to see what was going on. Since I was seated at the edge of the hut entrance, my face was only a few inches from his; he let out a terrified scream and went running to be comforted by his mother.

The chief asked about our trip and whether we were comfortable, but his tone was desultory, as if he were being polite rather than truly concerned. Given the presence of the padre, he wasn't directly responsible for our welfare, as he would have been in more traditional villages.

The chief next went through the usual Tirió litany of personal questions why I was here, my age, whether I had children, my father's name, my mother's name. . . . This constituted the Tirió version of a credit check.

Once the chief had exhausted his curiosity, he picked up a piece of whitish wood and an old machete and began whittling a toy canoe for his young son. While he whittled, I talked. Oral tradition plays a central role in Indian culture, and oratory is expected and appreciated. I started out by telling of my work among the Tiriós in Suriname. Next came an account of our hike through the savanna, replete with details of the animals we saw; the encounter with the electric eel elicited a chuckle from the chief. While I was concluding the story, several other Tirió men appeared and formed a semicircle, with the chief at the center. One member of the audience was Shafee, the Kaxuyana Indian I had met the night before. He winked at me as he took his seat.

Once again the chief asked, "So why are you here?"

"I have come to observe and to learn," I replied. "Having lived with and learned from the Tiriós in Suriname, I wanted to meet the people here and learn more."

"Hah!" remarked one older man in the group. "The Tiriós of Suriname! They aren't *real* Tiriós. They don't even speak the language correctly!"

This puzzling remark was later explained by Kamainja. "There are three major villages of Tiriós, two in Suriname and one in Brazil. Each village speaks the language a little bit differently—sometimes it's just a question of an accent, sometimes a different word. For example, several plants have names that vary from village to village."

I asked the chief whether, since they lived at the edge of the great grassland, they considered themselves people of the forest or people of the savanna. I knew this was a complicated question since it touched on philosophical issues, and several of the Indians got into a heated debate. The chief let the argument play itself out before he responded: "The Tiriós are people of the *itutah*—the forest. We live at the edge of the grassland and it is a good place to hunt, especially for birds. The forest, however, is where we make our villages and cut our gardens. *Mah, kudeh!*"

Roughly translated, the last two words mean "Yes, it is good" and are spoken at the end of pronouncements for emphasis. The other Indians nodded their approval at the chief's statement.

I then asked a more specific question: "So do you use more medicinal plants from the savanna or from the forest?"

The chief's reply was unexpected. "I don't know. When I am sick, I get medicine from the padre!" The circle exploded in laughter.

"Well, then who is the *piai*—the medicine man—here?" I asked, puzzled.

"*Piai?*" he asked. "We don't have any of that old-fashioned stuff here. The last one died several years ago!"

I was shocked at this unexpected news. "Aren't there any old people here who know the medicinal plants of the tribe?"

"Well," said the chief, "you should probably ask my father, but he is very old and rather forgetful."

As if on cue, an old Tirió walked slowly out of the hut to our right. His face was home to a thousand wrinkles, and he walked with the uncertain air of the aged and infirm. He wore the only breechcloth I saw the entire time I was in Palu. The old man squatted on his haunches and turned to face the sun like some primeval bird trying to absorb enough solar energy to make one last flight.

"Do you think he might be able to tell me about the local plants?" I asked.

"I don't think so," replied the chief. "He can't hear or see very well anymore. He hardly ever goes into the jungle. Most of the time he stays in his hammock, playing with his grandson or mumbling to himself."

No medicine man. No one who remembered the tribe's healing plants. No one who carried on the spiritual tradition rooted in the tribe's origins.

A deep sadness washed over me as I realized I was looking into the future. This surrendering of their culture was what awaited my Tirió friends in Kwamala; indeed, this was what awaited all Indians who, willingly or not, traded the old ways for the new.

Most of that day passed seated in front of the chief's house. People asked if I knew their relatives in Suriname or how many days' walk it was to my country. Much of the time nothing was said, as we enjoyed a cool breeze coming off the savanna. By midafternoon the sky had started to clear and the chief's wife came out of the hut to serve us cassava beer. She was much younger than the chief and wore an old calico dress, the standard uniform of the women in the village. Wrapped around her right bicep was a string of tiny orange beads; on her left arm she wore tiny blue ones. Red geometric designs accented her face. She handed me a vat of *cassiri* and looked deeply into my eyes; I was taken with her beauty. I managed to stammer out a Tirió greeting and, although she stared at the ground in response, I thought I saw a fleeting smile play across her lips.

After a few rounds of cassava beer, the sun came out in full force and it was too hot to sit in the direct sunshine. Kamainja and I excused ourselves and headed back to our room at the church. Soon after we departed, Shafee came trotting along behind us. "Hey, *pananakiri*," he said to me. "You see this plant over here? The Tiriós call it *wan-tah* and they used to use it to treat fevers."

"How do you know that?" I asked.

"I used to hunt with the son of the medicine man. His father sometimes came with us and he always tried to teach my friend about medicinal plants. I was more interested than he was, but the old man wouldn't teach me everything, since I was from another tribe."

"Do you know anything about the medicinal plants of the Kaxuyanas?"

"A little bit. Maybe about the same as I know of the Tiriós. Why don't we go into the forest tomorrow and see what we can find?"

This sounded great to me. I wanted to get away from the mission and into the forest, where I could be free of what the great nineteenth-century German naturalist Theodor Koch-Grünberg referred to as "the pestilential stench of Western civilization."

That night I decided to skip the mess hall rather than see Kamainja forced to eat in the kitchen again. We shared a can of tuna fish from my pack. I was lying in my hammock writing in my journal by the light of my flashlight when there was a knock at the door and the padre walked in. "Would you like to go for a stroll?" he asked.

I gingerly put a pair of shoes on my still-aching feet and we walked through the village. The light of the cooking fires cast a soft glow inside each hut. A dog howled at the edge of the village and the frogs of the savanna croaked loudly in unison.

"What do you think of our little village?" asked the padre.

"You have been very hospitable to me here. It is a lovely setting," I replied.

"And the Indians?"

"I like them very much. They are nice people."

He paused to light his pipe and the flare of the match illuminated his lined face.

"And their religion?"

I hesitated, not quite knowing what he was getting at. Choosing my words with care, I replied, "I'm a biologist, Padre. Religion is not my area of expertise."

He sighed and sat down on the tree stump in front of the dining hall. After a short pause, he continued. "I'll tell you what the problem is. It is not our religion. It is our religions. When the American missionaries lived with the Surinamese Tiriós, they taught that Protestantism was the one true path. Here, we are Franciscans, a Catholic order. So what you are left with is a tribe divided roughly in half, with each half believing the other to be heathens doomed to burn in hell. A tragic state of affairs, no?"

His candor was refreshing, even if his presence was obviously part of the problem. Rather than get into a theological debate in which I might lose my composure, I changed subjects. "Can you tell me a bit about the history of the mission?" I asked.

"Sure," he said, as he knocked the bowl of his pipe against the stump and pulled a worn brown leather pouch from his shirt pocket. He poured in fresh tobacco and lit his pipe.

"It all started with the Treaty of Tordesillas in 1494. Columbus had already discovered America, but the Portuguese weren't far behind. Both countries asked Pope Alexander VI to mediate. He drew a line on a map, dividing the New World in half at three hundred seventy leagues west of the Cape Verde Islands. Land west of the line belonged to Spain; land east of the line to Portugal."

"I'm familiar with the treaty," I said. "But what does that have to do with the mission?"

He smiled and puffed on his pipe. "If you look on a map, you'll see that the line of division passes through São Paulo. Officially the treaty gave Portugal the right to settle the east coast of Brazil. Everything to the west—which includes not only this mission site but most of the Amazon basin—supposedly belonged to Spain. The Spanish, though, were hindered by having to cross the mighty Andes, which form the western spine of the continent. In contrast, the Portuguese were able to sail due west along the Amazon River and then both northwest and southwest along its tributaries. By the time the Spanish were ready to establish large settlements on their property east of the mountains, they found the Portuguese had encroached on their land. They were already well ensconced near the foothills of the Andes, and the Brazilian border had been pushed far to the west of what had been agreed to in the Treaty of Tordesillas."

"Go on."

"At least partially as a result of this land grab—certainly no less audacious than much of the territorial acquisitions of the U.S., I might add—the Brazilians remain xenophobic, always fearing that their remote border regions may be overrun by settlers from neighboring countries. Since the turn of this century, the Brazilian government has proposed a series of ill-planned schemes to establish population centers at or near the border of each adjacent country, to reinforce their claim to the land. The army set up bases with the same purpose in mind. A far-sighted colonel anticipated the inevitable social problems that would result from encouraging large numbers of Brazilian peasants to settle on Indian lands. He asked the Franciscan Bishop of Óbidos to set up this mission to help the Indians deal with the inevitable process of acculturation as well as act as an intermediary between the Indians and the military. When we first came here, we learned the Indians' language, taught them Portuguese, and helped them build the airstrip nearby so that the military could construct its base. Let me assure you, I have seen what can happen when the military or the peasants come into contact with Indian cultures cold, without having the church acting as a go-between. It is not a pretty sight. It is the Indians who suffer most —prostitution, venereal disease, alcoholism, suicide. We don't have any of that here."

"What about their own religion?"

"The Tiriós had many gods, but one—Kan—was the most powerful. It was not too difficult to convince them that there is only one true God and that the others are only saints and prophets." Taking the pipe out of his mouth, he smiled at this last remark.

I was unable to tell by his expression whether he regarded this manipulation of the native beliefs as ingenious, slightly embarrassing, or both. Rather than dwell on this religious sleight-of-hand, I asked another question.

"What was it like when you first arrived?" I asked.

"Traditionally, the Tiriós did not live in large villages like we have here. Let me think—here we have over three hundred Tiriós and about eighty Kaxuyanas. Originally, both tribes lived in groups of thirty or so people. Each village consisted of little more than extended families living in two or three houses. Each site was settled and farmed for three years, until manioc yields declined because of the poor soils. As you know, this region is part of what the geologists call the Guayana shield, and it contains some of the poorest, most weathered soils in all of Amazonia. The Indians understand these soils and know how to farm them. If the government had succeeded in sending peasants here, they would have starved."

He talked on into the night. It was a vivid monologue, peopled with famous medicine men and hunters, all of whom are gone now. The padre recounted tales of hiking into the forest and coming face-to-face with Indians who had never before seen a white man, and the mixture of fear and curiosity evident in their expressions and gestures. He described how the evangelists had worked to convince the Indians that a better life awaited them at the mission. At the conclusion of the evening, he recited a tribal legend so extraordinary that I will never forget it.

"You have to remember," the padre began, "when I first arrived here in the 1950s, the scientific community did not agree on just where the Indians had originated. Today most people accept the theory that they came from Asia and crossed the Bering Strait during the last ice age, when a land bridge connected Asia and North America. But at the time of our arrival, people proposed all sorts of strange hypotheses. One of our bishops in Germany swore that the Indians were the descendants of the Lost Tribes of Israel!

"Anyway, when we were introducing the Indians to Christianity, we told them tales from the Bible, explaining that these were the stories of our ancestors. Since the Indians were a preliterate culture, all of their traditions were oral, passed from parent to child. When we told Biblical stories, we sometimes asked them to tell us about the accounts of their ancestors. One story, which I heard repeatedly from the old men of the tribe, was that in the distant past, the Tiriós crossed a land so cold that they had to wrap themselves in the skins of animals. The Tiriós live in the northeast Amazon, *senhor*. They do not see snow or experience cold weather, or wrap themselves in animal skins for warmth. They had never had any contact with white men who could have told them about these things. I believe that this tale is their tribal recollection of crossing the Bering Strait. If it is, that story is more than twenty thousand years old. Good night, *senhor*."

With that, he got up from the tree stump and walked off toward his house. The velvety darkness of the village swallowed him up, and I could see only the orange glow from the smoldering tobacco in his pipe growing smaller and smaller. Only a few days earlier I had been willing to lay all the Indians' problems at the feet of missionaries like the padre. Now I found myself thinking of what life might have been like for the Indians if the missionaries had not intervened. Mistreated by the peasants or the military—or both—the Indians would have lost not only their lands and their culture, but perhaps even their lives.

The next morning, when I peeled off the first bandage, the two toenails came with it. I stumbled down to the river to wash my wounds and there met Kamainja.

"What's up?" I asked.

"*Mmpah!*" he said. "Let's go!"

"Where do you want to go? I don't think I want to do much walking today."

He looked at my feet. "We'll take the canoe. I'll get a paddle."

A few minutes later, he returned with a paddle and his friend Shafee in tow. It took me a minute to recognize the Kaxuyana. He wore his trademark blue gym shorts, but he had added a special accessory: two large scarlet macaw feathers pushed through the pierced septum of his nose. They looked like giant mustaches and gave him a menacing appearance. He pointed to a canoe tied to a large, smooth-barked, columnar *walaba* tree and we both got in. Kamainja handed Shafee the paddle, then again walked back to the village.

He next returned carrying three hammocks, a shotgun, a cooking pot, and a large piece of manioc bread. He handed me everything and pushed our canoe away from the bank before hopping in.

As we floated slowly downriver, I once again marveled at the incredible wanderlust—and the spontaneity—of my companions. The presence of hammocks indicated that this was not an afternoon picnic but an overnight trek into the forest. Kamainja appeared to have planned this excursion in the course of borrowing a paddle.

Like the Sipaliwini River in Suriname, the Paru River is broken by a series of rapids; on several occasions, we had to get out of the canoe and carry it and our provisions along the riverbank until we were past the rough waters.

As we traveled farther away from the village, the seemingly endless stretch of cassava gardens gave way to stands of forest that crowded the water's edge. Often when passing the gardens, we could see women and their daughters peeling huge piles of cassava roots with their machetes. Occasionally canoes passed us going against the current as people returned to the village, their boats loaded to the gunwales with cassava or bunches of green bananas. As we cut smoothly through the water, iridescent blue *Morpho* butterflies darted in front of us.

We spent the first night with a Tirió family in a thatched hut at the edge of their garden. The next morning we were up early, tramping through the forest. At one point, Kamainja and Shafee went off to look for a Brazil nut tree they thought was nearby. They told me to stay put. I sat down on an old log and was enjoying the quiet when I heard a buzzing noise. I thought it was a bee, but when I looked up I saw a beautiful hummingbird with an appropriately lovely name: the blue-tailed emerald. The bird's iridescent green body contrasted sharply with its short black bill and blue forked tail. It perched briefly on a branch and then quickly darted down to a passion fruit flower, where it began feeding.

Hummingbirds occur only in the New World and although some make it as far north as Alaska, most are found in South America. By ornithological standards, hummingbirds are small. The largest, the so-called giant hummingbird, measures less than nine inches in length. By comparison, the tiny bee hummingbird of Cuba is slightly more than two inches long, and half of that is the bill and the tail. Just as unusual is the spectacular Andean sword-billed hummingbird, whose four-inch bill is longer than its three-inch body.

Although they also eat insects, hummingbirds have evolved specific adaptations for feeding on floral nectar. They have special bills to extract the nectar, and because many flowers cannot support the weight of feeding birds, hummingbirds have developed an extraordinary wing power—up to eighty beats per second—that allows them to hover near the flower to feed. They can fly up, down, forward, and backward like tiny helicopters. This exceptional mobility requires a high energy expenditure, which explains why hummingbirds consume nectar, which has a high sugar content and is a natural equivalent of high-octane fuel. Hummingbirds not only require this high-potency formula, they must feed frequently because their small size limits how much fuel they can store. Some hummingbirds need to feed every fifteen minutes.

Many of the Amazonian hummingbirds are neither threatened nor endangered, but a significant number of the Andean species are in serious trouble and some are probably already extinct. The colors of some hummingbirds are so breathtaking that their plumage was used to make hats, brooches, and belts. Literally millions of specimens were shipped to Europe during the nineteenth century to meet the demands of fashion. As a result, some species are known only from a few dried skins purchased from commercial dealers and have never been seen— and may never be seen again—in the wild.

The natural beauty lost due to the stupidity and greed of humans is best summed up in Robert Schomburgk's words describing a forest scene in Guyana:

Innumerable Humming-birds like scintillating meteors of many a color, again flit as quick as lightning from flower to flower and drink the nectar of the fragrant blossoms or sport with the dew-drops that, mirroring a world in themselves, are trembling on the leaves.

That night we stayed in another garden hut, and by the next day we had exhausted our meager provisions and hunger gnawed at our bellies. A few hours downriver we beached the canoe to look for game.

We trotted through the forest at a healthy clip until Shafee found signs of an agouti. Kamainja showed me the footprints and the half-devoured green *tonka* fruits the animal had left behind. We followed the trail, which bent back around toward the river. Turning into a small clearing created by a fallen fig tree, we saw the animal seated on its haunches, busily devouring a large reddish brown *walaba* fruit. Shafee raised the shotgun to his shoulder and fired; it appeared that the Indians were as accurate with shotguns as they were with bows and blowguns.

Kamainja went back to the canoe for the cooking pot while the Kaxuyana kneeled in the clearing and started skinning the animal. Related to the paca so beloved by the Maroons, the agouti is another member of the rodent family. Its fur is thick and reddish brown, and its body resembles a guinea pig with the head of a cat. Kamainja told me that agoutis incessantly bury fruit; like the squirrels of North America, they build up underground caches of food, storing Brazil nuts and palm fruits. This practice probably serves as an important seed dispersal mechanism as well.

Several hours later, after a filling if not overly tasty meal of boiled agouti—the creature was not the equal of the paca in flavor—we sat around a roaring fire listening to the croaking of the forest frogs. While the meat was cooking, Kamainja had assembled a temporary shelter of sticks lashed together with vines and then covered with the waxy green, ridged leaves of the *mu-ru-mu-ru* palm.

Shafee chose this tranquil moment to share some bad news: "I only brought one shotgun shell," he confessed. We were at least three days away from the mission and without food or any means to hunt it. Although I wasn't pleased by this lack of foresight, I decided to trust the resourcefulness of my companions and retired to my hammock.

The next morning found us out on the river again, still heading downstream away from the village. My companions seemed unperturbed by the lack of food and the absence of other people.

Since Indians are largely dependent on what they can find or kill for food, they are used to feeling hungry. By early afternoon, I was so hungry that I was getting dizzy. When I mentioned this to Kamainja, he steered the canoe over to the riverbank and disappeared into the forest, machete in hand. A few minutes later, he returned holding two *wapoe* palm hearts and what looked like two elongated orange lemons. The *wapoe* palm hearts were edible but not particularly appetizing, tasting something like asparagus that had been boiled for days. I devoured one and the Indians split the other. Then Kamainja offered me one of the orange fruits, telling me to peel it before I ate it. I did, and found that although it had large seeds and a dearth of edible pulp, the fruit was sweet. I asked Kamainja to show me where he got the fruit, and after looking carefully at the tree, I recognized it as a wild relative of chocolate.

Because Europeans first encountered chocolate at the court of Montezuma, botanists had long concluded that cacao was native to Central America. Yet according to Nikolay Vavilov, a Russian plant geneticist who died in Stalin's gulag, the center of origin of a cultivated species is most likely to be the area where most of the wild relatives of that species occur. Cacao's closest relatives are in the western Amazon. Many plants were domesticated by the Indians prior to 1492 and they were distributed throughout the Americas: corn, beans, and squash are just a few examples. Cacao may be another.

The paradox is that chocolate as we know it today is made from the seeds of the cacao plant, yet the Indians of the Amazon do not, as far as we know, use the seeds for any purpose. Perhaps cacao was planted from place to place for its sweet pulp. Only later did the Aztecs (or other Indians) find a use for the seeds. It was their genius that led us to a plant that scientists call *Theobroma cacao*, which translates as "chocolate—the food of the gods."

Later in the day, we found a narrow creek that emptied into the river from the east. Our canoe just fit into the creek, and we paddled upstream. As sunset approached, we pulled the canoe ashore and Kamainja built another temporary shelter. As I helped him hang the hammocks I noticed something strange: The Kaxuyana was cutting *wah-pu* palm fronds and using them to cover the canoe so that no one paddling down the stream would notice our presence.

Kamainja beckoned me into the forest with him to look for food. The results were discouraging; the best we could find were some half-rotten yellow *mo-pa* fruits—hog plums. Neither of us was feeling too finicky at this point, so Kamainja used his machete to slice away the moldy parts and we devoured the rest.

A terrific rainstorm hit the forest that night. Although the palm-thatched roof of our shelter proved watertight, we were awakened on two occasions by earsplitting thunderclaps, followed by lightning that lit up the entire forest. I was worried that the force of the storm might collapse our camp, but the lean-to held true and the steady tapping of the raindrops on the palm fronds eventually lulled me back to sleep.

The puddles of water that surrounded our lean-to in the morning were the only evidence of the previous night's storm. After washing up in the creek, I waited to see what would happen next. "*Mmpah!*" Kamainja said in his inimitable way. "Let's go!" Instead of taking the boat, however, we started off inland down a trail that for the most part was heavily overgrown. After several minutes, Shafee stopped and went back to camp. When he rejoined us, I asked what he had done.

"The storm blew the leaves off the canoe," he said. "I had to re-cover it so it could not be seen."

It all seemed a bit mysterious, especially when Kamainja told me to be as quiet as possible. "Don't even use your machete if you can avoid it," he cautioned.

The forest itself seemed unnaturally quiet. There was a remarkable lack of wildlife: no birds chirped in the trees, no monkeys chattered in the distance. I asked Kamainja the reason for this. His answer was typically terse: "Overhunting."

Several hours later, as we continued along the trail, we heard voices up ahead. As we came closer, I realized it was the sound of children at play. "Who is that?" I asked.

The Kaxuyana put his hand over my mouth and his finger to his lips, indicating that I should keep quiet. A bit farther on, we came to the end of the trail. From the cover of the trees, we could see a huge swath of deforested land. As we looked out at the naked expanse, Kamainja snickered. "*Pananakiri poy-deh-ken!*" he said slowly. "White man *dumb!*"

Shafee poked him in the ribs to shush him, but giggled as he did so.

"What's so funny?" I asked quietly.

"Look at that garden," Kamainja whispered. "I've seen better-looking agriculture inside a leafcutter ant's nest!"

To my untrained eye, the peasant garden did not look all that different from Indian agriculture. Once Kamainja stopped laughing, I asked him to explain.

"Look at that manioc! It is planted too far apart. You saw how we put ours close together; the leaves form a canopy like the forest's, which keeps the sun and rain from directly hitting the soil. And they have only one kind, whereas in our gardens we have more than twenty. That plantation is an invitation for the bugs to move in."

Kamainja was right. Since the manioc plants were all of one variety, insects that feed on that one variety might undergo a population explosion. I began to see what looked "primitive" to the two Indians.

"Look at the weeds!" Shafee chimed in.

"I don't see any," I said.

"Exactly! In our gardens, we always leave some behind because it binds the soil in the rainy season. That peasant's garden is probably cleaner than his house!"

"And another thing," said Kamainja. "You look at that plantation and you know the man doesn't understand the forest. A well-planned garden should look like a hole in the forest opened up when a giant *ku-mah-kah* tree falls over. Small openings in the forest are filled in by fast-growing weedy plants that attract game animals. When you cut down too much forest, the little plants can't seed in from the surrounding jungle and you don't have any birds or peccaries coming in that you can hunt."

"Besides," said Shafee, "this man put up fences at the edge of his garden. What a bad idea! Sometimes a peccary will come out of the forest to steal a green banana or a bite of manioc from my plantation. When that happens, my children eat peccary meat for a week!"

At the top of one of the blackened hillsides squatted a simple one-story wooden house with screenless windows and a small veranda. A clothesline draped with several old T-shirts and pairs of shorts spanned the veranda.

In front of the house, I could see several children—white children —and a sense of unease descended upon me as we stood there in the jungle looking out on the scene. When I had first seen the house and garden, my immediate thoughts were of food. Suddenly I wanted to be anywhere but here.

"Let's go!" I said.

"*You* go," said Kamainja.

"What do you mean, me? Let's *all* get out of here."

"Aren't you forgetting something?" he asked. "We don't have any shotgun shells. You're still hungry, aren't you?"

"What do want me to do? Sneak in the house and steal the shells?"

"Look, you speak Portuguese. Go and *ask* them!"

I pointed to Shafee. "He speaks it better than I do. Why don't you send him?"

"Because," said Kamainja, "*he's* an Indian. They'll *shoot* him. They won't shoot you."

I thought he was kidding, but the set of his face was serious. The Kaxuyana nodded in agreement. As if this weren't enough to convince me, Kamainja delivered the final argument.

"When we were on the savanna, I wanted to turn back but you didn't, so I continued. We are all hungry, but only you can get us some shells or maybe even a little food. I am asking you. *E-pah-wah-nah!*"

With this pronouncement, a smile spread slowly across his face. I turned, walked into the clearing, and headed toward the house.

As I approached the dwelling, one of the kids saw me and ran inside. It was time to announce myself. I halted. "*Boa tarde,*" I yelled. "Good afternoon." A man came out on the porch. He was five-foot-two and powerfully built, wearing faded blue cotton pants and a battered straw cowboy hat. I stopped and tried to give my friendliest smile. He just stared at me.

"*Boa tarde,*" I said again.

"*Boa tarde,*" he replied.

"I am an American biologist," I explained, my mind racing, "working at a museum in Belém studying Brazilian flowers. I was paddling up the river and my canoe hit a snag and I lost all my food. It's probably a two-day trip downriver where my friends are camped, so I was just wondering if I might buy some cassava or something to last me until I get back to camp."

"Come inside," he said.

I entered the house, which was little more than a simple shelter, lacking electricity and plumbing. A rough-hewn table and chairs furnished what passed for a kitchen. Hammocks were the only bedding visible.

He beckoned me into the kitchen, where a middle-aged woman I took to be his wife stirred a pot over a wood-fired stove. She turned and shook my hand, giving me the standard Portuguese greeting—"*Muito prazer*," or "A pleasure." Her husband told her my story and she gave me a pitying look, saying, "You poor thing! How long has it been since you had something to eat?"

"Uh, yesterday," I said, too hungry to be able to count the days.

She picked up a plate from a stack next to the stove, wiped it with her shirt, and ladled out a mound of beans and rice from the bubbling pot. When she sat it in front of me and turned to get a fork, I had to consciously refrain from grabbing a handful and cramming the food into my mouth. I thought guiltily about Kamainja and Shafee hiding at the edge of the clearing as I ate the hearty meal.

We made small talk about the weather and the mosquitoes, of which there were many. As I finished my meal with a steaming hot cup of jet-black, heavily sweetened Brazilian coffee, I asked how they came to be there.

The woman had been warm and hospitable from the outset, and as the man began to tell their story, he too dropped his defenses. "We are both from the state of Ceará in the northeast," he began. "It is the hottest and driest part of the country. My father was a *morador*, a poor farmer who grew cotton and manioc and collected the wax of the carnaúba palm, which he sold in the capital of Fortaleza. When he died, my brothers and I took over the farm, but it did not produce enough to feed all of us and our families. A few years after my first son was born, we heard about a program to assist the people of Ceará settle along the new highway they were building across the Amazon. Hospitals! Schools! Land! All this was promised when we first signed up. In the beginning, we enjoyed a better life. We had land and it produced more manioc than the soils of Ceará. The government told us that the schools and the hospitals would come soon but we had to be patient. 'You are pioneers,' said the president, speaking on the radio, 'helping to make Brazil a great country!'

"Well, we never did see the schools or the health care. We didn't like it, but we were better off there than on the farm. Until the third year, when our crops failed. Then we were desperate. One day a nicely dressed fellow showed up in a truck. He said he represented a big businessman in São Paulo and they had heard some people along the highway were having trouble. He told me that they wanted to buy half of my land and if I would just sign the contract, he would pay for it right then and there. Well, I don't read so well, but he told me exactly what it said and I signed. About a week later, the same truck showed up, but the nicely dressed fellow was gone. Instead, it was a *jagunca* —a band of thugs. They asked me why I was still on Senhor Coimbra's land. Didn't I know that I was supposed to be off it by now? I tried to argue, but two of them knocked me down and one started hitting me with a club. While I was on the ground, my wife came running out to see what was wrong and another thug grabbed her and said, 'The next time we come back, if you're still here, she comes with us.' With that, they left."

"What did you do from there?" I asked.

"We packed up everything we could carry and piled it by the roadside. We stopped the first truck big enough to carry our things and hitchhiked to town. From there we took a riverboat to the town of Oriximiná. There I heard about land upriver outside the grasp of the greedy land barons of the east. I pledged then and there that we would go upriver to this no-man's-land and claim it as our own. So here we are, *senhor.* Would you like another cup of coffee?"

Once again, as with the padre, I had been ready to dislike these people, to dismiss them as scheming trespassers on Indian land. Yet they were kindly and hospitable and, most touching of all, they were trying to eke out a better life on the barest terms possible.

The food had renewed and refreshed me and there was a warm, comfortable feeling in the little house. I wanted to learn more about them and their lives.

"Ever see any Indians around here?" I asked.

The man bristled and suddenly the air was electrified. "Indians! Indians! *Indians!*" My previously calm host had turned bright red and was screaming at the top of his lungs. "If I do, it will be too soon! Thieves! Animals! Those insects don't deserve the right to live! They kill my animals and eat my crops. The government is always talking about the poor Indians. What about the poor Brazilians? Those creatures aren't human. There is only one way to deal with them!" He held up his right hand and pulled the trigger on an imaginary pistol.

I was totally taken aback by his vehemence. Quickly changing the subject, I tried to get him to talk about his crops. We chatted a bit more, then I said I had to leave if I wanted to make camp before nightfall.

We stood up and shook hands. He smiled and said, "I thought you wanted to buy some food." Flustered, I'd forgotten that I didn't have any money with me. "I . . . I don't have any money! I lost it with my food."

He smiled and patted me on the shoulder. "Don't worry, amigo. We're not running a grocery. In this part of the world, white men have to stick together. I'll be right back."

With that he went out back. His wife gave me a large piece of cassava bread to take with me. "Don't pay any attention to Paulo's crazy talk. His brother was a gold miner on the Trombetas and he was killed by Sikiyana Indians. He gets really emotional sometimes."

Just then the man came back carrying two ripe pineapples and an enormous papaya. "Here," he said, handing them to me. "These should last you."

I was touched by their generosity. Among the poorest people on the continent, they were freely loading me up with provisions. I offered my watch in trade. He refused (not altogether convincingly), saying, "A gift is a gift." As I walked through his garden toward the jungle, he and his wife waved good-bye from the veranda. His seven children followed along behind me, a pied piper carrying pineapples, papaya, and cassava bread. When I got to the edge of the forest, I took off my watch and handed it to the oldest boy. "This is for your father. Tell him I said a gift is a gift."

We arrived back in Palu four days later. Kamainja and I spent one last night in the village, then strapped on our packs and once more hiked into the savanna.

As we slogged through the heat and the mud, I replayed many of my experiences in Palu, searching for meaning. I had indeed seen the savanna through the eyes of the Indians themselves, and it was apparent that they regarded it as more of a hunting ground and a highway between the forests than a rich repository of healing plants. That the Brazilian Tiriós had already lost much of their culture was not surprising given the presence of the Brazilian military, and hence the constant contact with the outside world; but seeing the Indians' lack of knowledge redoubled my determination to find ancient shamans who still remembered.

## CHAPTER 7

# Witch Doctor of the Wayanas

The [shaman] has power depending on his knowledge of the medicinal value of herbs . . . the importance of the shaman [is] that he deals both with body and with spirit, that he is both doctor and priest.

—Everard Im Thurn, 1883

● ● ● ● ● ● ● ● ● ● ● ● ● ● ● ●

It was August 1985 and I was back in Kwamala for a month to collect more plants. I had been in the village only a few days when Kamainja appeared at the door of my hut one evening literally shaking with fear. "It is not safe for you here at the edge of the village," he said. "Take down your hammock and sling it in my hut. The witch doctor of the Wayanas has put a curse on our village."

His alarm was contagious, and I quickly gathered up my belongings. Once I was safely in his hut, he told me what was happening.

"Last year," he began, "the son of the Jaguar Shaman went east to the Sipaliwini savannas to hunt parrots. One morning he woke up terrified, claiming that he had been cursed by the witch doctor of the Wayanas. The witch doctor lives in Tepoe, a village to the northeast, near the French Guiana border. As proof of the curse, the Jaguar Shaman's son showed us three small, pointed sticks he had found in his hammock."

"So what happened?" I asked.

"Three days later, he put a shotgun in his mouth and pulled the trigger. This evening his younger brother found the same types of sticks in his hammock, here in Kwamala. And tonight several hunters returning to the village saw an apparition of the Wayana at the edge of the river."

When I asked why the witch doctor would have cursed the young Indian, Kamainja could only speculate. "We believe that most disease is caused by evil spells sent by a rival shaman. Maybe the Wayana sent the curse because someone in his tribe was very ill and he thought the Jaguar Shaman had caused it." The village was in an uproar; the chief had said that only the most powerful black magic could break the deadly spell.

That night I hardly slept for thinking about the medicine man whose power had struck such fear in the hearts of my friends. I was torn between staying in the village to see what would happen next and heading east to Wayana country to meet the feared witch doctor. I had planned to research the Wayana tribe eventually, and the opportunity to work with such a potent shaman was enticing. Several days later my decision was made: when a bush pilot stopped in Kwamala to pick up a load of macaws, parakeets, and toucans to be sold as pets in the capital city, I paid him to take me to Tepoe.

The pilot headed due northeast for the Tapanahony River, which marks the boundary between the lands of the Tiriós and the Wayanas. We followed the brown ribbon of water until we saw canoes filled with Indians, then the thatched huts of the village. The little plane landed on a short, flat, grass-covered airstrip, about a hundred miles northeast of Kwamala.

I climbed out expecting to follow the routine established in Kwamala—find a hut, store my equipment, then meet with the chief. This whole process was short-circuited when an Indian who was about my age asked me in Surinamese why I had come.

I launched into an explanation of who I was, where I came from, and what I wanted. But I didn't mention the Tiriós and the curse.

"Oh, yeah, you're the guy Kamainja dragged across the savanna last summer—I heard about you. Look, my father is the chief. That's him over there." He pointed to a stout man with heavy-lidded eyes who, like the chief at the Brazilian village of Palu, wore Western-style clothes. The village was mixed—both Tiriós and Wayanas lived there—and the chief was a Tirió.

The young man went over to his father and spent a few minutes explaining things; I soon followed to answer any questions the chief might have. He looked at me for a brief moment, gave a disinterested wave of his arm, then turned and walked away. "He says it's okay," announced the son. A light rain began to fall as he showed me to the empty hut that was my new home.

"Anything else you need?" he asked as we finished hanging my hammock.

"Yes," I replied. "I'd like to meet the shaman of the Wayanas."

"Okay," he said, and then, abruptly, he was gone.

Several hours later the sun had set and the hut was lit by the soft glow of my kerosene lantern. The doorway filled with Indians who either just stared at me or peppered me with questions about my family, my country, and the Tirió village I had just left.

Suddenly there was a murmur from the back of the group and the crowd parted, revealing the single most frightening person I have ever seen. His long hair hung almost to his waist, and the color melted into the blackness of the jungle as he stood silhouetted in the doorway. An almost palpable, dark, pulsing energy flowed between him and the forest. His ebony eyes—deeply set and piercing—stared out of a thin, angular face. Although probably at least seventy, he carried his years with pride: he held his chin high and his muscled chest revealed him to be a master of the hunting bow.

This was the witch doctor of the Wayanas. In Kwamala, I wondered how a single man from a neighboring tribe could so terrify an entire village. Now I understood.

He was one of the last surviving heirs to a tradition born thousands of years ago in the wilds of Eurasia. In about 4000 B.C., the Aryan peoples occupying what is now southern Iran developed a cult based on ritual consumption of a hallucinogenic mushroom called the fly agaric. Those who ate the fly agaric believed it allowed them to journey to worlds inhabited by spirits. When descendants of these peoples invaded northern India two thousand years later, they carried their beliefs and customs with them. The mushroom cult flourished in its new home; the fly agaric and its mind-altering effects figure prominently in the sacred Hindu hymns known as the Rigveda, composed about 1350 B.C.

From India the cult swept eastward to the shores of the Pacific. In northeast Asia, it developed into a nature-spirit religion known as shamanism, with its own rites, traditions, and worldview. Adherents of shamanism believe that a continuum exists between the natural and the supernatural, and that the forces of the physical world and the spirit world exist in equilibrium. The shaman—a combination healer-priest —is at home in both worlds and is responsible for maintaining the balance between the two. Since even the weather is believed to be under the control of spirits, the very survival of a tribe or village depends on the shaman's prowess at communicating with the other world. The shaman is also the keeper of the tribe's traditions and lore, and as such offers guidance on proper spiritual conduct. But perhaps most important of all, the shaman is a powerful medicine man.

In the shamanic tradition, disease is thought to result from any number of causes, including the breaking of a taboo, the casting of a magic spell, the anger of the gods, or disharmony between the physical and spiritual worlds. Some illnesses have readily identifiable symptoms and traditional cures. But in cases that are serious or that resist treatment with plants alone, the shaman consults the spirit world to learn the origin of the disease and its cure.

Visiting the spirits typically involves entering a trance. In Eurasia the trance is induced by ingesting the fly agaric mushroom, while in Mexico the Huichol Indian healers eat peyote, a tiny, bulbous, hallucinogenic cactus. Still other shamans enter an ecstatic state by dancing, chanting magical words and phrases, or beating rhythmically on a drum. On such occasions, shamans may carry ritual objects such as rattles or mirrors and may wear symbolic clothing. In the Siberian tundra today, some healers wear a special parka with an iron chain sewn onto it so that helpers can pull the shaman back if he ventures too deeply into the spirit world.

While shamans invoke spirits and use sacred rituals to treat their patients, the process is not entirely magical. In addition to their broad and detailed knowledge of the healing properties of the local flora, shamans also employ such practices as relaxation and massage, hypnosis, visualization, and dietary prescriptions to treat their patients. Many of these therapies, including aromatherapy, massage, and stress management techniques, are now being "discovered" by Western health practitioners.

Throughout history, cults with a knowledge of powerful plants and potions have been frowned upon, first by proponents of Christianity and later by the Western medical establishment. Devastating events—from drought to floods to serious illnesses—were sometimes blamed on these cults to discredit them or to explain the inexplicable. The Black Death, for example, the epidemic of bubonic plague that swept through fourteenth-century Europe, was deemed by the church to be the fault of witches and Jews.

Witches were in many ways the shamans of medieval Europe; plants played a central role in their cults. In the opening scene of Shakespeare's *Macbeth*, the witches chant about a poisonous brew that blends "toe of frog" and "root of hemlock," among other ingredients. In fact, those two substances harbor compounds that are both toxic and hallucinogenic, which may explain how medieval witches were said to be able to "fly" through the air and have sex with demon lovers. Prior to their celebrations, or sabbats, the witches rubbed themselves with ointments that often included extracts of such alkaloid-rich plants as hemlock, aconite, belladonna, mandrake, and henbane, all of which are known to cause mental confusion, irregular heartbeat, delirium, and erotic dreams. According to one fifteenth-century account, "the witches confess that they anoint a staff and ride on it to the appointed place or anoint themselves under the arms and in other hairy places." Given the concentration of blood vessels and nerve endings in the vaginal region, the coated broomstick upon which they "rode" could have served as much as an applicator as a mode of transportation. It seems witches *did* experience flight, soaring across not the night sky but the hallucinatory landscapes of their minds.

These non-Christian practices represented a direct threat to the church. Western religion has often found it difficult to compete for new converts with belief systems that offer such vivid experiences and rituals. In nineteenth-century New Orleans, for example, the Catholic church was instrumental in banning the importation of slaves from Haiti when it learned that many local Catholics were converting to voodoo. Alternative religions, it seems—particularly those that have animistic and/or plant-based components—have been an anathema to Western religion for nearly two thousand years.

Witches soon became the victims of the church-backed Inquisition and were systematically put to death. This was just one manifestation of a Western tradition of intolerance of other belief systems. When Europeans first arrived in the New World, they accused the Indians of worshiping false idols and enslaved the natives. This amounted to direct attacks on shamans and shamanism, and the ancient religion was eradicated in many parts of lowland South America. According to one mid-sixteenth-century account, some of the Indians converted by the Jesuits in Brazil turned against members of their own tribes for clinging to the old ways:

> [One medicine man] claimed that he conversed with the sun, which established him as its son and as a god. He was brought back to the mission bound to a litter and gagged to stop him from preaching. The converts pulled him to the ground and started to kick him, pull him about, and puncture him with their arrows to such an extent that the Fathers had to intervene to save him. . . . Another sorcerer called Ieguacari, an old and twisted man, was forced to dance in front of the catechumens [converts]. The boys were frightened at first, but gradually lost their fear and finally came over and fell upon him, threw him to the ground, and mistreated him in every fashion. He ended by becoming the missionaries' cook.

The denigration of shamanism is by no means restricted to one area of the world. In Zimbabwe (then Rhodesia) shamanism was outlawed by the Witchcraft Regulations of 1895 and the Witchcraft Suppression Act of 1899. Guilty parties were subject to thirty-six lashes and/or seven years in prison. During the 1930s and 1940s in Siberia, the cradle of shamanism, medicine men were considered counterrevolutionaries. Government officials went so far as to compose poems celebrating the godlike qualities of Lenin and Stalin, which they distributed among tribespeople to convince them that communism's leaders were more powerful than their own. In Mexico, the conquistadors destroyed sacred temples and built churches on the same foundations, then melted down sacred gold and silver idols and turned them into coins and crucifixes. And throughout North America, American Indians, who have melded Christianity with their native beliefs, still struggle to be allowed to consume peyote, a traditional part of their religious rituals. The controversy over what is a sacrament in the eyes of the tribespeople prompted American anthropologist J. S. Slotkin to remark that "a white man walks into his church and talks about Jesus; the Indian walks into his tepee and talks to Jesus."

Even today the shaman's ways are ridiculed and belittled. In 1990 on the Indonesian island of Siberut, west of Sumatra, the Protestant church issued a declaration against the healers of that land. It states that the church

> considers the activities of the *Kerei* [medicine man] as heathen and blasphemous, and is determined to abolish the *Kerei* institution as soon as possible. It considers the *Kerei* activities as fraud at the expense of the people. The Protestant church forbids their church members to have anything to do with a *kerei*, and *kereis* are banned from the church.

But it is the American Indians who particularly seem to have had more than their share of suffering at the hands of the missionaries. In Venezuela, whole villages of Panare Indians were terrified into converting to Christianity when a Bible published in their language claimed that the Panare had crucified Jesus Christ and had better be prepared to suffer the consequences. Only by following the way of the one true God could they expect forgiveness. And in the Colombian Amazon, Protestant and Catholic clergymen set fire to holy longhouses and ornaments and exposed sacred musical instruments to the women and children of the tribe—a practice expressly forbidden by the tenets of the Indians' religion.

This is not to say that all missionaries are evil. Most have the best of intentions and the Indians sometimes benefit by their presence. Often, the missionaries bring Western medicines that are effective against imported diseases that ethnomedicines cannot cure. They usually teach the Indians how to read and write in the national language, which is essential for negotiating the legal rights of their traditional lands. And some, like the padre in Palu, teach the Indians a trade at which they can make a living in the outside world or ease the shock of initial contact with Western culture. But their major goal is still to "civilize" the Indians by supplanting their native beliefs with Christianity.

The "success" of our society in eradicating these cultures and their practices can be measured in the shrinkage of the range they once covered. When Columbus landed in the Bahamas five hundred years ago, shamans were busy practicing their sacred creed in bark long-houses on what is now Wall Street, in grass huts in what is now Hol-lywood, and in buffalo skin tepees on what is now Capitol Hill. To find medicine men still practicing their craft, I had to travel to one of the world's forgotten corners, all the while wondering how much time re-mained for these venerable old men and the wisdom they embodied.

I was lucky. The old Wayana was still at the height of his powers. (Like most Indians in this region, the Tepoe witch doctor has a secret name and it is taboo to use it; to do so is to wield power over him. Many Indians have "public" names that are used in everyday life, but the old Wayana did not.) I asked him to teach me about healing plants and he haughtily agreed. As I walked toward his thatched hut the morning after our meeting, I shivered with cold and anticipation.

The medicine man was waiting for me; without a word, he turned and headed toward the forest. The narrow trail wound through the jungle, twisting its way around giant, black-barked *batibati* trees and sharp-spined, low-growing *boegroe-maka* palms. The path was strewn with tiny starshaped purple flowers dropped by a liana that had woven itself into the canopy above. A squirrel cuckoo sitting on the liana cried *chee-kwah, chee-kwah,* and as I looked up, it scrambled from one branch to another with its peculiar rodentlike gait.

The old Wayana strode confidently in front of me. His back remained ramrod straight as his powerful legs kept up a rapid yet deliberate pace. I was admiring the noble figure he cut and congratulating myself on having tracked him down when I was hit by a troubling thought: we had been hiking nearly an hour and had yet to collect a single plant. I was puzzled, but decided to keep quiet and see what transpired. It was late afternoon when we passed a giant, moss-covered *Virola* tree growing at the edge of a stream; the tree looked vaguely familiar. A few minutes later, the path deposited us back in the village. The shaman gave me a halfhearted wave and ducked into his hut.

I headed down to the river for a swim and to consider my next move. Professor Schultes's dictum dominated my thinking: spend as much time as possible in the forest with the people. On the way back from the river, I stopped by the old man's hut and left word with his wife that I wished to return to the forest with her husband the next day. From there I would improvise.

The next morning was a virtual replay of the one before, and I knew the witch doctor had to be holding back. The Tirió shamans had found medicinal plants about every hundred feet along a trail, and it seemed impossible that the Wayana did not know as much as they did.

A little farther down the trail, I spotted a familiar purplish, low-growing herb with little red fruit, which the Tiriós used to treat fevers. "What about this one?" I asked, pointing it out. "Is it medicinal?"

The old man replied, "I have heard that it is."

"How is it used?"

He shrugged his shoulders. "I am not sure."

I repeated this experiment several times with other plants that I knew were valued as medicinal species by the Tiriós. The results were mixed: the old man either replied that he had heard the plants were good for something or that he didn't know anything about them. I wasn't getting anywhere, so I decided to try a stratagem developed by Schultes.

We walked for another hour in silence and then I stopped in front of a little green fern the Tiriós used to treat liver ailments. Plucking it from the ground, I examined it closely and said, "Grandfather, in my country we use this plant to treat ankle sprains." He did a double take as I carefully cleaned the fern and deposited it in my collecting bag. As we walked on I saw him look at me quizzically out of the corner of his eye. A bit farther down the path, I spotted a liana tangled around the trunk of a massive gray *Swartzia* tree. I recognized the vine as a species the Tiriós used to treat aching joints. "Grandfather," I said, "in my country we use this plant to treat cuts." Again he watched as I sliced off a section of the liana and dropped it in my collecting bag. We hiked on until we stood before a huge *bergibita* tree, its grayish brown bark characteristically pockmarked with small holes. *Bergibita* is used for a variety of medicinal purposes by both the Maroons and the Tiriós. I slashed off a piece of bark. "Grandfather," I said, "in my country we use this species to treat earache."

"Nonsense!" he thundered. "Everyone knows that tree is the cure for fever!"

"Earache!" I insisted.

"Fever!"

"Earache!"

"Fever!" His eyes glowed with anger. It was time to back down.

"Well, then," I asked politely, "what do you use for earache?"

"That liana, right over there. It's for earaches!"

He marched over to a giant fallen kapok tree and sliced off a section of a small yellow liana with a peculiar pentagonal stem. "This," he said, "is also good for when you are tired. You crush the leaves, soak them in cold water, and wash with the water. Soon you are refreshed. It is called *puh-nah-tah-wah*."

Then he sliced off a liana growing along the trunk of another large tree. "This one is *wah-kah-gah-mu*. If someone comes to me with a cold, I take the leaves and rub them over the chest."

From here he ventured off the trail to dig up a little green bamboo. "Good for when you don't feel so good," he began. "Soak the leaves in warm water and then wash with the water."

I struggled to keep up with the sudden torrent of words, grateful to Schultes for his stratagem. Its effectiveness is best explained by physiologist Jared Diamond, a professor of medicine at the University of California–Los Angeles, and the world's leading authority on the ornithology of New Guinea. Diamond claims that indigenous people will give little or no information about plants or animals if they sense that the questioner knows little about the subject. He tells the story of Ralph Bulmer, an anthropologist who devoted much of his life to the study of the Kalam tribe of New Guinea. After collecting detailed information on the ethnobiology of fourteen hundred species of plants and animals, Bulmer asked the Indians about the local rocks. The tribesmen insisted that they had only one word for all rocks. Diamond writes:

The next year, Bulmer returned to the Kalam area with a geologist friend whom he introduced to his Kalam informants. Within an hour, the geologist gave Bulmer a long list of words that the informants had volunteered for different rocks which they classified according to locality, hardness and use. At that point Bulmer exploded to his Kalam friends, "How could you lie to me? After all these years that I've been working with you! You kept insisting you didn't bother to classify rocks, and now you've embarrassed me in front of my friend." To which the Kalam replied, "When you asked us about birds and plants, we saw that you knew a lot about them, and that you could understand what we told you. When you began asking us about rocks, it was obvious you didn't know anything about them. Why should we waste our time telling you something you couldn't possibly understand?"

The Wayana taught me cures despite what he understood as my ignorance. He showed me a small liana that seemed to have gotten its start in the leaves of a wild pepper bush and then climbed up toward the canopy. "*Ku-nah-ne-mah*," he said. "You've got to get the whole plant and boil it in a closed pot. Then you let the steam escape under the hammock of the sick person. Good for 'electric eel disease.' "

During the course of my research I learned of treatments for many illnesses I never knew existed. The Wayanas suffer from "electric eel disease" (its symptoms, which resemble those of epilepsy, are similar to the effects of a shock by an electric eel); the Maroons are plagued by "cold-fat disease," the symptoms of which they could never seem to articulate; and the Tiriós claim to suffer from such a bizarre variety of venereal conditions, parasite ailments, and infectious diseases that I thought they were kidding me until I found that all the shamans had plants to treat them. Certain ailments seem to plague only certain cultures. For example, when some Mediterranean peoples eat broad beans, a popular food crop in China, they suffer from a condition known as favism, which causes fever, vomiting, and acute hemolytic anemia. In the case of many such diseases—and particularly psychosomatic ones —only the healers within a culture can successfully understand and treat the problem, another argument for preserving ethnomedicine.

The next species the Wayana found—a small bamboo that he called *wah-ru-mah*—underscored the importance of respecting indigenous ailments and healing practices. "Sometimes people in the forest come face-to-face with a jaguar," he explained. "Sometimes they are so frightened that I have to collect this plant and throw it in the fire. When they inhale the smoke, they begin to relax."

On the surface, it seems a Western researcher could safely ignore this find, since we have no use for a cure for people who have been frightened by jaguars. But Western medicine *does* need a better seda-

tive. Most of the sleeping pills currently on the market are either addictive or have troubling side effects: grogginess, weight gain, or nausea.
A willingness to listen to and record cures—no matter how outlandish
they may seem at first—might yield something far more important than
I could conceive of in the course of my fieldwork. Although nothing has
come yet of the *wah-ru-mah*, laboratory research is slated to begin soon.

By the time we had collected this last plant, the sunlight had begun
to fade inside the forest. Black-headed parrots began to roost for the
night and their harmonicalike notes laying claim to their territory
echoed through the trees. Although I hated to break the spell, I didn't
have a flashlight and suggested we return to the village. The shaman
shrugged, indicating his assent but implying that much remained to be
learned.

The next morning he gave me a personal wake-up call: He showed
up at my hut well before daybreak and declared it was time to get to
work. He was accompanied by an odd-looking fellow who I first took to
be a mestizo, a person of mixed Indian and white ancestry. The newcomer was about five feet tall and wore a faded orange Hawaiian print
shirt and an old pair of red gym shorts. He had parted his hair on the
left, which gave him a distinctly Caucasian appearance (most Indians
in the northeast Amazon part their hair in the middle), and slicked it
down with vast quantities of *tonka* seed oil. He told me his name, but
it was one of the few Indian names I could never remember or pronounce, so I took to calling him the first name that came to mind—
"Boss." He had a ready smile and a large paunch that added to his
general air of jocundity.

Boss explained that he was a Tirió who knew plants and that he
thought I might want some help. I felt I had begun to establish a relationship with the old medicine man and didn't want to lose it, but
Boss seemed to be there at the old man's invitation. Besides, I hadn't
had time to find someone who could climb trees to collect flowers in
the canopy. "Can you climb trees?" I asked.

"Better than an *ahdeme* monkey. Higher than a *mahkwe* monkey.
Faster than a *kwatta* monkey. Quicker than a—"

"Okay, okay," I said. "Mmpah."

The dynamic did change. The medicine man didn't talk as much, but
he continued to teach me about the plants. There was the *tut-pwa-muh*

fruit, boiled to form an ointment to treat genital rashes; the *o-ko-ne-de-kuh* tree, whose leaves are brewed into a tea and drunk for kidney problems; the *she-mah-ne* fern, crushed and rubbed on aching hands and feet; and the *ah-lah-wah-tah-wah-ku* herb, of which a cold-water infusion, light green in color, is drunk to expel belly worms.

Boss was as nimble as he had boasted. When the medicine man indicated that a giant forest tree with narrow buttresses and a furrowed trunk could be used to treat aches and pains, the Tirió started climbing before the words were out of the Wayana's mouth. He would rocket up most trees without even pausing to consider the best approach. If it was a particularly smooth tree, offering neither hand- nor toeholds, he would look around until he found a *pono* tree, a giant forest tree of the Brazil nut family with smooth brown bark and buttress roots. From this he would peel long strips of bark and tie them into a loop. He would insert a foot in either end of the loop and climb by pressing the bark loop down and against the tree trunk, creating a band of friction against which he could push himself up. When the old Wayana pointed out a truly mammoth fig tree as a source of a sap that was consumed to expel worms, I wondered what Boss would do. Its circumference was too big for a climber to wrap his arms around. The ever-resourceful Boss quickly scaled the tree next to it until he got high enough into the canopy—about a hundred feet—to break off several of the fig's flowering branches for my collection.

The plant data poured in as we trekked together for several days. There seemed no end to the ethnobotanical wisdom of the Wayana. Intriguingly, he often collected his own plants, ones he did not explain to me. Clearly he did not intend to share all of his potions and recipes with me.

The aloof Wayana obviously considered me a student or apprentice. He never asked me about my work. Boss, on the other hand, became a friend, and as I wrote my notes and impressions each evening, he would sit nearby and answer any questions or clarify any points I did not understand. It was he who explained to me the history of Tepoe.

"Here, we are at the eastern edge of the territory of the Tiriós and the western border of the land of the Wayanas. That is why both tribes live together in this village. Even though we overlap, each tribe has its own characteristics. In the old days, the Tiriós were known as the better warriors. The Tiriós are completely at home in forest and never were a river people. The Wayanas have always been good boatmen. We Tiriós are the best hunters; they are better fishermen.

"In the old days, the Wayanas lived mostly to the south, in Brazil. But they fought with a marauding tribe, the ferocious Wayapi, and when the Wayanas lost, they fled north across the Tumuc-Humac Mountains into Suriname and French Guiana.

"About twenty years ago, American missionaries working in Guyana came to the Tiriós in Suriname. My people were very sick with the white man's diseases and our medicine men could not cure us. The whites said that they brought the religion and the medicine of the one true God. We accepted both.

"The Wayanas accepted the white man's medicine, but not his religion. Most of the Wayanas live in French Guiana, where the national government has forbidden missionaries to practice. Many Wayana shamans moved across the Maroni River into French Guiana to avoid conflict with the missionaries. Now the missionaries have gone back to America. The Tirió shamans lost their powers because of the missionaries. That is why it is good for you to learn from a Wayana. They still live by the old ways."

"But there must be some old Tiriós in Tepoe who still know the plants," I said.

"Yes, there are several old ones who know the medicines. The most powerful is Mahshewah, who, they say, was once as strong as the old Wayana. Tomorrow I will take you to meet him. *Kokoropah!* Good night!"

The next morning the village pulsated with the sounds of music and laughter. "Come! Come quickly!" said Boss. "The Wayanas are leaving!"

As I looked out of my hut, a line of twenty young men slowly snaked by in a halting dance, taking two steps forward and one step backward. They wore the usual red breechcloths, but some wore belts made from the skins of small spotted cats—ocelot and margay. Long ropes of blue and orange beads had been wrapped many times around their necks to form thick necklaces, and small hand mirrors dangled from thin cotton cords around their necks. They all wore coronas made from the black, red, and yellow breast feathers of the toucan. Some had stuck white harpy eagle feathers under the coronas so that the feathers drooped down. More impressive, however, were the great headdresses that some of the Wayanas carried in their hands. These were over four feet high and made from a variety of spectacular bird feathers: white harpy eagle down topped with a layer of yellow parrot feathers, then green parrot feathers, then a layer of cobalt blue manikin feathers, and finally an explosion of scarlet macaw tail feathers. As the men danced down to the riverbank, they were accompanied by the trills of bamboo flutes played by some of the younger boys who were not making the journey.

I asked Boss if it was a special occasion for the village.

"There are not enough Wayana women in the village," he explained, "so these fellows are going upriver to attend a festival in another settlement. Everyone is wearing his finery to make the best possible impression. They are carrying their headdresses so as not to damage them before the big dance begins. It is not uncommon, especially in the smaller villages, to have too many men or women. In the old days, we used to go to war to capture more women," Boss mused. "We'd also fight to avenge the casting of an evil spell by a rival shaman."

Suddenly I had a troubling thought: if the Indians had fought over evil spells in the past, might my Tirió friends in Kwamala be getting ready to do battle against the old Wayana and this village? "Is there any warfare nowadays?" I asked casually.

"Not really," he said. "The Akuriyos to the east sometimes shoot people who wander into their territory, but that's not like warfare in the old days. Some say that shamans still cast evil spells, though, so you do have to be on your guard."

I started to ask about this, but he cut me off.

"Listen," he said, "the old man left early this morning to collect plants and he said he wanted to go alone. Tomorrow we can all go again, but today there is somebody you should meet."

"Who's that?"

"Remember, you wanted to know if any of the old Tirió *piais*, the witch doctors, were still around. Come on, I want to introduce you to Mahshewah, the shaman who hunted on his hands."

He led me through the village, past the timeless scenery. The women peeled and grated cassava while little girls cared for their infant siblings and little boys with small bows and arrows stalked lizards. At the edge of the village, on a bluff that rose above a bend in the river, sat a solitary figure in a wheelchair looking out over the water. One of the region's most powerful medicine men sitting in a rusty wheelchair: it is a sight that haunts me still.

As we approached, Boss quietly said, "*Tamo.* Grandfather," so as not to startle him. The old man turned the chair to face us. Silently he looked me over. As an act of respect, I kept my eyes on the ground and did not speak.

"Come closer," he said gently in Surinamese. His voice was soft but firm. He took my right hand and held it in both of his as he looked into my face. He wore a faded old cotton shirt and a red breechcloth. His arms and shoulders were huge, but his legs were shrunken and useless. As he turned his head to address my friend, I could see that the septum of his nose had been pierced, presumably to hold macaw feathers for ceremonial occasions.

"Tell him I want to know his name," said the old man to Boss.

"Why don't you ask him yourself, Grandfather? He speaks good Surinamese and terrible Tirió," said my friend, giving me a wink. The old man smiled and looked again at me.

"So, you like plants, I hear. Why do you come to my village and try and learn about plants from a *Wayana*?" Mahshewah asked.

I had to think fast. "Of course, Grandfather, I heard all about you from the Tiriós to the west. There your reputation precedes you. Uh . . . I spent many months there learning the Tirió plants. What I wanted to do, you see, was learn something from the Wayana and then compare it with your wisdom."

He nodded in agreement. "This was a good way to begin," he said, "but now I can help you."

"Leave us," he said to Boss, who immediately complied. The old man turned his chair to face the river again, and I sat beside him on the ground.

"Once I was the most feared man in the region," he began. "Everyone was terrified of my spells. All the plants and animals of the forest were mine to command and did my bidding. At night, I slept underwater and made love with the spirit of the river. Those days are gone. . . ."

We sat in silence for a bit, watching the river flow. Below, two women and a young girl climbed into a canoe and paddled upriver toward their garden. Their scrawny white dog stood proudly in the bow while a pet blue and yellow macaw squawked loudly in the stern. By now the sun had risen high overhead. The old man turned his chair around once more.

"Tomorrow evening," Mahshewah said, "I will come to your hut." Then he wheeled himself down the path to the village.

Once he was out of sight, I set off for the house of my friend to find out more about this extraordinary man. Boss was lying in his hammock carving wooden arrowheads with the blade of a small knife. "Tell me about him!" I implored.

"When I was a boy," Boss began, "he was the paramount *piai* of the Tiriós. Usually our medicine men and our chiefs were different, but so great was his reputation, he could have been both had he wanted to. I don't know whether he was born without the use of his legs or whether his lameness was caused by illness. What I do know is that he was already crippled as far back as I can remember. Some of the most vivid scenes of my childhood were of seeing him drag himself through the village, his bow and arrows clutched in his hand as he crawled into the forest to hunt. He not only fathered a family, he kept them fed, too, although his garden was cleared by his brothers.

"When the missionaries first came here in the mid-1960s, he was the person they most opposed. Several children of the tribe were suffering from diseases. He could not cure them, but the missionaries did. They said that they had both the religion and the medicine of the one true God. They brought him a wheelchair. Then one morning there was a big commotion down by the river. The old Tirió medicine man had wheeled himself down to the water's edge and said that the missionaries had convinced him to give up the old ways. He threw his magical charms into the river along with the *maraca*, the sacred rattle he used for healing ceremonies. The missionaries said this ensured that he would go to heaven and not burn in hell. The Wayanas, meanwhile, fled to French Guiana; they returned only after the missionaries had gone."

I thought of the old man, who had been talked into abandoning his long-held beliefs for the price of a wheelchair.

Boss spoke again. "He hasn't forgotten his plants; he just no longer uses them. There is much you can learn from that man."

———

As Boss had promised, the next day we resumed our work in the jungle. I hiked behind the old Wayana, wondering about the black magic attributed to him by the Kwamala Tiriós. Certainly a powerful, charismatic individual, his appearance was enough to give small children nightmares. But none of the plants he taught me seemed to have any magical applications. Was his reputation exaggerated, I wondered, or was he still holding out on me?

Our first find that day was a tall tree with a fragrant bark, vaguely reminiscent of cinnamon. The Wayana explained that a refreshing tea could be made from the dried leaves. I recognized the tree as a member of the *Lauraceae*, the cinnamon family, by the characteristic smell exuded by its essential oils. These same oils, widespread throughout this family of plants, were responsible for the abusive overharvesting of a species closely related to the tree we were examining.

One of the most sought-after fragrances from the plant kingdom is bois de rose oil, extracted from Amazonian rosewood. It is used to perfume a variety of high-quality creams, soaps, and lotions, and is a flavoring ingredient in candies, baked goods, and alcoholic beverages. The essential oil is extracted through steam distillation of the wood, which is most easily done by felling the tree. In Amazonian Brazil, from which most of the oil is exported, mobile stills are set up in the forest and workers fell every rosewood tree within a thirty-mile radius. Because no effort is made to replant, the tree is extinct over much of its former range. Although experiments indicate that the essential oils could be harvested from the rosewood's leaves and branches without damaging the tree, the harvesters have no plans to change their ravaging ways.

Our next find was a jungle giant known by the Wayana name of *ah-ku-de-tu-mah*. It is a wild species of chocolate from the same genus as the plant that gives us the cacao bean, used to make cocoa, chocolate, and cocoa butter. Boss quickly scaled the tree and dropped several branches to the ground; from their ends hung fragrant, yellowish green, slightly striated fruit that looked something like elongated lemons. The old man said the fruit was a favorite food of agoutis and noted that there was good hunting near these trees at the end of the rainy season. He peeled a piece of bark off one of the branches and a white resin oozed out; this exudate was painted on sores to accelerate healing, he explained.

The witch doctor observed that the tree's fruit was not considered particularly appetizing by the Wayanas. But Fusée Aublet, a French botanist who collected plants in neighboring French Guiana in the mid-eighteenth century, obviously felt differently about the wild chocolate's bounty.

The fruit, although milky, is good to eat. After peeling the skin, it is soaked in water; prepared in this manner, it has a pleasantly acidic taste and, because of its viscosity, it sticks to the teeth so much that the Creoles have named it "Quienbiendente" bastardizing the expression "Qui tient bien aux dents" ("which sticks well to the teeth"). They make jelly from both the peeled and unpeeled fruit. The jelly from the peeled fruit is a bit tart and refreshing, while that made from the unpeeled fruit is lightly purgative. It is prescribed here to cure dysentery.

Like the wild chocolate, the passion fruit liana is doubly nurturing, valued for both its edible fruit and its medicinal properties. The reddish fruit, which tastes a bit like key lime, is a favorite of the Indians, while the vine's sap is rubbed on the body to treat gonorrhea and taken internally to treat kidney stones. The name *passion fruit* stems not from any purported aphrodisiacal powers but from the plant's flower, which is said to symbolize certain aspects of the passion—the suffering—of Christ: the flower's fringed corona represents the crown of thorns; the style (its female reproductive parts) branch into three parts and symbolize the three nails; the five stamens (pollen-producing organs) stand for Christ's five wounds; and the length of time the flower blooms—three days—corresponds to the time between the crucifixion and the resurrection. I kept this religious iconography to myself, though, since the ancestors of my companions had undoubtedly been using this plant many thousands of years before Jesus Christ walked the earth.

Next we found a tall *wah-me-do* tree, a member of the myrtle tree family, growing along the riverbank. The old shaman claimed that a warm-water solution made from its tan-colored bark and washed over the body treats weakness, malaise, and lack of appetite. He offered me a taste of the small, reddish-purple fruit, but I found it a bit sour. Closely related species, I later learned, are much tastier: the jet-black fruit of the *jaboticaba* renders one of the most popular jams in Brazil. But perhaps the most extraordinary relative of *wah-me-do* is *camu-camu*. Most common in western Amazonia, this species produces a red fruit that is made into a tasty juice and a delicious ice cream in the Peruvian town of Iquitos. According to Dr. G. T. Prance, director of the Royal Botanical Gardens at Kew in London and one of the leading experts on Amazonian botany, the fruit contains thirty times more vitamin C than citrus. Preliminary analysis indicates that a forest stand rich in *camu-camu* is worth twice the amount to be gained from cutting down the forest and replacing it with cattle.

At one point on the trail, we entered a grove of the heavily spined *mu-ru-mu-ru* palms, a common understory species. Boss left the trail and searched the leaf litter for fallen fruit. He returned with only a handful of the small, roundish, brown fruit, then set about removing the tough outer casings. He gave me a *mu-ru-mu-ru* fruit to sample as he and the old Wayana devoured the remainder with obvious relish. It tasted insipid and I was puzzled as to why the two Indians regarded the *mu-ru-mu-ru* as such a delicacy.

Although the *mu-ru-mu-ru* palm is not particularly popular among other peoples, it has a close relative that is one of the Amazon's most promising species in terms of economic potential. The *tucúm* palm produces a tasty fruit that is a favorite of both Indians and peasants; it has the added advantage of containing three times the vitamin A of carrots. In the Brazilian town of Manaus, *tucúm* is made into a popular ice cream. More important in economic terms is the tree's fiber, one of the most durable known. Hammocks made of *tucúm* fiber are said to outlast those made from other natural fibers and synthetics, too.

I asked if fiber could be extracted from the *mu-ru-mu-ru* palm as well. Boss said no, but that fiber could be obtained from a different plant. But before I could ask any more questions, he and the Wayana were back on the trail and heading deeper into the forest.

About a half hour later, Boss located the fiber-yielding plant he had alluded to. It was a bromeliad, a relative of the common pineapple, and actually looked something like the top of a pineapple. Splitting a leaf, Boss showed me how to peel out the fibers inside.

In our technological society, we tend to overlook the importance of fibers for the survival of humankind, something impossible to do when living with tropical forest peoples. Without fiber, the Indians would have no clothes, bow strings, snares, fish nets, rope, baskets, backpacks, or hammocks. While plant fiber does not play the same central role in the industrialized world, it nevertheless is a mainstay in our daily lives. Although we can make clothing entirely from synthetic materials, most people prefer natural fibers, such as cotton. And despite all the talk about the "paperless office" promulgated by computer companies a few years ago, paper is still an indispensable part of our lives.

Other, little-known natural fibers figure surprisingly in American life. Abacá, also known as Manila hemp, looks very similar to the banana tree but produces an inedible fruit. However, the fiber extracted from the outer portion of the leaf stalks is flexible, durable, and resistant to both fresh and salt water. When it was introduced to the United States in the early 1800s, American sailors quickly realized its potential and wove it into marine ropes and cables. Abacá fiber quickly became a factor in the superiority of American sailing ships. Today this fiber continues to be used in the manufacture of marine cordage, fishing lines and nets, well-drilling cables, tea bags, and even dollar bills.

Our next stop was one of the strangest plants of all Amazonia: *Gnetum*, the Latin name for a vine that climbs in the branches of trees overhanging the river. It is a gymnosperm, a member of a group of mostly coniferous plants. Prior to the evolution of flowering plants, conifers like spruce and fir (along with ferns and cycads) probably dominated Amazonia. Today gymnosperms prosper only in temperate regions or at high elevations.

What fascinated me about this plant was not its intriguing paleobotanical history, but the Wayana healer's name for it: *kwe-i-ah-ku-wah-nu-puh*, which means "medicine man devil spirit." He used it to treat appetite loss, he said. For the first time, the old Wayana revealed that his knowledge or use of plants had something to do with belief in the supernatural.

I asked him to explain what the name meant, but he just glared at me and refused to answer. Out of the Wayana's earshot, I asked Boss the same question; he, too, remained tight-lipped.

That night the shaman, Boss, and I sat in my hut preparing to continue with the research. During our sojourns through the forest, I placed all plant collections in a giant cotton bag. In the evening, we would reconvene and I would empty the bag, recheck the medicine man's information, and then carefully arrange the botanical materials in a plant press before drying them over the cooking fire.

Curious villagers surrounded us as we looked over the day's booty prior to beginning the evening's work. Just as we were about to begin, the crowd parted and Mahshewah rolled his wheelchair into the hut. He and the Wayana did not look at each other, both revealing a streak of competitiveness and perhaps a certain amount of disdain.

"I have come," announced the old Tirió shaman, "to make sure you know how to use these plants correctly." Out of the corner of my eye, I saw the Wayana stiffen, as if his integrity had been impugned. My senses went on full alert: a powerful dissonance radiated from the two ancient wizards, who seemed as if they would hold nothing back if it meant that their rival would be made to look ignorant.

The Wayana picked up the first plant. "*Uh-pe* is the name of this one," he said. "It is used to make a wash to treat eye pain."

"Let me see that," said the Tirió. He looked it over carefully and then said, "In my language we know it as *weh-da-ka-la-ah-tuh-pe-lu*. A wash of the plant is good for fevers."

I was writing as fast as I could. The tension between the two men was palpable as the Wayana reached into the pile and pulled out a wild pepper bush with a light green flower cluster. "*Ko-no-lo-po-kan*," he said. "Very good for bleeding gums." He handed me the specimen and I attempted to pass it to the Tirió.

"I don't need to examine that one," Mahshewah said, dismissing it. "I'd know it anywhere. That's *no-lo-e-muh*, good for heart problems." He pointed into the pile of unsorted plants and said, "Hand me that one on top."

I gave him the one he had indicated, another species of wild pepper.

"This is also good for heart ailments. The entire plant is crushed and heated in a pot of water, which is then used as a wash."

Here the Wayana cut in. "I do not know either as a heart medicine. With this species, I treat black skin worm."

I picked up a branch with yellow fruit, which the Wayana called *pah-tu-ah*.

"What is the Tirió name for this one?" I asked.

Mahshewah replied, "In my language, it is called *kah-mah-ke*. I often used it to accelerate the healing of sores."

"How did you do it?" asked the Wayana, who was obviously surprised.

"The latex was painted on the sores."

"That is how I use it, too," said the Wayana. The two old witch doctors had found common ground and the tension began to recede a bit.

"What about that one?" a Tirió observer asked the Wayana, pointing to the wild chocolate. "Do you have a use for it?"

"I consider it a good treatment for swollen testicles. What do you do with it?" he asked Mahshewah.

"I always use it to treat ant stings. By rubbing the bark on the spot where you have been stung, you can stop the pain very quickly."

And so it went every night. Boss and I would come in from the forest with a load of plants chosen by the Wayana. Mahshewah would examine each one, telling me the Tirió name and whether a given species had a particular use. In many cases, the same species were used by both tribes; but more often than not, the use—or at least the part of the plant used—differed considerably. Sometimes, the Wayana would say that a particular species would be good for treating a certain illness and the Tirió would confess that he did not know this plant as good for treating that infirmity. But then he would give the Tirió name of another plant used to cure this malady and, with Boss's help, we would usually find it the next day. By following this approach, I recorded two to three times the amount of information I would normally glean from working with one shaman in the field. Those plants that had more than one application especially interested me. If a plant is used to treat a number of afflictions, it likely contains an active chemical compound and merits investigation in the laboratory.

Our trio crossed the river one morning to collect plants in a hilly area I hoped would harbor different species. The Wayanas had their gardens at the edge of the river and as we walked through them to get to the forest, I could see few differences from the plantations of the Tiriós. But in contrast to the gardens of the Brazilian colonists, the Indian plantations looked very sloppy. The manioc trees mingled haphazardly with papaya trees, while chile pepper bushes, sugarcane, and yams ran amok throughout the plot. The late botanist Edgar Anderson (whose most famous piece of writing was entitled "A Quiet Evening at Home with a Potato") wrote an insightful article analyzing a similar Indian garden in Guatemala. The plot was so wildly overgrown that he first believed it to be abandoned. Only after careful study did he realize the agricultural genius of the planting.

> In terms of our American and European equivalents the garden was a vegetable garden, an orchard, a medicinal plant garden, a rubbish heap, a compost heap, and a bee-yard. There was no problem of erosion though it was at the top of a steep slope; the soil surface was practically all covered and apparently would be during most of the year. Humidity would be kept up during the dry season and plants of the same sort were so isolated from one another by intervening vegetation that pests and diseases could not readily spread from plant to plant.

Like Charles Waterton a century earlier, Anderson reached a surprising conclusion:

> It is frequently said by Europeans and European Americans that time means nothing to an American Indian. This garden seemed to me a good example of how the Indian, when we look more than superficially into his activities, is budgeting his time more efficiently than we do. The garden was in continuous production but was taking only a little effort at any one time. . . . I suspect that if one were to make a careful study of such an American Indian garden, one would find it more productive than ours in terms of pounds of vegetables and fruit per man-hour per square foot of ground. Far from saying that time means nothing to an Indian, I would suggest that it means so much more to him that he does not wish to waste it in profitless effort as we do.

As we crossed the gardens, Boss pointed to a short herbaceous plant growing next to the charred remains of a fire-blackened tree stump.

"Look what we have here!" Walking over, I glanced at it and recognized it only as some species of legume. "What is it?" I asked.

He pulled the plant up by its roots and I had to laugh. It was a peanut bush! The nuts grow underground, so the plant is easy to overlook.

Although I had never seen them growing in the gardens of the Tiriós, peanuts originated in central South America, where they were domesticated by local Indians over three thousand years ago. Peanut remains have been found in pre-Columbian mummy bundles in Peru. Peanut motifs also occur on the pottery of the Mochica, a pre-Incan Peruvian culture best known for an extraordinary series of erotic ceramics. By 1492, the peanut had already spread north as far as Mexico. Although they apparently never attained the status of a major food crop in the northern reaches of their range, peanuts played an important role in the diet of the Indians of eastern Brazil. There the plant was discovered by the Portuguese; they in turn introduced it to West Africa, where it soon became a major crop. Because peanuts were inexpensive, not prone to spoilage, and nutritious (they have more protein than steak, more fat than cream, and more food energy than carbohydrates), these legumes were sometimes the sole source of nourishment for African slaves making the hellish voyage to the New World. The Bantu name for the peanut—*nguba*—was eventually Anglicized to "goober." Today it leaves traces of its world travel in many cuisines: the peanut is the base of the spicy satay sauce of Indonesian cuisine, the creamy peanut soup of west Africa, and the fiery Kung Pao dishes of Szechwan Province.

Although grown throughout the American South, peanuts were never highly regarded until hungry soldiers developed a taste for them during the campaigns of the Civil War. After the war, peanuts were sold by street vendors, at baseball games, and were peddled at the circus by P. T. Barnum. According to the botanical historian Frederick Rosengarten, peanuts were a popular snack in the less expensive sections of theater balconies, which became known as "peanut galleries."

The research of George Washington Carver (1864–1943) provided a boost to the peanut industry at a time when cotton production was falling prey to both soil exhaustion and the boll weevil. Peanut plantations enriched the exhausted soils and were not as prone to the depredations of pests. Carver developed over three hundred products from peanuts, including such diverse items as mayonnaise, shaving cream, and plastics.

The American peanut industry grew again after the Japanese captured Southeast Asia during the early years of World War II. Plantations in Asia had long provided the United States with natural rubber (from *Hevea* trees, native to the Amazon), quinine (from *Cinchona* trees, native to the Andes), and oils (from the coconut palm, native to the South Pacific). American farmers met the war shortage by expanding their peanut plantations, which provided both edible oil and glycerol for making explosives. Thus a plant domesticated by the South American Indians provided us with vital foodstuffs and ammunition during World War II.

Leaving the garden, we entered a zone of secondary vegetation where the forest had been disturbed during the clearing for agriculture. On either side of the path were several small trees, members of the St. Johnswort family, whose leaves were green on top but a vivid rusty brown underneath. With an efficient flick of the hunting knife he carried in his hand, the Wayana made a deep slice in the bark of one of these trees, a *wah-kah-pwe-mah*. After a brief wait, a thick yellow latex slowly oozed out of the cut. As it dripped down the bark, the sap was transformed from a pale yellow to an incandescent red.

The old shaman dabbed at the exudate and then rubbed it between his thumb and forefinger. "Very good for *oxi*," he said, a condition of white spots on the skin that seemed to be fungal in origin. I made special note of this, since deep fungal infections of the skin cannot be cured by Western medicine. Later that evening in the village, the old Tirió told me that his tribe used the same plant for the same purpose. This exudate, also collected by Professor Schultes in Colombia, is slated to soon undergo study in the laboratory of a California pharmaceutical company; according to preliminary test results, it may prove to be an effective antifungal treatment.

We collected enough plants to stock a drugstore: the leaves of the *nah-puh-de-ot* tree, good for foot cramps; the sap of the *tah-mo* liana, a treatment for earache; and the sap of the *kam-hi-det*, a cure for toothache. We found the huge *ku-tah-de* tree, whose bark was a good treatment for malaria; the sprawling *ah-kah-de-mah* liana, effective against coughs and colds; and the lithe *ah-tuh-ri-mah* vine, whose sap could be drunk to cure stomachaches. I considered my teacher to be a physician, a healer who could use the diversity of life around us to treat the ailments that afflicted humanity. But that recognized only one aspect of his abilities. The shaman stopped in front of a large, thick-stemmed liana and sliced it in half with a single chop. A clear liquid dripped out; he said it could be drunk. As I gathered a few drops in my palm to sample, he said, "If someone places a curse on you—the kind of spell that causes your belly to ache—then you wash with a cold-water infusion of the leaves."

Until then, every plant that we had collected was described as being used to treat a particular illness—and no causative agents had been discussed. Now, holding the liana section, the medicine man described a malady caused by evil spirits. Only the plant I had collected the previous week had a name that indicated a supernatural connection. I collected this new plant and waited for a chance to ask the Wayana more.

It was not long in coming. We crossed to the other side of the river to look for more plants. By late morning, we found a woody liana that the Wayana called *te-da-te-da*. "What is it for?" I asked.

"Well," he said, "when someone places a curse on you and it makes your stomach hurt, you must wash with the sap of the liana to get relief."

This ailment—and the remedy—sounded just like the one he had described earlier, so I tried to draw him out.

"In my country," I began, "we do not know any plants to treat this type of affliction. Our medicine men don't know how to cast an evil spell." Failing to take the bait, he walked on in silence.

"Do you know how to place a curse on someone far away?" I persisted, thinking of the Jaguar Shaman's son, who had found the sticks in his hammock and then committed suicide.

"Yes," he replied without stopping.

"How?" I asked, a bit frightened at my own forwardness.

The shaman slowed his pace, turned his head, and looked me full in the face, his eyes black with anger. "*Yolok*," he hissed, and he strode away.

"Don't keep this up," said Boss, almost bumping into me as he brought up the rear. "He won't talk about it and I don't want you to make him angry."

"But what did he mean? What is a *yolok?*"

"*Yolok* are the evil spirits of the Wayana shamans. *Yolok* is what they send to kill or sicken people who are far away. Let's not talk about this now; I don't like doing it while we're in the forest with him. When the time is right, I'll tell you what I know. Whatever you do, *don't* bring it up with him!"

We walked the rest of the way back to the village lost in our own thoughts.

One steamy afternoon, on the third week of my stay, I was coming back from a quick dip in the river when one of the Tiriós beckoned me into his hut. As I entered, he stealthily looked right and left as if to make sure no one saw me. Putting a finger to his lips to ensure my silence, he gave me a conspiratorial wink. Puzzled by the need for such secrecy, I looked around to see if I could solve the mystery. Tiptoeing, the Indian led me to the far side of the hut and pointed into a bowl fashioned from a palm spathe. As I looked in, he rubbed his stomach, rolled his eyes in gustatory delight, and said, "*Tupunyeh!*"—the most forceful way of saying "incredibly delicious" in the Tirió language. Unable to see what was so appetizing, I picked up the bowl and took it over to a crack in the wall where a shaft of sunlight shone through.

When the light illuminated the contents, I almost dropped the container. In it were a dozen or more palm grubs, three inches long, an inch thick, white, and slimy. They were still alive and writhed in the beam of light.

"*Tupunyeh!*" said my host as he reached into the pot and popped one of the squirming insects into his mouth. With closed eyes and a faraway smile on his lips, he swallowed his prize. Then he dumped the delicacies into a beat-up aluminum pot and put it directly on the cooking fire. As the pot began to hiss, he reached in and plucked out a juicy grub. To my horror, he held it up in front of my face, clearly intending for me to devour this tasty morsel. Suppressing the urge to gag, I mumbled something about having a terrible stomachache and walked as quickly as I could back toward the safety of my hut.

As I headed home, I recalled all I had read about palm grubs. The Indians propagate these creatures by felling palm trees and leaving them in the forest. A particular type of beetle lays its eggs in the decaying palm wood and the eggs hatch into the grubs so highly esteemed by the local people. Rich in both fat and protein, the grubs are said to taste like bacon. I realized then I had made a mistake. The successes that I had had in the course of my fieldwork had been due in no small part to my willingness to respect local beliefs and follow local customs— which included eating just about anything I was asked to try. Besides, I figured, the grubs were probably cooked by now and at least they wouldn't wiggle on the way down. Turning around, I returned to the hut of the worm chef.

When I arrived, the Indian was lying in his hammock with one hand behind his head and his other on top of his belly.

"Can I try one?" I asked.

The fellow gave me a sleepy smile. "*Awah*," he said, "*wakin.*" Nope, all gone.

"All gone?"

"*Tupunyeh!*" he said. "Delicious!" He rolled over and went to sleep.

While carrying a weighty bag of plants back to the village one day, I aggravated an old football injury in the triceps muscle above my left elbow. When the injury first occurred years earlier, I had visited a variety of physicians, who prescribed anti-inflammatory pills, heat therapy, ice therapy, ultrasound therapy, and even acupuncture, all for naught. One doctor shot my elbow full of cortisone, and my aching arm hung limp at my side for two days. Several treatments provided temporary relief, but usually within a week my elbow would start to ache again.

When my elbow problem flared up in Wayana country, my first inclination was to seek professional help. Of course, the only professional within hundreds of miles was the witch doctor himself. The morning after my elbow started hurting, he and Boss appeared at my hut as scheduled to begin the day's labors.

"Grandfather," I said, "I have injured myself and need some of your medicine."

He looked at me and raised his eyebrows as if he thought I was testing his powers. Turning to Boss, he said, "Tell him if he wants to be treated, he will have to pay."

I was a bit taken aback at this unabashed bit of capitalism. "How much?" I asked.

The old medicine man seemed surprised at my question.

"What?" he asked. "I don't know. Maybe some fishhooks. You don't pay until after I cure you."

After he had cured me? Here was a health care system with cost controls built in!

The old man asked for an explanation of the problem. After peppering me with a detailed set of questions, he examined my arm as skillfully as any orthopedic surgeon. Lifting my elbow away from my body, he watched the movement of the joint as I extended and bent my arm. Then he probed my elbow with his thumb as I flexed the joint. Finally he sat down, stroked his chin a few times, and said, "Today you will not work in the forest. I will go and collect the plants and prepare the curing ceremony."

With his usual abruptness, he left to gather his pharmacopoeia. Boss had a concerned look on his face. "Is this part of your investigation, or do you really have a problem? If you just want to know what the ceremony consists of, you could have asked me. It is not a good idea to have him consult the spirit world if you are making this up."

I assured him the problem was real and that I knew the old witch doctor was not a man to trifle with. Evidently satisfied, Boss left to do a little weeding in his garden.

The shaman returned in the late afternoon, his dark eyes glowing, as if anticipating the act of summoning his healing powers. In his left hand he carried a ball of cotton, freshly picked from someone's garden, coated with a mixture of aromatic plant oils. He rubbed this over the affected area and then massaged the oils in with his thumb. "What plants are you getting the oils from?" I asked.

He looked me in the eye, raised his eyebrows as if to say "Professional secret!" and maintained his silence. Tucking the cotton into the waistband of his breechcloth, he beckoned for me to follow. We walked for over an hour, out of the village, through the surrounding manioc plantations, and into the jungle itself. There we entered a small clearing in which he had built a simple shelter of *maripa* palm leaves. We both entered the lean-to and he indicated that I should lie down on the dirt floor.

I was getting a little nervous now. Since my trip to study the Maroons in late 1979, I had wanted to witness another healing ritual, and although I was anxious to participate in this centuries-old tradition, I couldn't help but remember the Wayana's reputation for casting evil spells. After all, I was still an outsider to him, and to compound matters, I had studied in the village that he had supposedly cursed. Even so, I argued with myself, this was what I had come to the jungle for—to experience life as the Indians did. Taking a deep breath, I stretched out on the floor.

Night was falling and the last shafts of sunlight filtered through the forest canopy and into the shelter. The shaman rolled a dry leaf of tobacco into a cylinder and placed it in a pipe made from the brown, woody, cylindrical fruit of the *po-no* tree, a relative of the Brazil nut. He then sprinkled several crushed herbs on top of the tobacco. Striking a match from a box I had given him earlier, he began to smoke the tobacco mixture as he sat down beside me. The musty smell of tobacco mixed with the sweet-smelling aromatic herbs filled the small shelter. With his right hand, he gently shut my eyes and then started to intone a series of chants in order to invoke the spirits (according to the explanation Boss later provided). A period of quiet then ensued as he awaited the arrival of the powers he had summoned. After a while, I heard one of the walls of the hut begin to shake violently as if something or someone were passing through it. Then the shaman moaned and began a dialogue between himself and a being that seemed to be speaking through him. This continued for what seemed like hours. I slowly drifted into a dreamlike trance, feeling as if I were sinking deeper and deeper into an enormous featherbed. Suddenly the wall shook again as if our visitor had departed. Silence enveloped us; then I heard the sound of a match being struck and the shaman relit his pipe. He gently took hold of my left wrist and raised my arm, then blew the magical smoke onto my elbow and massaged the area with his thumb. This was repeated three times and then he rubbed the area once more with the cotton swab.

The old medicine man began chanting again and I felt my body drifting farther downward, like a dry leaf caught in the autumn wind. Down I sank until I felt myself come to rest on a gentle bed of moss. Then I floated up to the top of the hut; from there, I looked down and saw the shaman blowing tobacco smoke over my prone body.

The shaman resumed his chanting and I felt myself drifting back down to the floor of the hut. The next thing I remember was him waking me gently by tapping me on the cheek with his fingers. He helped me to my feet; I felt a bit dazed and rather unsteady. The Wayana led me down the path toward the village by the light of a full moon, which gave the jungle an eerie iridescent silver glow.

"Wait here!" commanded the medicine man as he stepped off the path. In a moment he returned, his right fist in a ball. Slowly he uncurled his fingers to reveal three small, sharp, pointed sticks.

"Yolok peleu," he said. "The arrows of the evil spirits." He closed his fist and opened it again. There was nothing there. I was too frightened to ask any questions.

When I described my out-of-body experience to Boss the next day, he explained more about the curing ritual.

"The Wayanas believe that we all have a kind of spirit inside us that they call akawale—something like what the missionaries call a soul. The old Wayana said that you didn't have a hole in your akawale, which might have meant that someone had bewitched you, but that you had a weak spot in your 'spirit elbow.' The bad spirits that surround us every day were trying to get in. What he did was patch the weak spot in your akawale."

For me, the healing ceremony was a watershed event, second only to my dream of the jaguar three years earlier. As with the dream, I felt that I had been able to put aside my prejudices and predilections and enter the old Wayana's world. The ritual was not just about healing my elbow; it also allowed me a glimpse of a different reality, in which the shaman was at home and I was only allowed to visit. Yet I was a welcome visitor, I believe; the shaman proved that by showing me the arrows of the evil spirits—perhaps the same arrows that had appeared in the hammock of the Jaguar Shaman's son in Kwamala. Again I saw dark and light, good and evil, white and black magic integrated in a way that blurred the boundaries that had once seemed so clear.

The shaman's use of tobacco in my healing ceremony was very much in keeping with shamanistic traditions of other Indian tribes. Like so many of the plants first discovered and domesticated by South American Indians, tobacco's origins are little known by today's consumers of the plant. The modern history of tobacco began on November 5, 1492, when Spanish sailors Rodrigo de Jérez and Luis de Torres returned from a four-day exploration of the interior of Cuba to report to their captain, Christopher Columbus. They had witnessed a peculiar ritual practiced by the natives of the island. The Indians had rolled dried leaves into a cylinder, ignited them, and, according to these early accounts, commenced to variously "drinking," "swallowing," "chewing," or "sucking" the smoke. The verb "to smoke" did not yet exist in the Spanish language and the sailors were at a loss to describe the action.

The use of tobacco predated the arrival of the Europeans by thousands of years. When Europeans made first contact, almost every tribe in North America, Central America, South America, and the Caribbean employed tobacco in some form or another. The brown leaves were smoked, snuffed, licked, chewed, and even taken as an enema. Indians of South America and the West Indies smoked cigars. Peoples of Central America smoked cigarettes. In parts of Mexico and eastern North America, Indians smoked pipes.

The North American Indians' custom of smoking by passing a pipe from one person to another has its roots in botany. There are more than sixty species of the genus *Nicotiana*, but only two were ever cultivated by the Indians. In pre-Columbian times, tropical American Indians grew and smoked *Nicotiana tabacum*, the species that serves as the source of all commercial tobacco. The North American Indians cultivated *Nicotiana rustica*, which contains four times the amount of nicotine found in the other species. According to Professor Schultes, the high percentage of nicotine in the North American tobacco explains why the use of this plant was primarily ceremonial rather than recreational. So potent was a lungful of the North American tobacco that the pipe had to be passed from person to person in a group large enough to allow the smoker to recuperate between puffs.

Among South American Indians, tobacco was believed to have curative powers. As early as the mid-1500s, Europeans observed the use of tobacco in shamanistic healing. In 1565, Girolamo Benzoni, one of the first historians of the New World explorations, described such a ritual.

> In [Hispaniola] and the other islands, when their doctors wanted to cure a sick man, they went to the place where they were to administer the smoke, and when he was thoroughly intoxicated by it, the cure was mostly effected. On returning to his senses he told a thousand stories, of his having been at the council of the gods and other high visions.

Tobacco initially gained popularity in Europe as a medicine, where it was used as a remedy for everything from snakebite to malaria. It was chewed and snuffed in London for its supposed ability to ward off the Black Death.

As smoking rapidly became popular, the addictive nature of nicotine assured an ever-expanding market of consumers. To meet growing demand, the British shipped the *Nicotiana tabacum* plant to their Virginia colony, where it quickly became a leading cash crop. Ironically, this South American species was unknown in North America until the herb was introduced by Europeans.

With an increasing supply available, the use of tobacco continued to grow. Unaware of the harmful effects of tobacco, smokers waxed rhapsodic about it. Victor Bulwer-Lytton, Viscount Knebworth, wrote in the early twentieth century that tobacco "ripens the brain, it opens the heart, and the man who smokes thinks like a sage and acts like a samaritan."

Not all British royalty were as favorably impressed as the viscount, however. So great was British demand for tobacco that import costs threatened to exhaust Britain's silver supply. In 1604, King James I, determined to act on the silver problem, published the *Counterblaste to Tobacco*. In it he described smoking as:

> A custome loathsome to the eye, hateful to the nose, harmefull to the braine, dangerous to the lungs, and the blacke stinking fume thereof, neerst resembling the horrible Stigian smoke of the pit that is bottomless.

I don't know how important a role tobacco played in my treatment, but my elbow pain cleared up within a few days and did not return for another seven months. In return for my treatment, I paid the old Wayana two machetes and a file to keep them sharp. But when I asked him to explain the ritual and reveal which plants he used, he simply refused. Perhaps this was his way of telling me that no matter how much I studied, I could not begin to plumb the depths of his—or the jungle's—powers.

The next morning Boss appeared at my hut and told me that the old Wayana had gone hunting. My Tirió friend suggested that we head into the forest to look for game, since this was the time of year when the spider monkeys, who had been feeding on the abundant ripe fruit in the forest, were exceptionally fat. (He rubbed his stomach for emphasis.) Since spider monkeys were the favorite food of the Tiriós, it would have been impolite to refuse his offer.

Boss went home to get his bow and arrows and returned a few minutes later. As we set off for the forest, I reviewed my progress to date. Although I was pleased with all that I had learned from the medicine man, the old Wayana had let me know in his subtle way that there was much more information to be collected. I had a feeling, though, that the curing ceremony had been a climactic event: The treatment represented a vivid display of the witch doctor's abilities, botanical and otherwise, and he had tacitly admitted putting the curse on the Jaguar Shaman's son a year earlier by showing me the spirit arrows. Although I wanted to stay and continue my work with him, it was clear he would not divulge any information on my healing ritual or on the black arts. I also knew that a cargo plane was coming to collect birds and reptiles for market the next week. I decided it was time to move on.

Ethnobotanical studies are typically conducted during one long period of fieldwork. Generally, a graduate student goes into an Indian village and stays for a year, collects all the information that he or she can, and then returns home. When I originally arrived in Kwamala, I had been a curiosity and the healers were amused or curious enough to spend time teaching me. After several months, though, their interest began to flag. When I returned a year later, their enthusiasm had been recaptured; they showed me many new plants and fascinating applications, and added to my knowledge of familiar plants. As a Colombian colleague once told me, "If you are in my house for a week, you are a guest. Any longer and you become a pest." I decided to use the same approach with the Wayana: I would take my leave and plan to return the following year.

Boss proved to be a better tree climber than a hunter. We spent the whole day traipsing through *wah-pu* palm swamps without ever seeing or hearing any spider monkeys. By midafternoon, it was evident that we were going to have to turn around if we were going to make it back to the village before sunset. We took a short break before retracing our steps, and sat on a fallen branch of a fig tree next to a gurgling stream. From my pocket I pulled a handful of Brazil nuts that I had brought along for an afternoon snack. Boss deftly sliced off the shells with my machete and we ate in silence. Finally he asked, "How's your elbow?"

"Much better," I said. "It doesn't hurt at all."

"You shouldn't have any more problems with it. That old man knows his plants."

"How did he learn? Was his father a shaman?"

"I don't know; that was a little before my time," he said with a smile. "Although the Wayana shamans believe that everyone—even women—have the potential to be shamans and commune with the spirits, traditionally they preferred their sons as apprentices. The Wayanas say that we all have a sort of invisible blindfold over our eyes and this is what keeps us from seeing these other worlds. To become a shaman, one must learn to remove the blindfold."

"I've never seen a woman shaman. Are there any women apprentices to the medicine men of the village?"

Boss shook his head slowly and said, "My friend, haven't you learned anything during your time here? There are *no* apprentices, male or female!"

I had assumed that the old Tirió in the wheelchair had no apprentice; after all, he had made a public renunciation of his shamanistic practices. Thinking back to the Tiriós to the west, I realized none of those old healers had apprentices, either. And for someone as powerful and as skilled as the old Wayana to be without a student was a tragedy not only for his tribe—who, after decades of spurning Western missionaries and medicine, would become dependent on them—but for the human race.

In a conservation context, we stand at the edge of a precipice. We are scrambling to find ways to save the rain forest, yet thousands of years of accumulated human wisdom—the knowledge of how to use the forest, without destroying it, to benefit humankind—is going to vanish over that precipice within the next generation. Throughout the tropics species are disappearing, but the knowledge of how to use those species is disappearing at an even faster rate. Each time one of these medicine men (or women) dies, it is as if a library has gone up in flames.

Since Western medicine came to the Indians, young people have not been schooled in the old ways. The young do not learn and the old do not live forever. The Dutch botanist Lindemann noted this phenomenon among the coastal Arawaks in Suriname more than twenty-five years ago:

For the first trip four Arawaks were enlisted, and when we asked them who had the best knowledge of plants, three of them pointed without hesitation to the fourth and said: "He is much older than we are, he knows most." Why his being older should be a guarantee for a better knowledge of the flora was explained to me by one of the younger men. The children in the villages play all day until they are six years old, then they go to school and only after they have left school at about the age of twelve they start to learn the ancestral knowledge. As soon as they are obliged to earn a living for themselves, they have no time to assimilate the whole stock of knowledge of their parents. At the moment most of the younger Arawaks know only the more common trees and those plants that are in one way or another of use to them. [The older man] on the other hand appeared to know the names of a large number of trees and shrubs and also of some herbs, though like so many others, he confessed that his father knew a much larger number of them. In the Arawak tribe this decline proceeds fairly rapidly and they have lost several old handicrafts and are already losing their own language. In other tribes, however, the same trend is found.

This trend has taken hold throughout the tropics—indeed, just about anywhere in the world tribal people are found. Yet the medical profession, which has so much to gain through the study of these people and their plants, has not mobilized to take action.

There exists an unhealthy polarization in the Western world, in which the great majority believes that our medicine is the finest and most sophisticated anywhere and the sooner everyone adopts it, the better. The other group, admittedly much smaller, feels that our Western tradition causes more problems than it solves and that no good can come from synthetic medical compounds. Clearly, some sort of middle ground should be sought. Western medicine does *not* have all the answers— where is the cure for the common cold or for AIDS? By the same token, we cannot believe that the cures for all our ills lie in shamanistic practices. The fact is that no one system has all the answers, but a melding of the two might bring us closer to that goal. We need to learn from the medicine man ways to treat our incurable illnesses much as he needs to learn from our physicians how to treat introduced diseases like measles and whooping cough. The great problem is that our foolish belief in the total superiority of our technology, our culture, and our religion is destroying these other traditions faster than we can learn from them.

On one of my last nights in the village, I was up late pressing plants. Most of the Indians had retired to their huts and I was alone with the old Wayana, who seemed lost in thought.

"Grandfather," I asked, "does it bother you that the younger Indians do not learn the old ways? That you have no student to learn your plants? That your medicine is not given the respect it is due?"

The old man did not answer right away, and I wondered if he had even heard me, or if he found my question impertinent. Then he sighed deeply.

"It is true the youngsters do not want to learn. That is not my problem, but it will be theirs. One day the medicines that the missionaries send from the city will no longer arrive. The people here will come to me to relieve their pains, to protect their crops, to conquer the evil spirits that kill their children. But I will be gone and I will have taken my plants with me."

———

I spent the better part of the next twelve months in the United States plotting my return to Tepoe; I was obsessed with working with the old Wayana again and learning more about the Indians, their rituals, and their way of life. The medicine man constantly appeared in my dreams, silently beckoning me to return to the healing forest.

When I finally returned in June 1985, Boss was waiting for me at the edge of the airstrip. He enveloped me in a huge bear hug. *"Mati!"* I said. "Friend!" in Sranan Tongo.

*"Jako!"* he replied. "Brother!"

I was anxious to see the old man; I had heard from the Kwamala Tiriós that no one else had succumbed to his curse on the village and I wanted to ask him about it. But the old shaman was gone.

"Gone where?" I asked.

"Back to the forest, I guess."

No one knew exactly where he had gone or why. Perhaps he returned to live in the forest clearing where he collected his plants and practiced his most potent and secret medicine. Or perhaps he had gone to a more hidden place, a kind of elephant's graveyard, to await his own demise, knowing that the coming world holds no place for yesterday's beliefs and the powers that once dominated the earth.

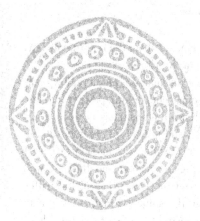

# CHAPTER 8
# The Semen of the Sun

Unlike the Colombian Indians, among whom the snuff is usually restricted to shamans, these tribes often take the drug in daily life. All male members of the group above the age of thirteen or fourteen may participate. The hallucinogen is often snuffed in frighteningly excessive amounts. —Richard Evans Schultes, 1979

● ● ● ● ● ● ● ● ● ● ● ● ● ● ● ● ●

When we entered the Yanomamo roundhouse, the exorcism was already in progress. At first it seemed as if pandemonium reigned. People yelled, cried, and ran about. Some chopped at the ground with machetes; others brandished axes, waving them in the air and screaming at the sky. The air was thick with the smoke of cooking fires and the scent of sweating bodies.

The roundhouse was a large circular dwelling about half the size of a football field. At its center, in an open area called the central plaza, the roof was cut away to reveal the sky; there a young Yanomamo Indian lay on the ground, naked except for a string around his waist. The man had been bewitched by a shaman from a neighboring village, we were told. A middle-aged man, whose torso was painted with black serpentine lines, ran feverishly back and forth swinging a machete and chanting at the top of his lungs; he was the local shaman working to rid the young Indian of the evil spirits that possessed him. On the sidelines, about ten women of the tribe, dressed in red cotton waistbands and black seed necklaces, watched the ritual in silence. All around the dwelling men sat in hammocks, watching the proceedings, carving arrowheads in silence, or exchanging comments about the unfortunate boy. Children played in the dirt, oblivious to the ritual taking place.

Periodically during the ceremony, a tribesman holding a hollow bamboo tube about a foot long sprinkled some reddish gray powder into one end of the tube, then blew it forcefully up the shaman's nose.

It was the first week of July 1987 and I had just arrived at the roundhouse, which sat on the banks of the upper Manaviche River. I was ready to spend some time studying the Yanomamo Indians, who live on the Brazil-Venezuela border, and the tribe's use of the hallucinogenic snuff called *epena*. To them, the snuff was nature's ultimate medicinal tool: it allowed them direct access to the spirit world, where all healing originates. This was a chance for me not only to study the plants that made up the magical snuff, but also to see shamanism in action once again, in a place where it was practiced more openly than among the other tribes I had studied. It was disconcerting, though, to show up in the middle of a curing ceremony of a tribe I had never visited. I asked my guide if I should wait outside until the procedure was over, but the ritual had reached such a fever pitch that he didn't hear my question. I put aside my doubts and watched the ritual.

The shaman stood over the sick man, waving his hands and shouting invocations to the heavens. Then he knelt next to the patient and appeared to seize the man by the throat. Looking closer, I saw that the healer never actually touched the patient, but made grasping motions as if he were pulling something out of the afflicted man's neck. The muscles in the shaman's back strained as he appeared to drag the evil spirits out of the bewitched Indian. He repeated this motion four times; then, with the mass of invisible evil heavy in his hands, the shaman gave a mighty roar, leaned back, and symbolically pitched his burden up and out of the roundhouse. Immediately the women rushed forward and gently flogged the patient with the stalks of a wild pepper plant to complete his cleansing. The shaman, exhausted by his labors, collapsed into his hammock.

With a population of about fifteen thousand, the Yanomamo are the last of the great South American lowland nations. Most forest-dwelling tribes, including the Tiriós and the Wayanas, seldom number over a thousand; more commonly, the tribes are only several hundred strong. Tribes living along the flood plain of such major rivers as the Amazon, with access to a large and steady supply of aquatic food resources, were more liable to grow into great nations. Most of these groups, including the Omagua of Peru and Brazil, were decimated by initial contacts with the first Europeans. The Yanomamo, who live in the remote recesses of the northern Amazon forest, were spared early contact with the outsiders and managed to survive.

But it was not only the tribe's inaccessibility that kept interlopers at bay. The Yanomamo are famous for their bellicose nature, a reputation detailed in a celebrated textbook published in 1968 by noted American anthropologist Napoleon Chagnon. Titled *Yanomamo, the Fierce People*, the book has become something of a cult classic and is widely used in introductory cultural anthropology courses in American universities. Chagnon wrote:

> The Yanomamo are still actively conducting warfare. It is in the nature of man to fight, according to one of their myths, because the blood of "Moon" spilled on this layer of the cosmos, causing men to become fierce. I describe the Yanomamo as "the fierce people" because that is the most accurate single phrase that describes them. That is how they conceive themselves to be, and that is how they would like others to think of them.

A debate rages in the anthropological community over whether this depiction of the Yanomamo is exaggerated and thus does them a disservice. In an intriguing paper on this question titled *Who's Fierce: The Yanomamo or Us?* American anthropologist Leslie Sponsel concludes it is not the Yanomamo.

Sponsel once explained to me that the brutality of the Yanomamo and the tales of their constant warfare have been blown out of proportion. I asked him about wife-beating, because many of the sources I read suggested that this was common among the Yanomamo.

"Well," he said, "many of the tales of abuse probably stem from rapes that happen after intervillage raids. Unfortunately, rape has often been a consequence of war, the world over."

The most disconcerting story of the tribe came from a Venezuelan physician I met briefly over a beer in Caracas; he had spent seven years among the Yanomamo. "I was working at a mission station in southern

Venezuela," he recounted. "A Yanomamo girl from a village near the mission fell in love with a Yanomamo boy from a faraway village who had visited her roundhouse during a festival. She wanted to leave with him and become his wife. Her father told her no and said that if she disobeyed she must never return because he regarded the people of that boy's village as his enemies. The girl left and married the boy, and shortly afterward war broke out between the villages.

"Several years later, word reached the girl that her mother was dying and had asked for her. Afraid and ambivalent, she finally decided to disregard her father's warning and return home. As a safety precaution, she asked if she could ride in our boat since we were heading there ourselves.

"As we pulled up at the beach near her village, she was hit by a hail of arrows. The Indians were such expert marksmen, not one arrow missed its mark. One of the missionaries tried to save her, but it was too late. The force of the arrows carried her out of the boat and she was dead before we could pull her out of the water."

These incidents paint a bleak picture indeed. But worth keeping in mind is that Yanomamo warfare is conducted by means of a raid, which generally involves surprising the intended victim in his garden or firing arrows at random into the top opening of a roundhouse until one—but usually not more than a few—of the enemy has been killed; ideally, the raiders then flee without being discovered. Thus the number of people killed in a battle is typically very low and often less arbitrarily selected than victims in modern technological war. In a Greek drama, a woman who ignored her father's warning would fare no better than the Yanomamo daughter the physician described. As Sponsel wrote in 1985, isolating aspects of Yanomamo aggression is roughly analogous to collecting newspaper clippings of gruesome crimes in a large U.S. city like New York and arranging them into a book entitled *New Yorkers: The Fierce People.*

I was fascinated by the tales of the tribe's warfare, but as an ethnobotanist, I was more interested in their plants. In Professor Schultes's class I had learned that the Indians of the northwest Amazon prepare and ingest a hallucinogenic snuff during annual religious ceremonies. Doing fieldwork among the Brazilian Yanomamo in the late 1960s, Schultes found that the Indians there snorted the snuff every day. According to Schultes, snuffing—which is the act of nasally inhaling a solid substance, as opposed to sniffing a smoke or vapor—was first practiced by the American Indian. It was not known in the Old World before the chronicles of the early conquistadors.

Amerindians are known to have taken hallucinogenic substances into the body in a number of ways, including orally and rectally, as enemas. The snuff method has an advantage over the others in that the nasal passages are full of capillaries that absorb the drug more rapidly into the bloodstream.

The earliest record of snuff in the New World comes out of the fifteen-hundred-year-old tomb of a medicine man in Andean Bolivia. According to an analysis of the tomb by Swedish ethnobotanist Henry Wassén in 1972, the healer was interred with what appeared to be a snuff made from the leaves of *guayusa*, a South American holly rich in caffeine. While the *guayusa* snuff was not hallucinogenic, presumably it was a powerful stimulant.

Schultes was able to record the ingredients of the Brazilian Yanomamo snuff during his work in the jungle, but the botanical components of the Venezuelan Yanomamo snuffs had never been fully documented. I had wanted to study the Venezuelan tribe since taking that first course with Schultes years earlier, but my work in Suriname collecting medicinal plants had taken precedence. Now much of my work there was done, and I wanted to see other areas of Amazonia and compare the lore of other tribes with what I had learned. In the back of my mind I hoped to contribute to research that Schultes had begun so many years ago; I wanted to know if the Yanomamo in Venezuela were using the same snuff made from the same plants as the tribe to the south. Here, I thought, was a place where Schultes's work and mine could complement each other. I packed my bags and headed for Venezuela.

I arrived in Caracas in June 1986. Through a series of inquiries, I learned that the best bush pilot in the country was a fellow named Boris Kapucinski. A Jew, Kapucinski had barely managed to survive in his native Yugoslavia when the Nazis overran that country in 1940. He did not fare much better under the regime that came to power after the war, and decided to flee to the West. As a world-class downhill skier, he was part of the Yugoslav national team in Helsinki for the 1952 Olympics. Kapucinski told me that when his turn came to race, he crossed the finish line and kept on going, disappearing into the Scandinavian crowd. He didn't stop, he said, until he reached Venezuela.

Living in Caracas, Kapucinski worked odd jobs until he had enough money to take flying lessons. Then he saved enough to buy a small plane and began making flights to the interior, building up a business ferrying supplies from the capital to little towns, mission stations, and oil exploration camps in the jungle.

By the time I knew him, Kapucinski had just turned sixty but was tall, lean, and as strong as a man half his age. Whether he was in the city or the jungle, he always wore a blue jumpsuit, which he described as "the official uniform of Kapucinski Airlines." He had been flying to Yanomamo country for thirty years.

Two days after I asked Kapucinski to take me to a Yanomamo village, we met at his hangar in a little domestic airport just outside the city limits. He checked the plane in excruciating detail: the fuel level, the oil level, the weight distribution of our equipment. After he was sure everything was in order, we stashed our belongings in a little storage compartment, climbed into the two-engine plane, and took off.

The sky was overcast, but through breaks in the clouds below us we could see savannas stretching in every direction. They soon gave way to rain forest, its verdant green expanse marred by areas that were being cut and burned for cattle pasture. This was something I had not seen in Suriname but that has become prevalent in most of Latin America. In Central and South America, a number of countries are experiencing rapid population growth, and the forests there are being cleared for timber, peasant gardens, pastures, and large-scale agricultural mono-cultures like bananas, coffee, or pineapples.

Through the wounded forest snaked the mighty Orinoco. One of the world's longest rivers, it is home to two-hundred-pound catfish and twenty-foot-long crocodiles. Presuming it to be the quickest route to the area's riches, such diverse explorers as Sir Walter Raleigh, the Spanish conquistadors, and Alexander von Humboldt followed it south into the depths of the jungle.

Once south of the river, the land begins to rise into forested foothills. Kapucinski observed that this was one of the least-explored regions of Venezuela and that a completely unknown Indian tribe had been found there less than a decade earlier.

"How could a group so close to the Orinoco be so isolated?" I asked.

"This tribe, the Hotis, never left the mountains to visit the Orinoco," he replied. "The conquistadors and the other explorers came up the river and totally bypassed this area."

I spied a village of thatched huts shaped like igloos.

"Are those the Hotis?" I asked excitedly.

"No," he replied. "They are Panare, a completely different tribe. The Panares are the sweetest, gentlest people on earth. You know, I think anthropologists study Indians so that they can learn about human origins, but all tribes are different. If you studied the Panare, you would say humans were originally a peaceful species, living in the Garden of Eden. If you studied the Yanomamo, you would reach the opposite conclusion."

We were now flying over undisturbed jungle. Directly in front of us rose the Lost World Mountains. These flat-topped sandstone formations are worshiped as the homes of the gods, much as Mount Olympus was revered by the ancient Greeks. According to Prussian explorer Robert Schomburgk, these mountains figure prominently in all of the creation legends of the surrounding tribes. As we flew over the formations, graced with beautiful names like Marahuaca and Huachamacari, we could see silver waterfalls plummeting into the deep green depths.

The pilot broke my reverie. "The airstrip we're headed for is on the south bank of the Orinoco," he said. "It was built by the missionaries."

"What kind of missionaries are they?" I asked.

"Oh, no missionaries are there now. The Yanomamo were too tough. The first missionary was an American, if I remember correctly. He decided that he was going to win the Indians over and put a stop to their intertribal warfare by trading Western goods for their bows and arrows. The Indians thought this was a marvelous arrangement. They traded their bows and arrows for machetes, mirrors, beads, knives, and radios. Then, as soon as the mission plane set off for Caracas, the Indians disappeared into the forest to find wood to make more bows and arrows. Eventually the Americans got discouraged and moved elsewhere."

Suddenly we found ourselves in the middle of a driving rainstorm. It pounded the windshield and tossed the little plane about as if it were a toy. The pilot said, "I hope this rain is just moving through the area. The landing strip is badly designed and gets very slippery when it is soaked."

Although I could make out little of the scene below us, Kapucinski lowered the wheels in preparation for landing. Slowly we descended and just as it seemed we would scrape the canopy, the plane touched down on a tiny airstrip. The runway was muddy and the brakes did little to slow the plane; we were closing in on the jungle wall at the far edge of the strip at an alarming speed. Kapucinski tried the brakes again and the plane fishtailed sharply to the right but began to gain some traction. We finally skidded to a stop near the edge of the runway. I climbed out of my seat and eyed the distance from the nose of the plane to the guava tree that marked the end of the airstrip: less than six feet.

The Indians quickly swarmed around us, shattering my illusion of the Yanomamo as primeval forest people. I was surrounded by Indians wearing filthy cast-offs: women in T-shirts that read ROLLER DISCO, boys in Puma gym shorts, even a man wearing an old dress. The Indians crowded around me, insisting in Spanish, "Give me salt! Give me a pot! Give me shotgun shells!"

Turning to Kapucinski, I said, "We're not staying here, are we?"

"No," he said. "I hate this damn place. Get your backpack out of the plane and load up. We will return in a week."

At that moment I was wishing he had explained the logistics—and that I had asked about them—before we left Caracas. I thought we would fly to a village and stay there for several weeks; instead we were going to leave the plane at the airstrip and backpack to the village the pilot had in mind. If I had known, I would have packed my things differently; as it was, I had an audience begging for each item I put into my pack.

Kapucinski seemed to know many of the Indians by name—at least by the "Christian" names given them by the missionaries. The Yanomamo have very strict name taboos, and as a show of respect and out of fear of breaking taboo, they do not refer to each other directly by name; instead, they use kinship designations called teknonyms: son of Xamaweh, or mother of Watorima, for example. One would never directly address Xamaweh by his name, but using his name to address his son is perfectly acceptable. And when a person dies, no one else may carry the name of the deceased; even to mention the dead person's name is a serious offense.

Kapucinski asked one young Indian called Pedro if he would accompany us on our trip and help carry our equipment.

"You must give me two flashlights, a shotgun, six shirts, and some salt. Then I will go," demanded Pedro.

"One flashlight, one shirt, and some salt," the pilot countered. "And you don't get it until we arrive at the village."

Pedro reluctantly agreed to Kapucinski's terms.

I finished packing, then sought shelter from the tropical sun under a wing of the plane. With all my belongings packed and out of sight, the Indians lost interest in me and focused on Kapucinski. I took this opportunity to get a good look at Pedro. He appeared to be a strange cross between a city boy and a forest Indian. His hair was cut in the typical Yanomamo tonsure, a bowl shape with the crown shaved completely bald. Both earlobes were pierced and the holes enormously stretched: in his right earlobe Pedro wore a 35mm film canister. He sported a black headband fashioned from the furry black tail of a brown-bearded *saki* monkey, an old blue tank-top shirt, and a worn pair of orange cotton shorts. Around his biceps were armbands made from the curly, ebony head feathers of the black curassow, a turkeylike forest bird. And in his mouth was a huge quid of rolled tobacco leaf, carried between his teeth and lower lip in typical Yanomamo fashion. Men, women, and children of the tribe all suck tobacco leaf, and according to Napoleon Chagnon and French anthropologist Jacques Lizot, the two leading experts on the Yanomamo, they are addicted to it. The Yanomamo word for poverty translates as "without tobacco," and Chagnon recounts that on several occasions he justified his reluctance to part with a machete or other possession because he was poor. In response, many of the Indians spit their tobacco into their hands and offered it to him.

Kapucinski had finished his preparations and we shouldered our backpacks. Pedro carried a pack full of supplies and led the way into the jungle. Pretty soon we were headed south on a trail through the peaceful forest and I could relax for the first time since we landed. Turning to Kapucinski, I said, "I hope all the Yanomamo are not like that." I spoke in English so as not to insult Pedro.

"No," he replied, "just there and maybe at some of the missions in northern Yanomamo territory. Actually, those fellows—the ones we just saw—have the worst of both worlds. They were introduced to our culture and became addicted to our material goods, and then they lost contact when the missionaries pulled out. It's bad enough when the missionaries give them guns and they hunt out all the game, but when the young ones can't get shotgun shells and didn't grow up using bows and arrows, it creates real problems. They've all been turned into beggars."

Soon Pedro turned around. "*Lluvia,*" he said. "Rain," and he pointed upward. We could hear nothing, but about ten minutes later there was the sound of distant thunder and rain pelted the canopy behind us. The storm we had flown through now overtook us, and we were drenched in a torrential downpour. There was no shelter to take refuge in, so we kept on going. Sheets of rain pounded us, but for me the thunderstorm was like a baptism: I felt cleansed. Once the rain ceased, the forest, too, seemed revitalized. Shafts of sunlight penetrated the thick fringe of leaves and bounced off the raindrops clinging to the foliage. The steady sound of dripping water provided an almost musical interlude. The forest floor exuded the smell of life.

The sandy-bottomed creeks of the jungle ran clear with sweet water. In what I later learned was Yanomamo style, Pedro stood in the shallow stream with his feet spread apart, leaned forward from the waist, and drank without getting his nose wet. After trying and failing miserably at this elegant maneuver, I settled for swigging water out of my canteen.

The streams were a vision, each like the focal point of a painting of an idyllic forest glade; the bridges, however, were a nightmare. On the surface, they looked quite impressive. Whereas the Tiriós simply fell a tree across a creek or a river to form a bridge, the Yanomamo not only fell a tree, they often engineer a railing by driving saplings into the riverbed every five to ten feet. The tops of these poles are then connected with a lengthy strip of vine as a handrail. The Yanomamo build their bridges during the dry season, but now it was the rainy season and all the rivers had risen. As we crossed the bridges carrying our full packs, the water sometimes came up to our chests. We gingerly picked our way along logs that were under three feet of water and were often slimy with algae. And although the current was slight, it made the footing all the more precarious. After the first crossing, I repacked all my belongings in order to keep my camera equipment and hammock above the waterline.

The trail was easy to follow and by the end of the day I had taken the lead. After climbing and descending a series of short, forested hills, I entered a small circular clearing that at first glance appeared to be an empty oasis in the forest. A voice speaking in soft tones off to my right broke the silence and, as my eyes adjusted to the growing darkness, I realized that we had arrived at a Yanomamo encampment. All around the edges of the clearing Yanomamo Indians lay in hammocks under temporary roofs woven from the large, flat leaves of the wild banana tree. So completely did they and their shelters blend into the forest background that the Indians seemed to be part of the landscape.

Although I must have been a strange and bedraggled sight, everyone remained tranquil. My companions were not too far behind and as Pedro entered the clearing, there were a few shouts of welcome.

"Tonight we stay here," he said, and pointed to an unoccupied shelter. Because the light was beginning to fade, I hung my hammock right away. A gaggle of little girls surrounded me. "*Nabe! Nabe!*" they yelled. "Foreigner! Foreigner!" and then burst into giggles. They looked like little forest nymphs: they wore red cotton bandoleers over each shoulder, which crossed at midchest. Their lustrous black hair was cut relatively short and the sides of their faces were painted with black serpentine lines. Wedged through a hole in each earlobe was a six-inch piece of yellow bamboo, and the front edge of the bamboo was decorated with bands of red and yellow toucan feathers. Most striking was that each girl's face had been pierced that so she could wear four wooden sticks: one through the nasal septum, two others in holes made at the corners of the mouth, and the fourth underneath the lower lip. It sounds painful and grotesque, but it looked exquisite.

Wanting to be as unobtrusive as possible, I climbed into my hammock and watched the action from there. The difference between these Yanomamo and the ones who had met us at the airstrip was like day and night. Among the new group, most of the men wore only strings around their waists under which they tucked the foreskin of the penis. Some of the younger men wore red breechcloths, a custom they had only recently adopted from other tribes, according to Kapucinski. Many of the men wore the same black armbands as Pedro, enhancing them by adding feathers of the emerald-green parrot or scarlet macaw. A few men, like the young girls, wore bamboo in their ears, decorating them not with toucan feathers, but with a single green and black parrot feather in either side. The women wore fringed red cotton belts around their waists and a band of cotton cloth across their chests, which they used as a sling to carry infants.

It felt wonderful to lie quietly in the encampment with the Yanomamo; I did not hassle them for ethnobotanical data, and they did not badger me for material goods, as the Indians at the airstrip had. Since I didn't speak their language, I wasn't even bombarded with the usual questions about where I came from and what I was doing there. If the Indians were curious about me, they asked Pedro for details. Soon two little girls came over, carrying what they indicated through a series of pantomime was my dinner. There was a large, creamy nut they called *kuwato*, which I recognized as the species the Tiriós know as *sho*, and a three-inch-long, greenish yellow palm fruit shaped like an acorn. The Yanomamo call this *rasha* and it is one of their agricultural staples. The little girls laughed when I tried to take a bite out of the fruit and indicated that I had to peel it first. Once I finally tasted the flesh, it was very appealing, something of a cross between a chestnut and a potato. Back in the States, I learned that *rasha* fruit contains carbohydrates, minerals, oil, protein, and vitamins in almost perfect proportions for the human diet. In cultivation, the tree produces more carbohydrates and protein per acre than corn. The Yanomamo not only eat the fruit as is, they boil it, dry it, and then grind it into flour.

The next morning, we prepared to go our separate ways. Many of the Indians were heading east to another village to attend a *reaho*, a funeral ceremony. After a Yanomamo dies, the body is either cremated in the roundhouse, which the Yanomamo call a *shabono*, or taken into the forest to decompose and then cremated there. The bones are believed to contain the essence of life, and the deceased cannot enter the afterworld if the bones have not been burned. Yanomamo women are known to threaten their children by saying, "If you don't behave, we won't burn you when you die." After the cremation, any fragments of bone are pulverized and the ashes are stored for a certain period of time. Then plantains are boiled into mush and the ashes are mixed in; during the *reaho* ceremony villagers and relatives from other *shabonos* drink the mush.

Pedro, Kapucinski, and I continued southward, hoping to reach before nightfall the roundhouse that the pilot had chosen as a waystation; the stop would mark the halfway point in our journey to the remote Yanomamo village he had in mind.

———

By the end of the day, we reached the village *shabono*. This circular edifice is shaped a bit like a circus tent: Its palm-thatched roof rises as if toward a peak but stops short, leaving a large opening in the roof that lets light shine onto a central plaza that serves as a village common. *Shabonos* vary in size; this one was about three hundred feet in diameter and was home to eight different families. Each family builds its own section of the roundhouse: the men do the heavy work, framing the structure with poles and lashing them together with vines, and the women and children collect the leaves that are woven together for the roof thatch. No walls separate the family groups. The *shabonos* last only a few years: either the roof begins to leak or, more commonly, the entire structure is abandoned or burned to destroy the cockroaches, scorpions, spiders, and other vermin that infest the roof.

We had to bend over and crawl through a small opening in the *shabono* wall in order to enter. When I asked Pedro why the entrance was so tiny, he smiled and said, "To keep enemies out." At night the Indians close the entrance and line the path to the *shabono* with leaves and brush so that strangers will be heard as they approach.

As was the case in the forest encampment, nobody seemed to notice our arrival and life went on in a leisurely fashion. Some of the Yanomamo were cooking, others were relaxing in their hammocks, and a troupe of naked little boys played in the central plaza.

We located an empty section of the *shabono* and set up our camp. I noticed that from the roof above the hammocks hung water gourds, baskets, tobacco leaves, green bananas, animal skulls, and an explosion of beautiful bird feathers. I climbed into my hammock to rest for a few minutes before getting something to eat, and fell sound asleep.

The next morning, I was awakened by a stocky, middle-aged Yanomamo man with a slight goatee, who stood directly over me and began speaking aggressively. His proximity, his nakedness, and his bulging lower lip stuffed with tobacco were intimidating. Before I could say I did not understand, Pedro rolled over in his hammock and translated: "He wants your machete."

When I hesitated, the man reached under my hammock and grabbed the machete. He then stood over me admiring his new tool. According to Pedro, he said "This is mine!" and smiled widely.

"Pedro," I said, "tell him he doesn't want it."

Pedro looked puzzled, but supplied the translation. The older fellow looked surprised and immediately responded.

Pedro said, "He wants it. It is his."

"Pedro," I continued, "tell him I cannot give it to him and he doesn't want it. Tell him a very old and powerful shaman gave it to me. The medicine man told me never to give it away. If I did, I would get sick, but the person I gave it to would die."

This, of course, was a complete lie, but the ruse worked. I knew from reading various studies of the tribe that some Yanomamo will use intimidation to get the Western tools and other goods they fancy. The fellow threw the machete back under my hammock and walked off, mumbling to himself.

I turned back to Kapucinski, ready to make plans for the day's research, when I saw that he was starting to pack up his belongings. "Why should we move?" I asked. "I'll bet these people know their plants."

"The chief at the other *shabono* is a friend of mine," the pilot replied. "That is where we are headed."

We left the roundhouse followed by a horde of boys and girls, darting in and out between us, holding our hands, and screaming, *"Nabe! Nabe!"* We soon reached the invisible line beyond which, for safety's sake, their parents would not allow them to go. They stopped and waved good-bye. I turned, waved, and said, *"Ciao!"*

Excellent mimics, they all started yelling *"Ciao! Nabe! Ciao!"*

We hiked through beautiful jungle studded with trees of enormous girth. From high in the canopy the cry of a red-billed toucan—*yo-yo-yo-yo*—echoed through the forest. About midday, two Yanomamo hunters came trotting down the trail toward us. They greeted us but did not break their stride. Shortly after that encounter, we paused next to a small river to eat. Kapucinski pulled a box of crackers and a jar of peanut butter out of his pack, but Pedro was more ambitious. Saying he would be right back, he followed the riverbank into the jungle. He soon returned with avocados and cashew "fruit."

What the Indians call cashew fruit, or *we-to*, is actually the swollen stem of the cashew tree. Unlike the cashew nut, which is toxic unless cleaned and roasted, the stems are edible right off the tree. These were unlike any other I had seen. Most Amazonian cashew fruit are bright red with a custard-yellow flesh, but these were red throughout. And where the other cashews were tasty but so mouth-puckeringly sour that you could not eat more than one or two, these were achingly sweet.

The avocados were about the size of tennis balls and tasted pretty much like commercial avocados. Avocados are native to the Neotropics, although there is some dispute as to whether they were first domesticated in Central or South America. The name *avocado* comes from the Aztec word for testicle, a reference to the shape of the fruit. It is one of the most nutritious fruits known, high in vitamins and protein and containing over 30 percent fat. Although they have been eaten in the United States since the late eighteenth century, the popularity of avocados is a relatively recent phenomenon. They are something of an acquired taste, and their thin skin makes them difficult to ship from the tropics without bruising the flesh. According to Dr. Beryl Simpson and Dr. Molly Ogorzaly in their 1986 textbook *Economic Botany*, at the turn of the century, horticulturists in the United States started paying serious attention to avocados and cultivated the fruit, developing the means to increase yields through grafting. Supply soon outstripped demand. In a textbook case of successful promotion, a marketing representative advised avocado growers to take out advertisements vehemently denying that avocados had any aphrodisiacal powers. Since then, demand has never flagged.

Pedro's find piqued my curiosity about the fruit trees around the area and, after we finished our snack, I asked him to show me the collection site. The avocado tree looked like avocado trees everywhere—about thirty feet high, with large, flat, dark green leaves and black bark. The cashew trees, on the other hand, were very distinctive, about the same height as the avocados, thus twice the size of any cashew tree I had previously encountered. Furthermore, the red coloration of the fruit was also unique. It did not appear that we were in a garden; the trees that surrounded us were huge. I asked Pedro, and he said we were in the forest, not a cultivated plot. But since the trees grew together in a group of at least thirty, I concluded that these trees had, in the distant past, been part of *someone's* garden, be they Yanomamo, pre-Yanomamo, or another group entirely.

Pedro and I hiked back to join Kapucinski, and then we all set out again, reaching the next *shabono* in early afternoon. Even before entering, we could hear the screams and wails heralding the exorcism that was being carried out inside. This was shamanism in all its raw power. Finally, I thought, a tribe untouched by Western culture and religion. Their plant knowledge and healing traditions would still be intact.

Once the ceremony had concluded, Pedro took us to the far end of the roundhouse to meet the chief. He struck me as young for a headman—probably no more than thirty-five. Although he spoke only a few words of Spanish, he welcomed us and told us where to settle in. The chief was missing his right eye, which Pedro explained he had lost in a *nabrushi* duel. The *nabrushi* are war clubs that resemble pool cues—they are thin and about eight to ten feet long, but heavy enough to pack a mighty wallop. Confrontations using war clubs take place frequently, between members of the same village and between villages; typically they involve disputes over women or the theft of food. Combatants try to hit each other on the top of the head, but when blows are flying, the warrior's aim is not always true. Most men have numerous battle scars on their crowns, which they proudly display by shaving away their hair.

The sky grew overcast as the sun began to set. Through a break in the canopy I could see blue-gray thunderheads drifting over us. The air thickened as the humidity intensified. We crawled into our hammocks and within a few minutes the only things visible in the *shabono* were the cooking fires that ringed the edge of the central plaza. Howler monkeys called briefly from the forest before settling down, and then the night belonged to the cacophony of sound unleashed by the jungle frogs. At the far end of the *shabono*, the village shaman suddenly let loose a wail that split the night; then his cry gave way to a simple but haunting chant. Just when it seemed as if the song would continue all night, a bolt of lightning creased the sky and a mighty rumble of thunder shook the *shabono* to its very foundation. A pounding downpour promptly ensued and the shaman ceased his lament, his apparent request for rain having been answered.

When I climbed out of my hammock the next morning, there was a screech and a swirl of feathers as my feet hit the ground. I had almost stepped on someone's pet *yebi*, an odd bird known by the common name of gray-winged trumpeter. This strange little black and white bird with gray wings looks something like a hunchbacked chicken. According to Pedro, the Yanomamo value them as pets because they kill snakes and because they cry out if they hear someone approach the *shabono* at night.

The *yebi* is an example of what biologists refer to as "incipient domestication." The process of domestication involves selecting and then breeding wild forms of plants and animals to produce a variety that meets specific human needs. Although a wild plant may produce an edible fruit, through generations of selection we may develop a variety with a much larger and/or more nutritious fruit. Amazonian Indians typically keep a variety of pets (usually birds or monkeys) captured in the wild. The distinction between previously wild pets and incipient domesticates lies in whether the captured animal produces offspring that can then be raised by people, eliminating the need to continue capturing wild ones. The pet birds of the Yanomamo may seem of little relevance to citizens of industrialized nations until we realize that the common chicken is a direct descendant of the red jungle fowl, domesticated by prehistoric tribes from the jungles of southeast Asia.

The sun rose slowly over the *shabono,* and its inhabitants began to stir. The women stoked the cooking fires and the men began to apply their body paint. To the Yanomamo, the body is a canvas to be painted afresh each day. The Indians drew blue circles, black dots, and red spots in every possible combination. One of the younger men mixed the blue genipa fruit with a handful of ashes and charcoal and painted his entire neck and face solid black, a fearsome sight.

Once the women had completed their preliminary chores, they, too, mixed their paints, and their designs and colors were no less spectacular. Even the children painted themselves or were adorned by others. So striking were the Yanomamo in their bold jungle finery that I thought our Western cosmetics industry could learn a thing or two.

Kapucinski left the roundhouse with soap in hand, in search of a watering hole. Pedro, meanwhile, showed me around the *shabono*. The Indians were friendly, outgoing, and curious, particularly the women, who, unlike the Tirió and Wayana women, were extremely forward and fired off a barrage of questions about my country, my family, and my home. I found it ironic that, although their place in Yanomamo society is one of complete subservience to the males, the women were not afraid to confront a stranger. The tone of male superiority is set early, with little boys being indulged by their parents and encouraged to become *waiteri*—a type of proud fierceness much admired within the tribe. Boys are not punished for peppering their sisters or parents with blows when they are angry. And while the boys spend their days playing warrior with their tiny bows and arrows, girls are pressed into performing useful tasks for their mothers, cooking, hauling water, helping to gather firewood, and minding younger children. By the age of ten, childhood is essentially over for a Yanomamo girl, and once she reaches puberty, she is ready to marry and maintain a home of her own. The girl usually has little say in choosing a husband; that decision is left to her father or brothers, who sometimes arrange her marriage before the girl reaches puberty.

Unlike the other tribes with whom I had lived, the Yanomamo made little use of benches, preferring to use their hammocks both as beds and as chairs. Most Amazonian Indians make their hammocks from either cotton or palm fiber, but the Yanomamo are unique: Although they can make cotton hammocks, they prefer to use the fiber of a liana. According to Pedro, the women will cut a six-foot length of a particular liana, dry it over a fire, and then pound it at the center of its length until the component fibers can be separated out and used to weave the hammock.

I admired the ingenuity required to create a bed from a single vine. Then my attention was caught by the shaman and another tribesman, seated around a huge banana leaf at the far end of the *shabono*. The shaman had dumped a small pile of reddish gray powder on the leaf. The other Indian held in his hands a hollow, yellow, foot-long tube made from the stem of a relative of the arrowroot and capped with a tiny hollowed-out nut from the *Attalea* palm. After blowing sharply on the tube to clear it, he handed the tube to the shaman, who filled the bowl with the powder—the legendary hallucinogenic snuff they call *epena*. The Indian placed the nut in one of his nostrils; then the medicine man fastened his lips around the other end of the tube and blew with such force that the other man's head snapped back. The shaman then reloaded the pipe and blew snuff into the other nostril.

A third man, his shoulders gaily decorated by bands of green parrot feathers, joined the pair. The shaman reloaded the pipe and handed it to the newcomer, who gave him two blasts of snuff. The medicine man let out a brief scream and then he and the first man rocked back and forth on their haunches, cradling their heads in their hands as if in agony.

I whispered to Pedro, "Why do the Indians take *epena* if it hurts so badly?"

With a slight sneer, Pedro replied, "The white man takes his whiskey, feels great, and then feels terrible. The Yanomamo takes *epena*, feels terrible, then feels great. Who is smarter?"

Soon the two men stopped rubbing their heads and the ceremony continued. The third man filled the tube and handed it to the shaman who blew the contents up the newcomer's nose and then gave another dose to the first man. This round-robin was repeated several more times and then the shaman slowly stood up and began to sing, his voice ranging from high quavers to low growls. He roared like an old jaguar and then began to slowly dance backward and forward with great dignity.

"What is he saying?" I whispered to Pedro.

"The shaman is summoning his *hekura*, the little men of the jungle. The shaman calls to them and asks them to come and live in his breast to help him cure and make magic. That is why he takes *epena*."

Here shamanism thrived in all its undiluted glory, and the snuff of a jungle plant was the catalyst. I was bursting with questions: What plants did they use? How did they make the *epena?* What was it like? And could I participate?

Before leaving the States, Schultes had given me one of his journals to read, which included an account of his taking *epena* with the Yanomamo in Brazil:

The dose was snuffed at five o'clock. Within fifteen minutes a drawing sensation in the forehead gave way to a strong and constant headache. Within a half hour, the feet and hands were numb and sensitivity in the fingertips had disappeared: Walking was possible with difficulty, as with beri-beri. I felt nauseated until eight o'clock and experienced lassitude and uneasiness. Shortly after eight, I lay down in my hammock, overcome with drowsiness, which, however, seemed to be accompanied by a muscular excitation except in the hands and feet. At about nine thirty, I fell into a fitful sleep which continued, with frequent awakenings, until morning. The strong headache lasted until noon. A profuse sweating and what was probably a slight fever persisted through the night. The pupils were strongly dilated during the first few hours of intoxication. No visual hallucinations nor colour sensations were experienced.

The Yanomamo snuff that Schultes sampled was prepared from the red sap of a tree of the nutmeg family. The Tukano Indians of the Colombian Amazon call this snuff *viho*. According to their tribal legends, the Tukano first received *viho* from the Sun's daughter, who obtained it through incest with her father. To the Tukano, *viho* is the semen of the Sun.

As I watched the snuff ceremony, I wondered whether the *viho* of the Tukano was the *epena* of the Yanomamo. Schultes's description of his experience taking the snuff did not lead me to conclude that it would be a pleasant experience, nor an illuminating one. Furthermore, he had told me that he had taken less than a quarter of the dosage used by the Indians. He had always prescribed participatory science, but somehow this moment just did not feel right for me to try to join the *epena* ceremony. I was still very much a stranger to these people and felt it was not yet time to participate in their rituals.

While I pondered the best method for learning about the botanical components of the *epena* snuff, Pedro pointed to the other side of the *shabono*. "Look over there!" he said.

An old man had stoked a cooking fire and it was burning brightly. He then chopped a banana leaf in half with his machete and quickly rolled it into a cone to make a funnel. He was obviously beginning to prepare some sort of potion—*epena*, I hoped. Pedro and I walked over to where the old man was working, totally engrossed in his project. After rolling the leaf into a cone, he tied a piece of a plant fiber around the midsection so that it would keep its shape, and fastened the leaf cone to one of the *shabono*'s supporting poles so that it hung one foot above the ground. He placed a small gray clay pot under the leaf cone and then put another clay pot directly on the cooking fire. Picking up his machete and a two-foot piece of liana, he began scraping the bark into the pot on the fire.

"*Epena?*" I asked.

The old man shook his head and said, "*Mamukure.*"

"What's that?" I asked Pedro.

"*Veneno*," he said. "Curare."

So much of science is serendipity. You search and search for one thing and as soon as you start looking for something else, you find the object of your original quest.

The water came to a boil and the old man added crushed leaves of several species of wild pepper. After the broth had bubbled for a while, the old man picked up the cooking pot using two sticks as a pot holder and poured the contents into the leaf-cone funnel. A dark blue-black mixture dripped into the pot under the funnel; cooked down, it thickened into a sticky paste into which arrow points would be dipped.

The addition of the wild pepper leaves excited me more than anything else about the old man's concoction. I had seen the same practice among the Tiriós more than five hundred miles to the east; another ethnobotanist had recorded the same phenomenon by the Wayapi Indians of French Guiana; and Edward Bancroft had observed similar practices among the Akawaio tribe of British Guiana in 1775. Once again I saw a pattern, not merely of different tribes using the same plant for *similar* purposes; it was different tribes using the same plants for exactly the same purpose. Whereas other biologists, such as the brothers Schomburgk, had dismissed curare admixtures as mainly superstition, I believed they were mistaken—even though I could not find any literature that supported my hypothesis that the admixtures can intensify or alter the curare's effects. It was not until several years later that I learned the answer from Dr. Norman Farnsworth, a leading plant chemist. He told me that recent laboratory research in India had revealed that injections of pepper extracts into the bloodstream increase bioavailability—or the ability of the blood to absorb foreign substances. Using wild pepper as a curare admixture would hasten the absorption of the curare's poisonous alkaloids into the bloodstream, amplifying its toxicity. Once again, the Indians proved to be better chemists than we are.

Kapucinski came over to say it was time for us to move on. We quickly packed our things and started out on a trail heading east, through the gardens of the Yanomamo, to the forest. Banana trees, *rasha* palms, papayas, and cashews—all common in Amerindian agriculture —vied for space in the gardens, but something was missing, and it took me a minute to figure it out. There was no manioc, *the* staple crop of most Amazonian tribes. I stopped to take a closer look and noticed that bananas dominated the Yanomamos' gardens, six or seven different varieties—large, small, green, red, and yellow among them. This was curious because bananas originated in the Asian tropics and were not brought to the Americas until the sixteenth century. What did this indicate about the origins of the Yanomamo tribe? Napoleon Chagnon, in his book *Yanomamo, the Fierce People*, states that the Indians once cultivated manioc but gave it up for bananas. In this regard, the Yanomamo are quite distinct from most Amazonian tribes.

Even their blood differs from the blood of nearby tribes. Mongoloid peoples (including Amerindians) have a compound known as the "Diego factor" in their blood. Of the major tribes whose blood has been tested, only the Yanomamo lack this protein. On the basis of this, scientists have put forth a number of theories about the Yanomamo. Some conclude that the Yanomamo may be the direct descendants of the first people to cross the Bering Strait, whereas all other Indians have descended from peoples who made the crossing at a later date. Others believe that the tribe somehow remained isolated from other Indian tribes during the migration. Still other scientists believe that the lack of the Diego factor is a mutation that cannot be explained by migration patterns.

In my studies with the shamans, I ask and re-ask questions. Often two people will give two different potential uses for a plant; sometimes the same person will give two different uses for a plant if asked on two separate occasions. It can be a mistake to start asking questions too soon, so I had made a special effort up to this point to refrain from asking Pedro about everything I wished to know.

Asking about "powerful" plants, species used by a variety of tribes throughout the Amazon, is a useful strategy. You sound less like the novice you would appear to be if you started out by saying, "Tell me about every medicinal plant you know and how you use it."

Shortly after leaving the garden, we passed a thirty-foot-tall *kumu* palm, one of the more common Amazonian species. The Maroons had showed me how to use the sap to stanch blood from deep cuts, the

Creoles had mentioned that consuming the fruit reduced hypertension, the Tiriós had made a refreshing and nutritious drink from the fruit, and I had heard that tribes in Colombia believed the oil to be an effective cure for tuberculosis. "What do you call this one?" I asked Pedro.

"*Sharabe*," he replied.

"How do you use it?"

"We eat the fruit."

"In my country, we use it as a medicine."

"We don't," he replied.

As we walked on, two Yanomamo women came down the trail toward us. Each carried on her back a large basket, colored a deep brownish red and decorated with large black circles. A wide strap that was looped around the mouth of the basket and over the forehead of each woman supported the load of firewood to feed the ever-hungry cooking fires. As in almost all Amerindian tribes, Yanomamo women spend several hours each day hunting for firewood, sometimes traveling several miles outside the village to collect it. The women smiled but did not stop.

A little while later, I recognized an ant tree like the one that I had first seen while working with the Maroons. "Do you know this one?" I asked Pedro.

"Yes. That's *kanahyeh*. Be careful of the ants!"

"Don't worry," I said. "I already made that mistake. Do you use it for anything?"

"Like what?"

"Well," I said, "some people to the east take a tea of the bark for stomachaches. Others use it for headaches. To the west, a tribe called the Makunas use it to cure aching muscles. What about the Yanomamo?"

"No, it is not a medicine," he replied.

"Do you think the old men might have a use for it that you are not familiar with?"

"I don't think so," he said. "My uncle was a famous *shapori*—a shaman—and I used to watch him cure people. He never used this tree."

My next find was a *goebaja* tree, one of the most common denizens of the Amazon forest. *Goebaja* stands about eighty feet high and has a distinctive cylindrical bole. The uppermost part of the tree, blending into the canopy above, was hung with bright violet flowers.

"What do the Yanomamo call this one?" I asked Pedro.

"The name is *shetebahre*," he said.

"What do you use it for? Is it a medicine?"

"Let me think," he said. "I once hunted with a Makiritare who said his tribe put the leaves in the cooking fire to repel mosquitoes. The Yanomamo don't use it as a medicine, though."

I found this extraordinary. Almost everyone in the Amazon—white settlers, Creoles, Maroons, Indians—has a medicinal use for *goebaja*. The Brazilians employ it as a treatment for syphilis; both the Creoles and the Maroons believe it effective against leishmaniasis, a dreaded Amazonian parasite; and numerous Indian tribes use it as treatment for coughs and colds. Yet the Yanomamo did not consider this species medicinal!

The ramifications of this intrigued me. Ethnobotanists generally assume that all Amazonian tribes use a wide variety of plants for medicinal purposes, yet a recent study of the Waorani Indians of Ecuador reached a very different conclusion. In some ways they parallel the Yanomamo: famous for their bellicosity, many Waorani remained uncontacted until fairly recently. When scientists finally studied them in 1984, they found that the Waorani knew little of curative plants, leading the researchers to conclude that they represented the state of Indian pharmaceutical knowledge prior to 1492. The scientists theorized that it was only after the arrival of the Europeans with their new, lethal diseases that the native Americans began to experiment with the healing properties of local vegetation.

I disagree with this conclusion. It seems to me that the tribes who lack an ethnopharmaceutical tradition (such as the Yanomamo or the Lacandon Maya of southern Mexico) rely heavily on shamanistic contact with the spirit world for healing purposes, and they use *epena* as the bridge between worlds.

Kapucinski spoke up. "We don't have far to go now. It's just over the next bridge."

"What's so special about this *shabono?*" I asked. "Why did you select it?"

"Several years ago, when the mission was still open near the airstrip," he said, "I had just landed with a plane full of supplies for the missionaries. Several Yanomamo walked up, half carrying, half dragging a woman who looked as if she had not long to live. She was the wife of the headman, who was one of the bearers. The padre and the nuns examined her and found that she had a bad case of malaria, and hepatitis as well. They did not have all of the medicines necessary to treat her and asked me to fly her and one of the nuns to the hospital in the town of Puerto Ayacucho. When I brought her back several weeks later, the chief told me that I was always welcome in his *shabono.* I have been there several times over the years and it is far enough away both from the mission and the airstrip not to be contaminated by Western culture. That is why, when you said you wanted to find a place that wasn't too 'civilized,' I decided to bring you here."

By now we had reached the bridge. Several Yanomamo children saw our approach and began yelling *"Nabe! Nabe!"* A few, obviously frightened, turned and ran into the *shabono* for protection. I took this as a positive sign, indicating that few foreigners had reached this place.

Pedro asked for the headman but was told that he had gone hunting. A small elderly man climbed out of his hammock and smiled a greeting. Kapucinski explained that he was the shaman. The Indian unbuttoned the front of my shirt, patted the hair on my chest, and said *"Basho, basho,"* which I thought meant "Welcome, welcome." Later I learned it meant "Spider monkey, spider monkey!"

Taking me by the hand, the shaman led me to his part of the *shabono.* Looking into the rafters, I saw his bow and arrows, which were quite a bit longer than the five-foot-tall medicine man. A bamboo tube held curare-dipped arrow points for the next hunting excursion. Then I saw a snuffing tube. *"Mokohiro,"* I said, calling the tube by its Yanomamo name. The shaman reached into the rafters, pulled the tube down, and offered it for my examination.

*"Epena,"* I said, demonstrating that I knew some words in his language. He smiled and nodded his head in agreement. The medicine man was probably seventy but looked as if he could have been more than a hundred years old. He had a slightly receding hairline—unusual for an Indian—and an ancient face brightened by a perpetual smile. He wore only a penis string around his waist, and the unadorned sticks

that protruded from holes in his earlobes gave him a slightly ominous appearance.

We sat down at the edge of the central plaza. He pointed the *mokohiro* at my nose and made motions as if he were blowing snuff up my nostrils. I smiled and pantomimed receiving it. He said something to one of the men standing behind us, who then reached up for a little bag hanging from the rafters. Suddenly things were happening a bit faster than I had planned.

"*Yopo!*" said Kapucinski, calling the snuff powder by its Spanish name. The man passed the bag to the shaman, who then dumped the reddish gray powder onto a banana leaf that had been placed on the ground between us. "Now you've done it!" chided Kapucinski, who looked as uncomfortable as I felt.

I tried to tell the shaman that I would like to try the snuff but not until tomorrow, but he spoke no Spanish. He just smiled and began loading the pipe. I looked desperately for Pedro to translate my message, but he had melted into a crowd of Indians at the far end of the *shabono*. When I turned back to the shaman, he was pointing the tube at me. With equal parts anxiety, excitement, fear, and anticipation, I placed the tube's bowl in my right nostril. The shaman held the other end between his lips and blew, starting off slowly and finishing with a mighty blast.

The force of the blast blew me backward from my squatting position. Immediately a warm sensation flooded me—my nostril, my sinus, my head, my limbs were all aflame. I picked myself up and the pain began to register.

The crown of my head started to throb as if I'd been hit with a war club. My vision blurred and I was overcome by dizziness; I struggled to breathe as both my throat and nose filled with a mucuslike discharge.

In the midst of my discomfort and confusion, I looked over and saw the shaman refilling the tube. He pointed it at me again and gently eased the palm nut at the end of the tube into my left nostril. My first inclination was to refuse, but before I could gather my wits to speak, the shaman let go another powerful blast.

The force seemed to propel the drug from the shaman's tube directly into my bloodstream and then into my very soul. Although my heart pounded painfully in my chest, a subtle sense of exhilaration accompanied the pain that wracked my body. At the edge of my field of vision, tiny figures began to appear.

My nose started to run, but my vision cleared a bit. I saw Indians in other parts of the *shabono* point at me and break into enormous grins. Some of them stopped what they were doing—chatting to each other in their hammocks, carving arrow points for the hunt, making their own batch of snuff—and sat in a circle with me at the center.

I felt a warm bond of brotherhood with them. As the snuff coursed through my body, the Indians spoke in their native language, which I now seemed to understand. One of them patted me on the back as another stroked my arm. Overwhelmed by this sense of belonging, I pointed to the *epena* on the banana leaf in front of me. "More," I said to the shaman, although it sounded as if it were someone else's voice speaking.

The shaman loaded the pipe and blew the *epena* into my right nostril, refilled, and blew it into my left. I sensed he was giving me subnormal doses and blowing the snuff much more gently than the Indians did among themselves. Even so, I was beginning to hallucinate.

"More," I said. I wanted the full experience.

By now my senses had been severely altered. My hearing was especially acute; I felt as if I could hear everything in the *shabono*. My field of vision had been greatly expanded: it was as if I were looking at the world through a wide-angle lens. At the edge of my field of vision, the little figures began to dance.

The shaman raised the snuff tube again, and I took several more blasts, each larger and harder than the one before. The final blast knocked me backward again and I lay flat on my back. My throat was burning; the top of my head felt as if it would explode; I cradled my head in my hands.

Another old shaman sitting next to me saw my distress and began massaging one of my arms. A warm, relaxed feeling flowed through me, and I let go of my head as the pain abated. He placed his hand on my scalp and began to squeeze, ever so slightly. Almost immediately the pain was gone, and the effects of the snuff rolled through my body like a wave—from my head down to my feet and back again. A great peace seemed to settle over me, my friends, the *shabono*, the surrounding jungle. The dirt floor of the *shabono*, swarming with ants, lice, and other vermin, now felt as comfortable beneath me as a bearskin rug. I was extremely relaxed, yet remarkably alert. My head and my heart seemed to be pulled in two directions at once—I was struck by the futility of the hatred, injustice, jealousy, and warfare that ran rampant in the world, yet at the same time I was filled with a sense of my own power and invulnerability, and a desire to be *waiteri*—fierce and brave in the best Yanomamo tradition.

After taking a few more blasts from the shaman's pipe—some of the Indians were starting to take the snuff as well—I seemed to gain a greater awareness of the world outside the *shabono*. Whereas I had originally wondered why the Yanomamo chose to leave a gaping hole where the roof belonged, it now made perfect sense: no matter where you were in the village, you only had to look up to see the bluest of tropical skies.

In the distance, I heard a giant crocodile slowly slide off a riverbank into the water in search of fat fish; in the hills to the east, several male cock-of-the-rock cried *Mewh, Mewh* to attract females; a huge harpy eagle sailed under the canopy in search of capuchin monkeys, while a giant jaguar emitted a series of deep guttural grunts. To the north I heard the far-off waters of the Orinoco flowing toward the rapids that churned the river as it made its way to the coast. To the south a soft rain gently pelted the canopy covering the mountains that formed the border with Brazil.

Then my attention focused again on the images. The little figures at the edge of my field of vision multiplied in number as they danced faster and faster. I tried to get a better look, but it was like standing backward in front of a mirror and trying to turn around fast enough to see the back of your head: every time you look, the image is gone. I asked the shaman who the little men were.

"They are the *hekura*," he replied, "the spirits of the forest."

At this point I must have lost consciousness. I felt that once again I was slipping through a crack in the wall, moving from what we in the West perceive as reality into a different world—one that is an integral part of the Indians' reality. Like the visit of the jaguar and the curing ceremony of the old Wayana, the *epena* had given me a glimpse of a world that, for the Western scientist, is not supposed to exist. Such an experience almost inevitably leaves you with more questions than answers. But it also opens your mind and forces you to ask what is real and what isn't, what is primitive and what isn't, what we know and what we have yet to learn.

Several hours later I woke up in—and spilling out of—a small Yanomamo hammock. Pedro was standing over me.

"How do you feel?" he asked, with a lopsided grin.

"Okay, I guess." I stood up and stretched. "Quite good, really." My head was clear, although the back of my throat was a bit raw.

"Come on," said Pedro, and we headed out of the *shabono* accompanied by the shaman and some of the younger men who took part in the snuff ceremony. "We'll show you something I think you'll find interesting."

We walked quickly down a narrow trail, passing a lovely spray of *Oncidium* orchids whose little yellow flowers looked like a flock of butterflies frozen in time. We stopped at a *nyakwana* tree, tall with straight buttress roots and horizontal branches. The shaman used his machete to make a circular cut around the tree about four feet above the ground. He then pried off a strip of bark directly under the original cut, which he peeled down to where the roots began. He collected several strips of bark in this manner; then we returned to the *shabono*. Just before we entered, the old man pointed to a large leguminous tree growing just outside the palisade. "*Hisiomi*," he said.

"What's that?" I asked.

"*Hisiomi* is the source of the second snuff you took," explained Pedro.

"Then what was the first?" I asked.

"That was *nyakwana*. It is made from the bark sap of the *nyakwana* tree and lets you see things like the *hekura*. *Hisiomi* is made from the seeds of this tree and it helps you to hear things. The tree does not grow in the forest; it grows on the savanna. We plant it here near the *shabono*."

Inside the dwelling, the shaman held the bark strips over a cooking fire, where they began to ooze a viscous red sap that dripped onto a metal plate. Once all the liquid had been extracted from the bark, the medicine man scraped out the inner bark with the machete and added it to the plate. Using a banana leaf as a pot holder, he held the metal plate over the fire until the mixture was dry. During the drying process, the leaves of two plants, *mashohara* and *ama-asi* were added; according to Pedro, these plants "make the snuff stronger and make it smell good."

The botanical components of the two snuffs once again demonstrate the chemical sophistication of Amazonian Indians. These two hallucinogens are prepared from two different parts (sap and seeds) of two different trees (a nutmeg relative and a legume). The biochemical contents of the two trees responsible for the hallucinogenic effects are tryptamine alkaloids, which are almost identical. Living in the heart of the world's greatest forest, surrounded by tens of thousands of different trees, these "primitive" people had found the two plants that gave them direct access to the world of their spirits.

In historical terms, the legume, source of the *hisiomi*, is the better known of the two snuff plants. Originally native to the savanna regions, it was so highly valued for religious purposes that it was transported to many different areas in pre-Columbian times. Even in Andean regions where it could not be grown, highland tribes traded for the seeds with Indians of the Amazonian lowlands. Inca shamans in Andean Peru and Muisca medicine men in Andean Colombia are known to have used the seeds for divination well before 1492. When Europeans first arrived in the New World, the use of the plant as a hallucinogen was already widespread in the West Indies, where it was known as *cohoba*. There it was observed by the missionary Bartolomé de las Casas:

The Indians sucked up the powder and sniffed it up the nose, receiving that amount of it they had determined to take. The powder thus snuffed up went to their brains, almost as if they had been drinking strong wine. In this manner the Indians become intoxicated, or almost intoxicated. The powder, the ceremonies, and the procedure, they called "cohoba" . . . . in their language. This intoxication, caused them to babble confusedly, or talk like the Germans.

A more biased view was provided by the Jesuit missionary José Gumilla, who worked with the Indians of the Orinoco in the early eighteenth century. (So "successful" was missionary work among the Otomacs of the central Orinoco that this tribe is now extinct.) Of the Otomacs, Gumilla wrote:

They have another most evil habit, to wit: to intoxicate themselves through the nostrils, by using certain wicked powders . . . [which] totally deprives them of their reason and they will furiously take up arms.

He then added a description of how they prepared the snuff and concluded by noting:

Before a battle, they would throw themselves into a frenzy with "Yupa," wound themselves and, full of rage, go forth to battle like rabid jaguars.

The history of the use of the wild nutmeg sap, the "semen of the Sun," has only been elucidated over the last forty years. Schultes discovered the ritual consumption of the sap of this tree among tribes of the Colombian Amazon in 1954. Unlike the legume hallucinogen, this is a true rain forest species that occurs throughout most of Amazonia. Because the secret of this tree was kept hidden in the depths of the Amazon for so long, it is seldom mentioned in the historical accounts of this hallucinogen.

I lay in my hammock that night listening to the sounds of the *shabono*—the snuffling of the hunting dogs, the snoring of the Indians —and reflecting on the events of a glorious day. Participating in a ritual I had read about for over a decade is the kind of experience I had hoped for but could never plan. I was delighted to find the basic answers to my questions about *epena:* what it was made from and how many variants the Yanomamo used. Furthermore, being able to see the plants grown and used in their native habitat reminded me of the pilgrimages art students make to the great museums of the world to see for the first time the paintings and sculptures that for them had previously only existed in their textbooks.

I had read about the legume but never seen an actual specimen. The wild nutmeg, on the other hand, was an old friend; the Tiriós had first shown it to me. The sap served as an effective treatment for their fungal infections, toothache pain, and mouth sores. In the northwest Amazon, it is used as a treatment for fungal infections of the skin, as well as a hallucinogen.

Western medicine, for all of its miracle cures, does not have an effective treatment for these skin infections. This is a particularly serious problem with many cancer and AIDS patients, since some are literally devoured by fungal infections. These ailments are common in the humid rain forest environment and tribal peoples have no shortage of herbal treatments. The sap of the wild nutmeg, however, seems to be the most effective. Schultes collected the tree bark, dried it, and sent it to pharmaceutical labs in both the United States and Western Europe in the 1950s. They found nothing. However, at the University of São Paulo in Brazil, recent investigations in the laboratory using fresh material uncovered three compounds previously unknown to science. These compounds are of a chemical type known as lignans, complex molecules that are known to have a variety of effects on the human body. Two of the lignans discovered in the lab apparently have antifungal properties. Even if these are cures for the effects of our most insidious diseases, it is ironic that we are finding them in cultures we continue to disrupt and forests we continue to destroy.

The next morning Kapucinski left with an Indian guide for the airstrip and his return to Caracas. In two weeks, he would come back to pick me up at the airstrip. He packed his things, we shook hands, and I was left with my new Yanomamo friends.

I had decided to use the time to collect all the information about the snuffs I could find—exact dosage, variations in methods of preparation, associated myths and taboos. As I unpacked my field notebooks to record interviews with the Indians, a great commotion erupted around a newcomer in the *shabono*. Pedro translated what the man was saying: He had crossed over the Parima Mountains from Brazil after his *shabono* had been attacked by Brazilian gold miners. Some of the Indians had been shot and the women abducted. The Yanomamo had known for some time that the gold miners were in their area; they did not like having them nearby but decided that killing them would only bring retribution from the Brazilian army.

Gradually the problems began to build. Terrible epidemics of malaria and other fevers killed many of the children. The miners released mercury, a by-product of the gold mining process, into the water, which made many people sick. Two of the women had been seduced by the miners and developed venereal diseases for which the shaman had no cure. Finally, some of the younger men decided they had had enough: they donned their war paint and went to tell the miners to leave their lands. Frightened by their fierce appearance, the miners fired at them and wounded one of the Indians. The Indians sent forth a hail of arrows, killing one of the miners. The next day, the miners attacked the *shabono*.

Some of the Indians in my *shabono* wanted to retaliate, but the old shaman counseled otherwise. "It is not our battle," he said. "The village is over a six-day walk from here. Besides, we once went to war against that *shabono*. This is not our battle."

I reflected on the situation. Despite my efforts to find an "unspoiled" village, despite my efforts to escape the omnipresence of my own culture, despite the fact that I had finally found a place untouched by Western society, Brazilian gold miners had arrived as the ugly agents of change less than a week's walk to the south. There, the final chapter of the conquest that had begun in 1492 was still being played out. As I looked around the *shabono*, I realized how incredibly fortunate I was to have found one of the few places left on the planet where there were no vestiges of Western civilization. No clothes, no plastic, as far as I could see; only the machetes had come from the outside world. One of the Indians beckoned me to join in an *epena* session that was about to commence. As the warm powder burned its way deeper into my brain, I relaxed and prepared myself to commune once more with another reality. As I surrendered to the drug and felt myself drift away, somebody turned on a cassette tape player, and Cab Calloway's "Hi-de-ho" burst out in the *shabono*.

The music dampened my elation over my discoveries. Though I had found out what plants the Venezuelan Yanomamo use in their snuff, and confirmed that they were the same plants Schultes had reported on so many years before, I was crushed to find that even in this remote corner of the Amazon there seemed to be no avoiding Western influence. As I had seen and heard time and time again, once modern ways gain a toehold in Amazonian culture, it is usually only a matter of time before Western diseases coupled with an obsession with Western culture and material goods overwhelms the traditional way of life.

CHAPTER 9

# Return to
# Kwamala

It is curious to note that tribes who become acculturated fastest also
disappear quickest. —Henri Coudreau, 1886

● ● ● ● ● ● ● ● ● ● ● ● ● ● ● ● ● ● ● ●

The visit to the Yanomamo had been a rude reminder that the clock
was ticking for the Amazonian Indians. I had been unexpectedly and
deeply disappointed to find Western material goods, such as cassette
tapes and players, and illnesses such as malaria and venereal diseases
permeating even one of the most remote tribes. If the Yanomamo were
feeling the effects of the outside world, I worried that the Tiriós might
now be overrun. I decided to return to Kwamala in January 1988, after
an absence of three years.

I not only wanted to visit old friends, I also had a debt to repay.
During my first visit to the Tiriós in 1982, I had given the chief my
solemn word that any medicinal plant knowledge I learned from the
tribe would be returned to them in written form. This had been our
agreement, yet I did not know if the results of my studies would have
any impact. The headman had made it clear during our first meeting
that he regarded the white man's medicine as superior to his own tribe's
and he had never shown any interest in my research.

Yet as indigenous cultures continued to be disrupted or destroyed
through contact with the outside world, the conservation community was
beginning to wake up and pay attention to the importance of ethnobotany for rain forest preservation and utilization. International conservation groups were learning that a focus on the kind of appealing

animals that philanthropists rally around—what Russ Mittermeier referred to as the "charismatic mega-vertebrates"—was simply too narrow for organizations trying to protect tropical ecosystems. Somehow, both plants and indigenous peoples had to be factored into the equation. Unfortunately, most people are not intrigued by plants; and many conservationists regard them as something that goes in one end of a panda and comes out the other. You cannot save the animal, however, unless you also save the plants it feeds on.

Ethnobotany takes a holistic approach to conservation and proves the vital importance of the role indigenous people can play in the ongoing struggle to protect, use, and sustain the rain forest. In Central America, the most pristine tracts of rain forest that remain are strongholds of indigenous culture; in other words, where you have forests, you have Indians—but, more importantly, where you have Indians, you have forests. Traditionally, conservationists have regarded people as the problem: people kill animals, eat plants, and in general destroy habitat. But indigenous peoples have spent lifetimes coexisting with the forest, living off the forest while at the same time sustaining a fragile ecosystem by not overhunting its creatures or exhausting its soil. The beauty of ethnobotany is that it brings people into the forest picture, showing that tribal peoples can help provide us with answers on the best ways to use and protect the forest.

Yet even as the conservation community has begun to pay more attention to indigenous peoples in general and ethnobotany in particular, the overall picture continues to worsen. Population growth spirals unabated, multinational companies encroach on indigenous lands, and forests continue to be cut down. A Peruvian conservationist once said, "Roads are the cancer of the rain forest"; they indiscriminately destroy vegetation and invite "civilization" into the virgin wilderness. Roads provide access to markets, thus making it economically viable in many cases to start felling trees and selling the logs. Roads also bring in peasants, who inevitably engage in land squabbles with indigenous peoples and bring new and virulent diseases to the tribes. And missionary activity continues unabated among the Indians; conservationists have been unable to convince the crusaders that their efforts often result in a negative impact on the people *and* the environment. The missionaries' penchant for concentrating the Indians in "supervillages" of several hundred may make their job of converting the Indians a little easier, but at the same time, the surrounding forest is depleted by overhunting or destroyed by cutting gardens in the same places for decades, which ravages soils and never allows the forests to regenerate. I had little hope that my friends in Kwamala had managed to remain unscathed.

From the air, the village appeared much the same. The only difference immediately apparent was the corrugated aluminum roofs that had replaced the traditional palm thatch. I did not realize at the time how accurate a symbol of cultural disintegration this was.

As always in these remote regions, the sound of our plane created a stir in the village. Many of the Indians stood outside their huts, shading their eyes from the afternoon sun to watch our arrival. After a bumpy landing, I climbed out of the plane and looked around. Kamainja was standing at the edge of the airstrip; he gave a gasp of recognition, chuckled, and enveloped me in a big bear hug. "*Jako, joe doro,*" he said. "Brother, you've returned." He spoke a mixture of Tirió and Sranan Tongo.

"*Ai, Jako. Mi doro, sasame wae,*" I replied. "Yes, it's good to be back!"

We unloaded my meager supplies—hammock, backpack, plant press, and a few canned goods—then watched the plane take off. As we walked through the village, I smiled as I took in all the familiar sights, sounds, and smells: women combing each other's hair, spinning cotton, and grating manioc; the smoke and crackle of cooking fires; the shrieks of little boys playing hunter with their child-sized bows and arrows. But now new sights jarred me. Most of the young men had exchanged their red breechcloths for secondhand Western clothing. The older men, most of whom had worn their hair long in the back, had cut it short to resemble pictures of Westerners they had seen in magazines left behind by the missionaries. Gone were the beaded bracelets, toucan-feather headpieces, and the body painting, those symbols of a timeless culture, and with them all sense of pride in that culture. Several of my friends boasted that they no longer made curare or hunted with bows and arrows; they preferred instead to use the shotguns that they had traded parrots for in a village in Brazil. I felt sick to my stomach. Although I knew intellectually things had likely been changing while I was gone,

I wasn't prepared for my emotional reaction to seeing how quickly their culture was ebbing away.

We dropped my things in an empty hut. Forgoing the usual trip to the hut of the headman, who was off on a hunting trip of several weeks, we went to Kamainja's to relax in the cotton hammocks slung from the rafters. Tirió hospitality had remained the same, I thought, as Kamainja's wife quickly brought me a calabash full of cassava beer. I drank the warm, sour beverage and she sliced a piece of meat from the charred carcass of a peccary being smoked over a smoldering fire.

The next morning, I heard a voice calling out the traditional Tirió morning greeting: "*Jako, kude manah?* Brother, are you well?"

My hammock was still swathed in mosquito netting, so I couldn't see who was speaking. "*Ai, jako, kude wae!*" I replied. "Yes, brother, I am well."

Suddenly the voice shifted into English. "Good morning, my friend, how are you?" Koita! I rolled out of bed to embrace him. If I hadn't heard his voice, I might not have recognized my old friend right away. No red breechcloth, no beaded belt, no wristbands of *sho-ro-sho-ro* seeds. In their place Koita wore a green and blue Hawaiian shirt, blue denim jeans, and black high-top sneakers.

"Where did you get all this?" I asked. "You look like a *pananakiri.*"

Koita's broad smile faded. "You mean you don't like them?"

I realized I had hurt his feelings and tried to recover. "Well," I stammered, "it's just that . . . just that you look very different, that's all. I hardly saw anyone wearing breechcloths yesterday, either. What happened while I was gone?"

"There have been some changes," he said. "The missionaries were here and they brought the clothes with them. Also, the wildlife trader who used to give us flashlights and fishhooks for the animals we caught now gives us clothes."

"What else?" I asked, at the same time dreading to hear the answer.

"Well, our friend Yaloefuh isn't here anymore. He was caught in the hammock of another man's wife and the missionaries and the chief had him whipped in front of the whole village. Then he was expelled and he went to live in the village in Brazil that you visited with Kamainja."

"He can never come back?" I asked incredulously.

"Chief says no," Koita replied.

"What about his wife and children?"

"Oh, they are still here."

Astonished by this piece of news, I wondered whether the beating given my friend was initiated by the missionaries or by the Indians themselves. When some of the missionaries first came to Suriname, they insisted that each man could have only one wife. This caused a great deal of heartache among the tribes that practiced polygamy because several old women were cut adrift without husbands to care for them.

"Any other changes?" I asked.

"Yes," said Koita. "The chief told us no more singing the old songs and dancing the old dances. They are part of the old ways."

This, too, was heartbreaking news. The Tiriós were famous for their dances, which re-created such everyday occurrences as hunting scenes, jaguars chasing a herd of peccaries, and cock-of-the-rock males displaying their feathers and strutting about to attract the females of the species. American explorer William Farabee visited these Indians at the turn of the century and their dances made a vivid impression on him. The moves were "all so well done that we understood perfectly." I couldn't believe the Tiriós had been forced to give up such an essential part of their culture in exchange for an imported religion.

"So what do you sing now?" I asked.

"The missionaries taught us new songs," he replied excitedly. "Here, listen to this." The tune he sang sounded vaguely familiar, but it took me a minute to recognize it: a Tirió version of "Jingle Bells."

I found that the effect of missionary activity reached far beyond the Indians' music and dance. Traditionally, the Indians had been given names drawn from nature. The true name of the Jaguar Shaman meant "Bone," while Koita was named after the *koi* palm. Now the newborns were being named after people in the Bible. The missionaries also set up a generator, hooked it up to a 16mm projector, and showed the sequence from Cecil B. deMille's *The Ten Commandments* in which Moses parts the Red Sea. When I later met one of the missionaries who had been responsible for this, he told me that he had carefully explained to the Indians that this was not the *real* event but an enactment. A fine trick; show a film to people who have never seen a film before; tell them that what they are seeing isn't really happening but really did happen in the past, and that it is proof that everything in the Bible actually

occurred. And the missionaries claim that Indians choose Western religion of their own volition!

Religious belief, however, was not one of the reasons the tribe's chief
so wholeheartedly embraced the missionaries; it was the access to Western goods and the idea of joining such a superior culture. He received
the best clothes, more machetes and flashlights than anyone else,
canned goods, salt, and a prize that he alone possessed—a radio that
picked up stations in Brazil. On top of that, he occasionally traveled on
a plane to Bible meetings in the capital city.

An upheaval in the village interrupted Koita's tale of the events of
the last few years. We followed the noise and soon saw Ijuki, the old
shaman, carrying on his back a giant anteater that he had killed in the
forest. The beast was so large—about six feet long from the tip of its
snout to the end of its tail—that its limp body all but covered the old
man: we could see little else but Ijuki's two strong, skinny legs laboring
under their burden. The shaggy gray creature with the elongated snout
looked as if it weighed more than its slayer.

Koita explained that the giant anteater is a dangerous animal to hunt;
if you do not kill it straightaway, the wounded beast gathers its considerable strength and, when the hunter approaches, strikes out with its
claws to deliver a final, often fatal blow. As nineteenth-century British
naturalist Charles Waterton reported, "The Indians have a great dread
of coming in contact with the ant-bear; and after disabling him in the
chase, never think of approaching him till he be quite dead."

The nineteenth-century British explorer Barrington Brown recorded
a telling incident in Guyana involving a local hunter who made a fatal
error in judgment:

These large Ant-eaters are very dangerous customers and have
been known to kill men. [My guide] told me that an Indian, living
near Roraima, was hunting in the forest to the north of that mountain with some others, armed with his long blow-pipe. In returning
home, considerably in advance of the rest of the party, it is supposed he saw a young Ant-eater, and, taking it up in his arms, was
carrying it home, when its Mother gave chase, overtook, and killed
him; for when his companions came up, they found him lying dead
on his face in the embrace of the Ant-bear, one of its large claws

having entered his heart. In the struggle he had managed to stick his knife behind the back into the animal, which bled to death, but not before the poor fellow had succumbed to its terrible hug. . . . So firmly had the animal grappled him, that to separate it from the corpse the Indians had to cut off its forelegs.

Ignoring the crowd that had assembled to watch his return, Ijuki struggled on toward his hut, where he finally relaxed and allowed his burden to slide off his back onto the ground. The old medicine man was covered in sweat and the clotted blood of his prey, and flies buzzed around him. He gave the crowd a thin-lipped, triumphant half-smile, then slipped into his home to collapse in his hammock. Meanwhile his young wife came outside and began skinning her husband's prize.

Only after the shaman had a day to recover did we learn what had transpired. As was his custom, Ijuki was out in the forest hunting alone, accompanied only by two of his hunting dogs. Suddenly, both dogs started barking excitedly and racing ahead down the trail. Ijuki, hoping they had found a tapir, hurried after them. As he entered a small clearing in the forest, he was surprised to find a giant anteater, more commonly found on the savanna. The beast was seated on it haunches, flailing away at the two dogs with its powerful front claws. The braver of the two dogs went on the attack, trying unsuccessfully to dodge those deadly hooks. The giant anteater grabbed it around the neck and held it in a lethal hug. The old man quickly sent a poisoned arrow deep into the anteater's heart and within a few minutes the huge animal rolled over and died. It was too late to save the dog, though; the anteater's claws had cut its throat. Waiting until he was sure the anteater could not do to him what it had done to his dog, Ijuki hoisted the beast onto his back and shoulders and started for home. Although giant anteater is not a preferred food item (the Indians claim it has a "stinky" taste), the old man believed in eating what he killed, and lugged it three to four miles back to the village.

Because Ijuki was the oldest of the shamans and reputed to be the most powerful, he was just the person I needed to help unravel the mystery of ku-pe-de-yuh, a small shrub to which I had been introduced by the Jaguar Shaman on my two previous expeditions.

When I asked the Jaguar Shaman what it was for, he had replied

cryptically, "We use it to talk with the ancestors." This had excited my
interest because it implied some form of hallucinogenic usage; I had
never seen evidence of drug use among the Tiriós, and I was eager to
learn more about this mysterious plant.

"How?" I had asked.

"We soak the plant in cold water, and then we wash with it," he had
replied.

This wasn't quite the answer I had expected. Typically, hallucinogens
must be ingested—that is, swallowed, snorted, or smoked—to induce
a physiological response. Thus, from the Jaguar Shaman's response, I
couldn't be certain that this plant was hallucinogenic. Furthermore, although I collected specimens, I was unable to identify them in the
herbarium because they had no flowers or fruits. To be able to make an
identification within the framework of Linnaean taxonomy, I needed to
see the plant's reproductive parts.

Little is known of hallucinogenic plant use by the Indians of the
northeast Amazon. The coastal Caribs of Suriname are believed to consume the sap of *takini*, a member of the fig family (and thus a not-too-
distant relative of marijuana) as part of the shamanistic initiation. But
prior to my research with the Tiriós, there was no record of any hallucinogenic plant use among the Indians of Suriname. The repeated references to the *ku-pe-de-yuh* plant as a method for "contacting ancestors"
or "becoming a shaman"—accounts given to me by all the medicine
men with whom I worked—indicated that further research was war-
ranted. As a student of Schultes, I had been taught that hallucinogenic
plants can serve as a window into Amazonian culture since that is how
the Indians commune with the spirit world. I also knew from the example of psilocybin and visken that hallucinogens can yield therapeutic
compounds useful in our own society. The fact that it had taken me
several expeditions to begin to unlock the mystery of Tirió hallucinogens
meant that I was getting into some of the shaman's most powerful medicinal plant knowledge and applications.

But I would have to wait a few days for Ijuki's attention. He was too
worn out from his encounter with the anteater.

In the village that night, I had dinner with Koita and Kamainja. A frog
that had a call like a jackhammer croaked in the nearby forest. We

finished our meal of boiled *hoko*, a forest turkey, then sat and stared into the cooking fire as we talked. We discussed the usual topics: hunting, the weather, when the pineapples would be at their ripest. My friends recited the list of births and deaths that had occurred during my absence. I was saddened to learn that Kaloshewuh, the shaman who had been named after the plant his mother had used in childbirth, had passed away. After a bit, I broached the topic of *ku-pe-de-yuh*.

"What is *ku-pe-de-yuh*?" I asked.

"That is a dangerous plant," warned Kamainja. "Didn't we find that the last time you were here?"

"Yes, but I want to find it with flowers or with fruit."

This request always mystified the Indians. They could identify any plant by its appearance, without needing the fruit or flowers—its reproductive organs—as clues. Living in a tropical forest, surrounded by hundred-foot trees whose tiny fruits or flowers would appear a hundred feet from the forest floor only one week each year, they had developed the infinitely more practical ability to identify a species by the sight or smell of its bark.

When Ijuki had recovered, Koita, Kamainja, and I headed for the shaman's hut. We explained our purpose and asked if he would guide us. True to form, he declined, claiming that he was too tired, too old, his head hurt, his knees hurt, he had a sore back from carrying the giant anteater home.

When it seemed as if all was lost, Koita rose to the occasion. "Come on," he said to Kamainja and me, "poor Grandfather is too old for this sort of thing. Let's go ask Nahtahlah. He's a few years younger and, besides, he knows a lot more about plants. Some say his medicine is more powerful."

The old shaman jutted out his lower jaw. "Nahtahlah," he snorted, "*I* trained *him*. You think he knows more than me? Where's my machete? *Mmpah!*"

I hastened to keep up with the old medicine man as he strode purposefully into the jungle. Two hours later, we entered the forest clearing I had visited with him and Yaloefuh on my last trip. Yaloefuh had told me that this was where the old man came to work his medicine.

The shaman stood at the entrance to the clearing and pointed to the far side. "There!" he said triumphantly. It took a few minutes for my eyes to focus and to distinguish just what it was he was pointing at. As I walked closer for a better look, I inadvertently gasped. At the other edge of the clearing stood several *ku-pe-de-yuh* bushes, three feet tall and hung with yellow-green fruit. The fruit resembled the common tomato, indicating that this was a species of *Brunfelsia*, which is widely used in the western Amazon for a variety of purposes. A cold-water infusion of the roots is used to treat yellow fever, snakebite, rheumatism, and syphilis. And one species has been used as a fish poison by local tribes.

"Grandfather," I asked, "may I collect these plants?"

"You may take two," he said, "no more."

Following his instructions, I gingerly uprooted the plants, digging up the roots with the blade of my machete. When you collect specimens of a tree, you usually take only a few branches and maybe a piece of bark. When dealing with an herb or a small shrub, you collect the entire plant so that you can see its root structure and growth pattern. Whether or not I decided to sample the hallucinogen myself, I wanted to have a good specimen for the herbarium.

We headed back to the village in a festive mood, and I asked Ijuki how *ku-pe-de-yuh* was used.

"You must take the bark and the root of *ku-pe-de-yuh* and soak it in cold water. The next day, you must wash with some and drink most of the rest. You will vomit. Soon you will see the evil spirit. He wears a red breechcloth. In one hand he carries a war club; in the other, plants. You must drink more of the *ku-pe-de-yuh* until the demon begins to speak. He will teach you how to cure by singing and by using healing plants. That is all."

The hallucinogenic properties of *Brunfelsia* have been analyzed twice: in the late 1960s by Professor Schultes, and again in the late 1970s by ethnobotanist Tim Plowman at the Field Museum in Chicago. Both men found that while the plant contains alkaloids, those compounds do not appear to be responsible for the plant's hallucinogenic activity.

Ijuki was tired, so we left him, but the next morning, we returned to his hut. He looked surprised and slightly annoyed. "What is it?" he asked.

"Grandfather," I said, "what if I wanted to take the potion?"

"*Awah*," he said. "No. This is a very dangerous plant. Many apprentices have taken it and some have lost their minds. Some did not survive." He paused for a minute and then continued. "If you take it you will die." That settled, he announced he was going hunting.

I was surprised by his stern response. Outside, I bid my friends goodbye and walked back to my hut. I reviewed what I knew about the *Solanaceae*, the plant family to which this species belonged. In terms of economic plants, the *Solanaceae* is unquestionably one of the most important families in the plant kingdom. It includes such edible species as potatoes, tomatoes, chile peppers, and bell peppers. In addition to those benign species, however, the family contains belladonna and henbane, poisons that figured heavily in the witches' brews of the Middle Ages. Upon my return to the States a few weeks later, I read a classic early work on hallucinogenic plants by the German toxicologist Lewis Lewin titled *Phantastica: Narcotic and Stimulating Drugs—Their Use and Abuse.* Lewin wrote:

> Besides other disagreeable symptoms, these *Solanaceae* and their active elements, give rise to hallucinations and illusions of sight, hearing and taste, which differ, however, from those produced by the other Phantastica. They are not of an agreeable but, on the contrary, of a terrifying and distressful kind.

Many newcomers who knew to be cautious with the poisonous members of the *Solanaceae* family did not always trust that some species were nontoxic. Such was the case with tomatoes, as reported in 1989 by eminent economic botanists Beryl Simpson and Molly Ogorzaly:

> Tomatoes were brought to temperate North America by the British, but they were initially grown only as ornamental plants. Until 1800, the fruits were relegated to a role as a pustule remover. According to an old farm journal, doubts about the fruit's edibility were dramatically removed in 1820 when Colonel Robert Gibbon Johnson announced that at noon on September 26, he would eat a bushel of the dreaded fruit. Two thousand people thought him mad and turned out to witness the event. To their astonishment, he survived.

Johnson was a braver man than I; I heeded the shaman's advice. I knew that a different species of *Brunfelsia* had a long history of ethnomedical use in the western Amazon. It is said to be a powerful additive to the highly hallucinogenic brew known as *ayahuasca*, which is consumed as a religious sacrament in Amazonian Colombia, Ecuador, Peru, and Brazil. Some reports indicated that this western species of *Brunfelsia* was hallucinogenic in and of itself. These reports led to laboratory analysis in the late 1970s at the Field Museum in Chicago, which uncovered a compound new to science—brunfelsine. This compound caused convulsions but not hallucinations. Further chemical work is needed if we are to fully understand the biochemical secrets this plant harbors.

The day after we had collected the plant, I awoke to find the village awash in a tropical downpour. A solid wall of water poured off the thatched roof of my dwelling; thunder rumbled in the distance, and I heard a series of small splashes coming toward the hut.

Koita burst through the doorway, dripping water, out of breath, and white as a sheet. "What's the matter?" I asked.

"Old Ijuki. He has really done it this time. He woke up this morning grumbling that he wanted some honey and wasn't going to let a little rain stop him. He was climbing an old *we-de* tree to look for a hive when a branch broke beneath him and he fell to the ground. Someone heard him yell and several people went out to get him. They say he cannot move his legs."

We arrived at the shaman's hut just in time to see him being carried out of the forest. He writhed in excruciating pain and the men carried him inside and gently laid him in his hammock, a spot he would never leave. Even the combined powers of the local medicine men proved ineffective, as did the modern medicine tendered by a physician who visited the village a few months later. Apparently Ijuki had fractured several vertebrae and damaged the surrounding nerves. The doctor wanted to bring the old man to the city and operate; he acknowledged, however, that although the surgery might relieve the pain, Ijuki still would not be able to walk. The old shaman refused.

As I gazed at Ijuki lying in his hammock day after day, realizing that I was not only watching the life drain out of him but also out of his culture, I remembered the pessimistic words of the nineteenth-century

German explorer Theodor Koch-Grünberg. During his final visit to the northeast Amazon, he wrote:

> The Indians of Rio Branco are close to their end. Those who escaped influenza, which killed entire [villages], are now being liquidated forever by balata gatherers, gold prospectors or diamond seekers. The region around Roraima is thoroughly invaded by whites, blacks and detribalized mestizos from British Guiana, Brazil, Venezuela and God knows how many other countries. The few Indians who survive have been deprived of their rights and reduced to slavery. Their ingenuous happiness has gone, their solemn dances have ceased . . . the joyful playing of children on the sandy center of the village by moonlight has ended. Happy are those who died in time.

Koita and I were still sitting in Ijuki's hut when Kamainja ducked in out of the rain. He shook the water out of his hair and said, "*Jako*, the chief has returned from his hunting trip. He wants to see you later this evening."

That evening the sky cleared and a fiery red sun dropped behind the glistening trees. The village was preternaturally quiet; it seemed as if people were enjoying the silence after listening to the roar of the rain pounding the canopy of the surrounding forest and pelting the village ground.

Koita and Kamainja waited for me at the entrance to the thatched hut. Inside sat the chief, wearing a red Hawaiian print shirt and a pair of red cotton pants. I sat down on a low bench across from the chief; Koita and Kamainja sat on either side of me.

As was his wont, the chief was inscrutable, saying nothing and betraying no emotion for the first few moments. Then he began: "We welcome you back to our village. I am pleased to see you cause us no trouble. Some of the people who have been here, mostly those working for the wildlife trader, have caused problems. They bring in liquor, tobacco, and marijuana, and then try to seduce our women. You have not done this and for that I thank you."

His appreciation pleased me, but being thanked for stupid things I *hadn't* done struck me as a backhanded compliment. I stood up and gave him a three-ring binder containing a two-hundred-page manuscript detailing everything I had learned about the medicinal plants of his tribe. Again showing no emotion, he accepted the binder and thanked me for living up to my end of the bargain. The next day, he called a meeting of all the Indians in the forest, a gathering to which I was not invited. I was a bit puzzled by that, but not concerned.

Afterward, Koita showed up at my hut. "Did you go to the meeting?" I asked.

"Yes."

"What happened?"

"Chief said this information might be important in the future. He asked me to work with you and the old shamans to translate it into our language. The information will then be used in the little schoolhouse set up by the missionaries to teach our children."

A shaman's apprentice had been found! The traditional knowledge would now be passed on *within* the tribe, from shaman to apprentice, elder to student. No longer would it be necessary for a researcher from another land to preserve the tribal lore.

The answers to a dilemma that had troubled me all along were becoming clear. I had gone to the Amazon to search for healing plants, magic bullets that could cure some of our incurable ailments. I had quickly learned from the Indians that these plants worked—they soothed my wasp sting, cured my ear infection, and eased my tendinitis. But then I found myself in a quandary: How best to proceed? How might my work help the people from whose kindness and knowledge I had so benefited? Of all the wonder drugs already derived from tropical plants, worth hundreds of millions of dollars in world trade, not one penny had been paid back to any of the indigenous peoples who taught us the plants.

When I began my work, no pharmaceutical firms had any interest in ethnobotany. But given the increasing concern and publicity devoted to the rain forest issue, I was confident the situation would change—and I was right. In February 1989, an article describing my field research appeared in *Smithsonian* magazine.

Within two weeks of the article's appearance, I was besieged by venture capitalists who saw ethnobotany as a fail-safe route to quick riches. "We'll raise some capital," one would-be tycoon said, "set up a lab, find some cures, and synthesize the compounds. Then we'll sell it all off to a big drug company and pocket a ton of money." My most serious objection to their schemes stemmed from the take-the-money-and-run approach; they had virtually no interest in the people who were teaching me about the plants, or about the fate of the forest in which these plants were found.

Just as I was about to give up on the idea of working with the business community, a woman named Lisa Conte visited me. Trained in pharmacology and biochemistry, Lisa had given up a promising career in science to go to business school. She was young, hip, and inexperienced enough to try something no one else had the gumption to suggest. After she pitched her ideas to me, I replied, "You've told me what is in it for me, but that is of less interest to me than what is in it for the Indians." Instead of being taken aback, as I had expected, she smiled knowingly, as if I had fallen into her trap.

"Look," she said, "you've emphasized the need to return some money to the indigenous peoples who gave you the knowledge and to the countries where the plants are found. Why not earmark a percentage of any profits resulting from the development of new pharmaceuticals for the indigenous peoples, be it for education, purchase of their traditional territories, or what have you? Another percentage could go to the national government of the country to support development and management of national parks and other protected areas. Finally, a percentage would also go to support further ethnobotanical research."

This conversation was one of the factors that led to the birth of Shaman Pharmaceuticals in San Carlos, California. Lisa has been able to garner the support of indigenous rights advocates and venture capitalists, as well as recruit a staff that includes ethnobotanists, biochemists, and physicians. She set up a board of scientific advisers, with Professor Schultes serving as honorary chairman, who work with staff scientists to help identify priorities and to offer advice on which countries, tribes, or plants to pursue. An Amazonian tree extract code-named SP-303 proved so effective in the laboratory for treating herpes viruses, as well as viruses causing flu and respiratory conditions, that the extract was being tested on humans just sixteen months after the company started— a success story almost unheard of in the pharmaceutical industry, where it takes an average of five years for a drug to advance to human testing.

And true to her word, Lisa has established a nonprofit organization called the Healing Forest Conservancy, set up expressly to return a percentage of all profits that flow from these potential medical products back to the indigenous peoples who teach us the plants and to the countries in which the plants grow. The Tiriós have asked me to begin re-collecting their medicinal species in quantities large enough to begin testing for potential new medicines. (I had collected only voucher specimens up to this point—usually a branch with flowers—for deposit in the Harvard herbarium.) Meanwhile, major pharmaceutical companies are now jumping on the bandwagon. Merck Pharmaceuticals has given a $1 million grant to the Costa Rican government to launch a project to develop new medicines from local plants. Bristol-Myers-Squibb has begun negotiating with Conservation International to work collaboratively with Amazonian Indians in the search for new therapeutic compounds. And Eli Lilly, the firm that markets the rosy periwinkle alkaloids, which is still the most effective treatment for certain cancers, has decided to undertake a joint venture with Shaman Pharmaceuticals to search for new antifungal compounds from rain forest plants; they have also agreed to earmark a percentage of any profits to be returned to the native peoples.

More important from my point of view is what has happened among the Tiriós. Although two of the shamans have died—Ijuki and Tyaky—Koita and Kamainja have been chosen by the chief to serve as shaman's apprentices, working under the tutelage of the Jaguar Shaman. They are responsible for fact-checking my data, adding any new information to the book, and teaching the younger Indians about the healing plants. Over the past three years, I have periodically returned to the village to help them translate the information I collected back into their language. We completed this effort, and as I write this, I am also busy typing up the *Tareno Epi Panpira*—the *Tirió Plant Medicine Handbook*. I feel strongly that this effort has helped validate their culture in the eyes of the Indians. Prior to this work, the Tiriós had only one book written in their language: the holy Bible. This research constitutes a true partnership between Western and Indian cultures; both share in any potential material benefits, but more important, this approach to ethnobotany helps the indigenous peoples understand the potential global importance of a fundamental aspect of their culture.

At the historic United Nations Conference on the Environment held in Rio de Janeiro in 1992, the most contentious issue discussed was "intellectual property rights"—that is, who benefits from the commercialization of natural resources, especially those found in the tropics. Most attendees (with the notable exception of former President George Bush and his U.S. delegation) agreed that some legal framework had to be designed to ensure that a percentage of profits flowed back to the country where the healing plants originated and to the people who first discovered the plants. Nonetheless, the indigenous people present were challenged by then-Senator Albert Gore:

> We agree that the system has not worked fairly in the past and we must seek ways to reimburse our indigenous colleagues for new products developed from plants they teach us. Yet if the people of these cultures do not perpetuate and pass on this knowledge, if these people do not keep growing the 15 or 24 or 56 varieties of corn or manioc or rice that may possess resistance to some new pest or disease, they will *not* have the option of commercializing them in the future. Whether indigenous peoples want to share or commercialize this germplasm or information in the future is entirely up to them. If, however, this knowledge and/or germplasm is not passed on, that option will be forfeited forever.

In an attempt to see whether the shaman's apprentice approach would be replicable, Conservation International sponsored a similar effort in 1991 among the Bribri Indians living in the village of Coroma, located in the foothills of the Talamanca Mountains of southern Costa Rica. The project has succeeded beyond our wildest expectations. Four shamans have chosen a class of four apprentices and a four-year training program is under way. More importantly, this effort has sparked a whole cultural revival in the sense that customs that were being allowed or even encouraged to die out are now being revived. The Indians have built a traditional thatched meeting house, the first ever seen by the youngest members of the tribe, who only knew the wooden houses in which they now live. And traditional dances are once again being performed.

A neighboring tribe has accused the Bribri of trying to go back in time, of returning to antiquated ways. I believe this dissonance is a good thing: the Indians are now debating their own culture and deciding their own destiny, where in the recent past, life as they knew it was dying out without *any* discussion at all.

Representatives of eight other Indian villages have visited Coroma to decide for themselves whether to initiate similar programs. Most encouragingly, representatives of the Guyami Indians of Panama walked tens of miles through the jungle, over the mountains, and across the border into Costa Rica to evaluate the shaman's apprentice program. They were favorably impressed. And in Bolivia, the Chimane tribe heard about the program through Dr. Guillermo Rioja, an anthropologist who works with them and is affiliated with Conservation International. When he asked the tribe if they would be interested in setting up such a program, they enthusiastically agreed.

As I did with the tribes in Suriname and Costa Rica, I have been working with the Guyamis and Chimanes, along with local scientists, to help organize their shaman's apprentice programs. Once the programs are up and running, sometime in 1994, they will be administered for the most part by the Indians themselves.

In the face of these successes, there is still no shortage of doom and gloom in the environmental movement. Toxic waste, ozone depletion, deforestation—sometimes it seems so overwhelming that it is easy to lose hope. Yet these problems are *caused* by people and therefore I believe the problems can be *solved* by people. Yes, forests are declining, species are disappearing, and cultures are disintegrating. But all is not yet lost; simple, creative solutions can and do make a difference. For most of the time I spent working with the Tiriós, I felt the cultural integrity of these people would not in any way survive. But my pessimism was premature. Koita, Kamainja, and the Jaguar Shaman are living proof that there is hope. A missionary once asked Professor Schultes, "Why do we want to know all the plants on the earth? When the final trumpet is sounded, we'll know everything anyway." That may or may not be true, but until then we cannot sit still. If we are to safeguard the rights of the indigenous peoples, protect endangered species, find new foods to feed the hungry and new medicines to cure the sick, now is the time to act. We must develop a proactive, holistic approach to the environmental problems we face, realizing that previously overlooked or even ridiculed worldviews like shamanic wisdom can help us find answers to some of the questions we face. If we don't, our children and grandchildren will inherit a world infinitely less diverse biologically and culturally than the one into which we were born.

# Recommended Reading

● ● ● ● ● ● ● ● ● ● ● ● ● ● ● ● ● ●

## Chapter 1

Jacobs, M. 1988. *The Tropical Rain Forest.* Berlin: Springer-Verlag. An indispensable introduction to rain forest evolution, ecology, and conservation.

Kreig, M. 1964. *Green Medicine.* New York: Bantam Books. An excellent overview of ethnobotany, including a superb biography of Schultes.

Plotkin, M. J. 1988. The Search for New Jungle Medicines. *The Futurist* 25, 9–14.

Schultes, R. E., and R. Raffauf. 1990. *The Healing Forest.* Portland, OR: Dioscorides Press. This technical work is the standard reference for ethnobotanists working in the Amazon.

————. 1988. *Where the Gods Reign.* Oracle, AZ: Synergetic Press. A photographic essay on the ethnobotany of the northwest Amazon—a gem!

Simpson, B., and M. Ogorzaly. 1986. *Economic Botany.* New York: McGraw-Hill. Although a textbook, *Economic Botany* is an extremely enjoyable introduction to the history and botany of useful plants.

Soejarto, D., and N. Farnsworth. 1989. Tropical Rain Forests: Potential Sources of New Drugs? *Perspectives in Biology and Medicine* 32(2), 244–256. A classic paper that is widely cited in the conservation literature.

Wilson, E. O. 1992. *The Diversity of Life.* Cambridge, MA: Harvard University Press. The best conservation overview available, written by the leading biologist of our time.

## Chapter 2

Forsyth, A., and K. Miyata. 1984. *Tropical Nature*. New York: Scribner's. A superbly written introduction to the ecology of both Central and South America.

Forsyth, A. 1990. *Portraits of the Rainforest*. Camden East, Ontario: Camden House. An underappreciated sequel to *Tropical Nature*.

Goulding, M. 1980. *The Fishes and the Forest*. Berkeley: University of California Press. The classic account of the ecological interdependency between fish and the riverine vegetation written by the leading Amazonian ichthyologist.

————. 1989. *The Flooded Forest*. London: BBC Books. A popular account of Amazonian ecology that is well written and profusely illustrated.

Miles, A. 1988. *Devil's Island*. Berkeley: Ten Speed Press. A readable history of the penal colony.

Neil, W. 1971. *The Last of the Ruling Reptiles*. New York: Columbia University Press. A useful and well-researched introduction to the ecology and evolution of crocodilians.

Plotkin, M., F. Medem, R. Mittermeier, and I. Constable. 1983. Distribution and Conservation of the Black Caiman. In A. Rhodin and K. Miyata, eds., *Advances in Herpetology and Evolutionary Biology* (pp. 695–705). Cambridge, MA: Museum of Comparative Zoology.

## Chapter 3

Hemming, J. 1978. *The Search for El Dorado*. New York: Dutton. The best account of the colonial European search for gold in tropical South America. Not only is it superbly illustrated, but it reads like a novel.

Price, R., ed. 1973. *Maroon Societies*. Baltimore, MD: Johns Hopkins University Press. An anthology of studies of Maroon communities throughout the New World, edited by the leading authority on the Maroons of Suriname.

Price, S., and R. Price. 1980. *Afro-American Arts of the Suriname Rain Forest*. Los Angeles: Museum of Cultural History. An excellent overview of Maroon history, culture, and art.

Stedman, J. 1796. *Narrative of a Five-years' Expedition Against the Revolted Negroes of Surinam*. London: J. Johnson and J. Edwards. An extraordinary account of a British mercenary sent to Dutch Guiana to capture runaway slaves and who not only begins to sympathize with the slaves, but falls in love with one of them. Someone should make a movie of this book.

## Chapter 4

Hames, R., and W. Vickers, eds. 1983. *Adaptive Responses of Native Amazonians.* New York: Academic Press. Anthropological essays on how different tribes utilize tropical resources.

Im Thurn, E. 1967. *Among the Indians of Guiana.* New York: Dover. Originally published in 1883, this travelogue teems with vivid accounts of the plants, animals, and Amerindians of British Guiana.

Maxwell, N. 1961. *Witch Doctor's Apprentice.* Boston: Houghton-Mifflin. A female ethnobotanist's travels and travails in Colombia and Peru.

Plotkin, M. 1988. Ethnobotany and conservation in the Guianas: The Indians of southern Suriname. In F. Almeda and C. Pringle, eds., *Tropical Rainforests: Diversity and Conservation* (pp. 87–109). San Francisco: California Academy of Sciences.

## Chapter 5

DeFilipps, R. 1991. The History of Non-timber Forest Products from the Guianas. In M. Plotkin and L. Famolare, eds., *Sustainable Harvest and Marketing of Rain Forest Products* (pp. 73–89). Washington, D.C.: Island Press.

Plotkin, M. 1990. *Strychnos medeola:* A New Arrow Poison from Suriname. In D. A. Posey, ed., *Ethnobiology: Implications and Applications* (pp. 3–9). Belém, Brazil: Museu Goeldi.

Thomas, K. 1963. *Curare.* Philadelphia: Lippincott. A readable survey of the history, botany, and chemistry of curare.

Waterton, C. 1984. *Wanderings in South America.* London: Century Publishing. Still fun to read almost two centuries after it was first published.

## Chapter 6

Bodley, J. 1982. *Victims of Progress.* Menlo Park, CA: Benjamin/Cummings Publishing. A scathing indictment of the treatment of tribal peoples by western society.

Frikel, P. 1973. *Os Tiriyos: Seu Sistema Adaptivo.* Hanover, Germany: Kommisionsverlag Munsstermann-Druck. A good ethnographic study of the Brazilian Tiriós that, unfortunately, has not been translated into English.

Hemmings, J. *Red Gold.* Cambridge, MA: Harvard University Press. An often heartbreaking history of what has happened to Brazil's original inhabitants since the arrival of the Europeans.

Sarmiento, G. 1984. *The Ecology of Neotropical Savannas.* Cambridge, MA:

Harvard University Press. The standard reference on Neotropical savannas.

## Chapter 7

Eliade, M. 1974. *Shamanism*. Princeton, NJ: Princeton University Press. An important survey of shamanism around the world.

Middleton, J., ed. 1982. *Magic, Witchcraft, and Curing*. Austin: University of Texas Press. Sixteen articles on the subject, based on studies of over ten different tribes.

Reichel-Dolmatoff, G. 1975. *The Shaman and the Jaguar*. Philadelphia: Temple University Press. Classic study of shamanism in the northwest Amazon.

Vogel, V. 1970. *American Indian Medicine*. Norman, OK: University of Oklahoma Press. An encyclopedic account of Amerindian curing practices.

Wilbert, J. 1987. *Tobacco and Shamanism in South America*. New Haven, CT: Yale University Press. A detailed account by a leading anthropologist.

## Chapter 8

Chagnon, N. 1992. *Yanomamo: The Last Days of Eden*. New York: Harcourt, Brace, Jovanovich. A substantially revised version of *Yanomamo: The Fierce People*, the standard college text that led so many students to choose careers in anthropology.

Donner, F. 1982. *Shabono*. New York: Delacorte. An enthralling account of a woman who leaves Western civilization behind to live life as a Yanomamo. Although some anthropologists consider it fiction, it is a wonderful read.

Lizot, J. 1986. *Tales of the Yanomamo*. New York: Cambridge Press. Along with Chagnon, Lizot is the leading authority on the Yanomamo. This excellent book details the life of these Indians through the eyes of an anthropologist who lived with them for well over a decade.

Schultes, R. E., and A. Hofmann. 1992. *Plants of the Gods*. Rochester, VT: Healing Arts Press. Well-written and beautifully illustrated popular book on hallucinogenic plants.

## Chapter 9

Caufield, C. 1985. *In the Rainforest.* New York: Knopf. The best popular account of rain forest conservation around the world.

Goodstein, C. 1992. Is There a Doctor in the Jungle? *Elle* 8(2), 146–147. A brief account of the Shaman's Apprentice Program in Costa Rica.

Plotkin, M., and L. Famolare, eds. 1992. *Sustainable Harvest and Marketing of Rain Forest Products.* Washington, DC: Island Press. An anthology on the past, present, and future of sustainable harvest, featuring articles by leading thinkers on the subject, such as J. Clay, D. Posey, R. E. Schultes, and V. Toledo.

## ADDITIONAL REFERENCES

de Acuña, C. [1641] 1859. Nuevo Descubrimiento del Gran Río de las Amazonas (Madrid). Translated by C. R. Markham. In *Expeditions into the Valley of the Amazons* 24 (pp. 41–134). London: Hakluyt Society.

Anderson, E. 1954. *Plants, Man and Life.* London: A. Melrose.

Aublet, F. 1775. *Histoire des Plantes de la Guiane Françoise.* Paris: Didot.

Avé, W., and S. Sunito. 1990. *Medicinal plants of Siberut.* Report to World Wide Fund for Nature, Gland, Switzerland.

Bancroft, E. 1769. *Essay on the Natural History of Guiana and South America.* London: Becket and De Hondt.

Bates, H. 1863. *The Naturalist on the River Amazons.* London: J. Murray.

Benzoni, G. 1565. *Historia Del Mondo Nuovo.* Venice: F. Rampazetto.

Brown, B. 1876. *Canoe and Camp Life in British Guiana.* London: E. Stanford.

de las Casas, B. 1909. *Apolegética Historia de las Indias.* Madrid: Baily, Bailliere e Hijos.

Carr, A. 1940. A Contribution to the Herpetology of Florida. *Biological Science Series* (University of Florida) 3(1).

Caufield, C. 1982. *Tropical Moist Forests.* International Institute for Environment and Development, London.

Coudreau, H. 1886. *La France Équinoxiale.* Paris: Librairie Hachette.

Crevaux, J. 1879. Voyages d'Exploration dans l'Intérieur des Guyanes. *Le Tour du Monde* 37, 337–416.

Diamond, J. 1989. The Ethnobiologist's Dilemma. *Natural History* 6(89), 27–30.

Farabee, W. C. 1924. *The Central Caribs* (Series No. 10). University of Pennsylvania Museum Anthropological Publications, Philadelphia.

Furst, P. 1976. *Hallucinogens and Culture.* San Francisco: Chandler and Sharp.

Gottlieb, O. 1981. New and Underutilized Plants in the Americas: Solution to Problems of Inventory Through Systematics. *Interciencia* 6(1), 22–29.

Gumilla, J. 1745. *El Orinoco*. Madrid: M. Fernandez.

Hemming, J. 1987. *Amazon Frontier*. Cambridge, MA: Harvard University Press.

von Humboldt, A.; and A. Bonpland. 1852–53. *Personal Narrative of Travels to the Equinoctial Regions of America*. Edited and translated by T. Ross. London: H. G. Bohn.

Juma, C. 1989. *The Gene Hunters*. Princeton, NJ: Princeton University Press.

King, James I. 1604. *A Counterblaste to Tobacco*. London: R. Barker.

Koch-Grünberg, T. 1909. *Zwei Jahre unter den Indianern*. Berlin: E. Wasmuth.

Lee, R. J. 1982. Charles Waterton's First Journey Throuh Guyana. In G. Watson, ed., *Charles Waterton* (pp. 32–33). Wakefield, U.K.: Yorkshire Communications.

Lewin, L. 1964. *Phantasica*. London: Routledge and Kegan Paul.

Lewis, W., and M. Elvin-Lewis. 1977. *Medical Botany*. New York: Wiley-Interscience.

Lindemann, J. 1953. The Vegetation of the Coastal Region of Surinam. *The Vegetation of Surinam* 1(1), 1–135.

Lovejoy, T. 1984. The Tropical Rain Forest—Greatest Expression of Life on Earth. In R. Mittermeier and M. Plotkin, eds., *Primates and the Tropical Forest* (pp. 45–48). Pasadena, CA: Leakey Foundation.

Moore, H. 1973. The Major Groups of Palms and Their Distribution. *Gentes Herb.* 11, 27–141.

Naipaul, V. S. 1962. *The Middle Passage*. London: A. Deutsch.

Plotkin, M., R. Mittermeier, and I. Constable. 1980. Psychotomimetic Use of Tobacco in Surinam and French Guiana. *J. Ethnopharm* 2, 295–297.

Plowman, T. 1977. *Brunfelsia* in Ethnomedicine (Botanial Museum Leaflet no. 25 [10], pp. 239–309). Cambridge, MA: Harvard University.

von Roosmalen, M. 1985. *Fruits of the Guianan Flora*. Utrecht, Holland: Institute of Systematic Botany.

Roth, W. 1924. *An introductory study of the arts, crafts and customs of the Guiana Indians*. Thirty-eighth annual report of the Bureau of American Ethnology, Smithsonian Institution, Washington, D.C.

Schomburgk, O. A. 1931. *Robert H. Schomburgk's Travels in Guiana and on the Orinoco During the Years 1835–1839*. Translated by W. Roth. Georgetown, British Guiana: Argosy.

Schomburgk, Richard. 1923. *Travels in British Guiana 1840–1844*. Translated by W. Roth. Georgetown, British Guiana: Daily Chronicle Office.

Schultes, R. E. 1973. Orchids and Human Affairs: What of the Future? (Bulletin No. 42, pp. 785–789). American Orchid Society. Cambridge, MA.

———. 1974. Palms and Religion in the Northwest Amazon. *Principes* 18, 3–21.

Slotkin. J. 1956. *The Peyote Religion.* Glencoe, IL: Free Press.

Smith, N., J. Williams, D. Plucknett, and J. Talbot. 1992. *Tropical Forests and their Crops.* Ithaca, NY: Comstock Publishing.

Wallace, A. 1853. *Palm Trees of the Amazon.* London: J. van Vorst.

# Plant Glossary

**Acalypha**—*Acalypha hispida* Euphorbiaceae (Rubber family): Also known as the monkey's tail plant because of its hanging fuzzy inflorescences, this species is cultivated throughout the tropics. Acalypha probably originated in tropical Asia.

**Aconite**—*Aconitum napellus* Ranunculaceae (Buttercup family): Aconite (also known as monkshood because of the shape of the flower) is native to Central Europe. Rich in alkaloids, it was previously used to treat fever and pain. Aconite was also a standard ingredient in witches' brews in medieval Europe.

***Agrobigi***—*Parkia nitida* Leguminosae (Legume family): Trees of this species typically exceed one hundred feet and have huge buttress roots. The bark of trees of this genus is said to be rich in tannins, which would explain why people in various parts of the Amazon are said to take a bark of the tea to treat dysentery. About twenty-five species of this genus are known from Amazonia.

***Ah-de-gah-nah-mah***—*Theobroma subincanum* Sterculiaceae: This tree is usually found growing on or near riverbanks. The Tiriós value the twigs as kindling to start fires.

***Ah-kah-de-mah***—*Cissampelos sp.* Menispermaceae (Moonseed family): *See* CURARE.

***Ah-kah-nah-pah-to-do-to-do***—*Herrania kanukuensis* Sterculiaceae (Cacao family): The fruit of this species is one of the tastiest in all of Amazonia. The Latin name of the species indicates that it was first found by Western scientists in the Kanuku Mountains of southwestern Guyana. *Kanuku* means "rich forest" in the Macushi Indian language.

***Ah-ku-de am-pe-de***—*Casearia pitumba* Flacourtiaceae (Flacourtia family): The Tirió Indian name for this plant means "agouti smell," though to me and many other biologists agoutis have no characteristic aroma. This is yet another example of how acute is the Indians' sense of smell—many times I have been on some jungle trail in search of plants when my Indian guide would say "Smell that? A tapir [or a jaguar or a giant armadillo] just passed here!" and I couldn't smell anything unusual.

**Ah-ku-de-tu-mah**—*Theobroma sp.* Sterculiaceae: Native to the Neotropics, this genus (which means "Food of the Gods") includes about thirty species, the best known of which is *T. cacao*, the chocolate of commerce. *Cupuacu* (*T. grandiflorum*) is extremely popular in Brazil and some compare it favorably to chocolate. To me, however, it smells of old gym socks.

**Ah-mo-de-ah-tuh**—*Tanaecium nocturnum* Bignoniaceae (Catalpa family): According to Dr. Ghillean Prance, director of the Royal Botanic Gardens outside London, the Paumari Indians of southwestern Brazil prepare a hallucinogenic snuff from this species.

**Ah-tuh-ri-mah**—*Gurania sp.* Cucurbitaceae (Cucumber family): This genus contains seventy-five species, all of which are found in the Neotropics. As far as I know, the Tiriós are the only tribe reported to use this vine for medicinal purposes.

**Al-lah-ku-pah-ne**—*Piper sp.* Piperaceae: This small vine is usually found growing near streams. Although it is usually employed as a curare admixture, the Brazilian Tiriós claim that this particular species is poisonous. Slipped into a drink like cassava beer, it is said to cause somnolence and, eventually, a painless death.

**Al-lah-wah-tah-wah-ku**—*Piper sp.* Piperaceae (Black pepper family): This genus contains approximately two thousand species, most of which are climbing shrubs or small trees. The roots of several species are used in the northeast Amazon as analgesics for the relief of toothache, the crushed root being applied directly to the aching tooth. These roots are probably rich in essential oils, which would explain their painkilling properties (much as clove oil is used in this country).

**Allspice**—*Pimenta dioica* Lauraceae (Cinnamon family): Allspice is the only major spice grown almost exclusively in the New World. The name *allspice* is said to be derived from the fact that it tastes like a combination of cinnamon, cloves, and nutmeg. Although it is best known because of its use in baked goods, allspice is an important pickling spice (it's the tiny black spheres at the bottom of every jar of pickles) and a major flavoring in Benedictine liqueur.

**Ama-asi**—*Elizabetha princeps* Leguminosae: Although Schultes has stated that this beautiful tree is not common, it lines the banks along some sections of the Manaviche River in southern Venezuela. The Yanomamo in both Brazil and Venezuela add the burned bark of this tree to one of their hallucinogenic snuffs.

**Assaí**—*Euterpe oleracea* Palmae (Palm family): The purple fruit of this palm is the source of a major forest industry in the Amazon estuary. Not only is the fruit mixed with water and sugar and made into a gruel that may be eaten up to three times a day by local peasants, but it is also made into cakes, ice cream, and even a liqueur in some of the better restaurants in Belém, the major port city at the mouth of the river.

**Attalea**—*Attalea maripa* Palmae: Often found on riverbanks in the northeast Amazon, the fruit of this species is one of the most sought-after by local Indians. The ripe fruit has only a thin pulp (botanically, a mesocarp), but it tastes something like a Creamsicle!

**Avocado**—*Persea americana* Lauraceae: Native to Central America, avocados range in size from that of a hen's egg to over four pounds. At least three distinct commercial varieties are recognized: Guatemalan, Mexican, and West Indian.

**Ay-ah-e-yah**—*Lonchocarpus sp.* Leguminosae: This yellow-wooded liana is used as a fish poison by the Indians of the northeast Amazon. The active principle is rotenone, which is used around the world as a biodegradable insecticide.

**Ay-mah-rah-e-wah**—*Eschweilera corrugata* Lecythidaceae (Brazil nut family): The 120 species known from this genus are restricted to tropical America. This particular species has buttress roots and often reaches over a hundred feet.

**Balata**—*Manilkara bidentata* Sapotaceae (Sapote family): This common tree produces both a high-quality wood and a high-quality inelastic latex. Because the latex (unlike rubber) does not stretch, it was previously used for making machine belting, but has since been replaced with synthetics.

**Bamboo**—*Bambusa sp.* Gramineae (Grass family): This genus contains about seventy species, which are distributed throughout the tropical and subtropical regions of both the Old World and New World. Bamboo's characteristic strength and light weight make it one of the world's most useful groups of plants.

**Banana**—*Musa paradisiaca* Musaceae (Banana family): Bananas are native to Southeast Asia and occur in a wide variety of shapes, colors, tastes, and textures. Over seventy varieties are known from the Philippines alone.

***Banisteriopsis***—*Banisteriopsis caapi* Malpighiaceae (Malpighia family): See CAAPI.

**Bark cloth**—*Broussonetia papyrifera* Moraceae (Fig family): Peoples of Polynesia prepared their cloth by peeling the bark off this tree, soaking it in water, and then pounding the strips together with a wooden mallet.

***Batibati***—*Ambelania acida* Apocynaceae (Dogbane family): This tree is common in the rain forest understory of the northeast Amazon. The fruit is edible.

**Belladona**—*Atropa belladonna* Solanaceae (Potato family): The name *belladona* means "beautiful lady." In medieval Europe, women would use eyedrops made from this plant that would dilate their pupils, giving them a wide-eyed look then considered to be the height of fashion.

***Bergibita***—*Geissospermum argenteum* Apocynaceae: The bitter bark of this rain forest tree is rich in alkaloids. Both the Maroons and the Indians of the northwest Amazon employ this tree for medicinal purposes, usually as a treatment for fevers and/or stomachache.

**Black palm**—*Bactris sp.* Palmae: The wood of this species of palm is used throughout the Amazon to make both blowguns and hunting bows.

**Black walnut**—*Juglans nigra* Juglandaceae (Walnut family): Native to eastern North America, the black walnut is one of our tallest species, capable of reaching a height of over 140 feet. Not only is the nut edible, but the wood is extremely valuable.

**Blueberry**—*Vaccinium* spp. Ericaceae (Heather family): In light of the fact that apples are native to Eurasia, it might be better to say "As American as *blueberry* pie," since blueberries are one of the few fruits native to North America. Today they are grown commercially in the United States, Belgium, Germany, and the Netherlands.

***Boegroe-maka***—*Astrocaryum sciophilum* Palmae: This genus contains fifty species found in tropical America. Several species produce a high-quality fiber and a useful oil. This particular species sometimes forms pure stands in southern Suriname.

**Bougainvillea**—*Bougainvillea spectabilis* Nyctaginaceae (Four o'clock family): This ornamental is grown throughout the tropics. What most people consider to be the characteristic red flowers are actually modified leaves known as bracts.

**Brassavola**—*Brassavola martiana* Orchidaceae (Orchid family): In Suriname, this species is usually found growing on or near riverbanks. A better-known species is *B. nodosa*, which is found from Mexico south to Peru and in the West Indies. In the Choco region of western Colombia, I found this species growing above the waterline on boulders in the Pacific!

**Brazil nut**—*Bertholettia excelsa* Lecythidaceae: Brazil nut trees may reach a height of 150 feet. The specialized fruit, known as a pyxidium, looks like a coconut and may weigh over four pounds. Inside the fruit are up to twenty-four seeds, what we know as "Brazil nuts."

**Breadfruit**—*Artocarpus altilis* Moraceae (Fig family): Native to Southeast Asia, this tree is now planted throughout the tropics. The notorious "Mutiny on the *Bounty*" in 1789 occurred during a voyage carrying breadfruit tree seedlings from the South Seas to the Caribbean. The British believed the breadfruit would provide a cheap source of food for slaves.

**Buckwax**—*Symphonia globulifera* Guttiferae (St. Johnswort family): This large tree has stilt roots and is found throughout the Amazon. Its copious yellow latex was once dried and used as a form of currency among Indians in the northeast Amazon. In Amazonian Brazil, peasants sometimes make furniture from the wood.

**Caapi**—*Banisteriopsis caapi* Malpighiaceae: Caapi, also known as *Ayahuasca* ("vine of the soul" in the Quechua Indian language), is the most common hallucinogenic plant in use among tribes of the western Amazon. A detailed account is given in Schultes and Hofmann, *Plants of the Gods* (see Recommended Reading section).

**Camu-camu**—*Myrciaria dubia* Myrtaceae (Myrtle family): With the highest known concentration of vitamin C known in the plant kingdom, this species holds real economic promise for the future. It is already made into a popular ice cream in Iquitos, Peru.

**Caraná**—*Mauritia carana* Palmae: The leaves of this palm are used for thatch in the Río Negro region of the Brazilian Amazon.

**Cardamom**—*Elettaria cardamom* Zingiberaceae (Ginger family): Cardamom is native to south India and Sri Lanka. It is perhaps best known to the Western world as the ingredient in Arabic coffee that provides its unique flavor.

**Cassava**—*Manihot esculenta* Euphorbiaceae: Cassava is one of the world's most important crops. Native to the Amazon, it is as popular in tropical Africa as it is in its native land. Ironically, although the young leaves make a delicious green vegetable, many Amazonian tribes do not eat them.

**Cassia**—*Cassia alata* Leguminosae: This six-foot shrub is typically found in the Guianas either in secondary vegetation or along riverbanks. The Maroons rub the crushed leaves on skin infections, considering them a highly effective treatment.

**Chicle**—*Manilkara achras* Sapotaceae: Known as the *sapote, sapodilla,* and *nispero* in its native Central America, the fruit of this tree is exceptionally sweet and tasty. The wood was used by the Mayans in the construction of their temples and the latex was chewed by them and other pre-Columbian tribes as a masticatory.

**Chocolate**—*Theobroma cacao* Sterculiaceae: Chocolate is native to the Amazon, although it was transported to Central America thousands of years before the arrival of Columbus. Although the Amazonian Indians tend to eat only the white seed coat, what we know as chocolate is made from the roasted fermented seeds.

**Cinnamon**—*Cinnamomum zeylanicum* Lauraceae: The cinnamon tree is native to south India and Sri Lanka. The spice is prepared from the dried inner bark.

**Cloves**—*Syzygium aromaticum* Myrtaceae (Myrtle family): Native to the Moluccas, the so-called "Spice Islands" of Indonesia, cloves are dried flower buds. Cloves have been part of international trade for thousands of years and have been used as a spice, a medicine, a breath freshener, a fumitory, and a perfume. Today the largest producer of cloves is the island of Zanzibar.

**Coca**—*Erythroxylum coca* Erythroxylaceae (Coca family): Native to western South America, coca leaf is one of the world's most effective medicinal plants, particularly valuable for the treatment of stomachache and altitude sickness. Unfortunately, the alkaloid cocaine when taken in its purified form (which the Indians never do) is highly addictive.

**Coffee**—*Coffea arabica* Rubiaceae (Coffee family): This species, known commercially as "arabica coffee," along with *C. canephora*, known as "robusta coffee," are the most common commercial species. The island of Madagascar is home to dozens of wild species, all of which are naturally caffeine-free.

*Copaiba*—*Copaifera sp.* Leguminosae: About twenty-five species of this genus are found in tropical America. The clear yellowish resin is valued in the Amazon to treat a variety of ailments, including coughs, psoriasis, and gonorrhea sores.

**Copal**—*Copaifera* spp. *See* COPAIBA.

**Corn**—*Zea mays* Gramineae: Native to middle America, corn is one of the world's most important crops. The United States is the top producer, growing more than two hundred thousand tons in 1989 alone.

**Cotton**—*Gossypium* spp. Malvaceae (Cotton family): Cotton is now grown throughout much of the tropics and subtropics. The fibers are actually seed hairs.

**Cranberry**—*Vaccinium macrocarpon* Ericaceae: Although native to northeastern North America, the cranberry is also produced commercially in Germany and Scandinavia.

**Curare**—Amazonian curares have traditionally been divided into two major types, based (oddly enough) on the types of containers the Indians stored them in: pots and tubes. Pot curare predominates in the eastern Amazon and usually features *Strychnos guianensis* of the Loganiaceae or Strychnos family as the toxic component. Tube curare is mostly made from *Chrondrodendron tomentosum* of the Menispermaceae or Moonseed family and is the curare of choice in western Amazonia. The curare used in modern medicine is made from the latter species, hence the trade name *tubocurarine*.

**Duroia**—*Duroia aquatica* Rubiaceae: This genus consists of about twenty-five species, all of which are trees native to South America. Many of these trees are myrmecophilous—that is, inhabited by stinging ants that protect the plant from other organisms like herbivores.

**Eh-ru-ku-ku**—*Dracontium asperum* Araceae: Thirteen species of this genus are found in tropical America. At least three different species are employed as snakebite remedies.

**Fly agaric**—*Amanita muscaria* Agaricaceae (Fly agaric family): This hallucinogenic mushroom has a long history of use by shamans in Siberia. It may also have been used in ancient India for similar purposes.

**Foxglove**—*Digitalis purpurea* Scrophulariaceae (Foxglove family): Native to Europe, these beautiful plants are the source of the heart stimulant digitalis.

**Ginkgo**—*Ginkgo biloba* Ginkgoaceae (Ginkgo family): Native to China, the ginkgo is the most ancient species of plant alive today. Long used in Oriental folk medicine, it is now being marketed in Europe to treat a variety of ailments. Although its exact effect on the human body is incompletely understood, some believe it may prove useful for treating even more ailments than it is already used for.

**Goebaja**—*Jacaranda copaia* Bignoniaceae: This hundred-foot tree is common in the Guianas. Several related species are cultivated throughout the tropics for their showy flowers.

**Go-lo-be**—*Gloeporus sp.* Polyporaceae (Polypora family): Species of this genus are found in both the tropics and the subtropics. Alkaloids are known from this family.

**Gongora**—*Gongora sp.* Orchidaceae: The twenty species of *Gongora* orchids are native to the American tropics.

**Gooseberry**—*Ribes* spp. Grossulariaceae (Gooseberry family): The 150 species in this genus tend to be found in cooler climes. Gooseberries are related to currants.

**Guanabana**—*Annona muricata* Annonaceae (Annona family): Native to the New World tropics, this fruit has a green skin and a milky white flesh. It is grown commercially in Spain, Israel, Thailand, and Brazil.

**Guava**—*Psidium guayava* Myrtaceae: Originally from the New World tropics, guava is now widely grown in Asia and Africa as well. The fruit is said to harbor more vitamin C than citrus.

**Guayusa**—*Ilex guayusa* Aquifoliaceae (Holly family): The leaves of this species, native to South America, are rich in caffeine.

**Gutta percha**—*Palaquium gutta* Sapotaceae: The latex from this tropical Asian species was once used to fill root canals, cover golf balls, and insulate underwater cables. Its use has been largely superseded by synthetics.

**Heliconia**—*Heliconia psittacorum* Musaceae: The 120 species of this genus are found in the tropics. The species name for this one refers to its parrotlike coloration: green, yellow, and red with black spots.

**Hemlock**—*Conium maculatum* Umbelliferae (Carrot family): The four species of this genus are all very poisonous. This particular species was the one that Socrates drank.

**Henbane**—*Hyoscyamus* spp. Solanaceae: Native to Europe, the species of this genus known as henbane contain the alkaloids atropine, hyoscyamine, and scopolamine.

**Hisiomi**—*Anadenanthera peregrina* Leguminosae: This genus contains two species native to tropical America. Indians grind the seeds—which are rich in hallucinogenic alkaloids—to make a potent snuff.

**Hogplum**—*Spondias mombin* Anacardiaceae (Poison ivy family): Hogplum is widespread in the Neotropics and is generally considered to be one of the world's best-tasting fruits. In Brazil, where it is known as *tap-erebá*, the fruit is made into both an ice cream and a liqueur.

**Inga**—*Inga edulis* Leguminosae: There are over two hundred species of *Inga* in tropical America. This species is widely cultivated.

**Ixora**—*Ixora coccinea* Rubiaceae: This species is native to Indonesia. Ironically, it is the national flower of Suriname.

**Jaboticaba**—*Myrciaria cauliflora* Myrtaceae: This thirty-foot tree produces a sweet black fruit. In Brazil, it is made into a popular jam.

**Jará**—*Leopoldinia pulchra* Palmae: The fruit of this species is made into an edible paste. The closely related *piassaba* palm (*L. piassaba*) produces one of the best of all plant fibers.

**Jarakopi**—*Siparuna guianensis* Monimiaceae (Monimia family): This thirty-foot tree is widespread in Amazonia. In the Guianas, both the Maroons and the Indians take a tea of the leaves to treat fevers.

**Jeajeamadou**—*Virola sp.* Myristicaceae (Nutmeg family): There are sixty species of *Virola* in South and Central America. Some species provide excellent timber while others produce a hallucinogenic resin used ceremonially by several Amazonian tribes (see Schultes and Hofmann, 1992, in the Recommended Reading section).

**Jerusalem artichoke**—*Helianthus tuberosus* Compositae (Daisy family): Neither from Jerusalem nor an artichoke, this sunflower relative is native to North America. This plant was first taken to Europe in the early seventeenth century and ever since the edible tuber has been more popular there than here.

**Kah-lo-she-wuh**—*Rollinia exsucca* Annonaceae: This fifteen- to twenty-five-foot tree is not uncommon in the rain forests of the Guianas. Other species of this genus are said to have edible fruit.

**Kah-mah-ke**—*Ambelania acida* Apocynaceae: See BATIBATI.

**Kakabroekoe**—*Swartzia benthamiana* Leguminosae: This seventy-five-foot tree is common in the Guianas.

**Kam-hi-det**—*Syngonium sp.* Araceae (Philodendron family): The twenty species of this genus are found in tropical America. All are large, climbing herbs.

**Kanahyeh**—*Triplaris surinamensis* Polygonaceae (Buckwheat family): All twenty species of this genus harbor stinging ants. This particular species is often found near rivers.

**Koi**—*Mauritia flexuosa* Palmae: This is the most beautiful, the most widespread, and the most useful of the Amazonian palms. In Brazil alone, where it is known as *Buriti*, this palm serves as the source of wood for canoes and houses, thatch for roofing, edible fruit, edible starch, and a high-quality fiber for weaving hammocks.

**Ko-no-lo-po-kan**—*Piper sp.* Piperaceae: *See* AL-LAH-WAH-TAH-WAH-KU.

**Ko-noy-uh**—*Renealmia exaltata* Zingiberaceae: The seventy-five species of this genus are restricted to tropical America and west Africa. In the Guianas, species of this genus are used both by the Maroons and the Indians as a tea to treat fevers.

**Konsaka wiwiri**—*Peperomia pellucida* Piperaceae: This common South American herb is used by the Creoles, the Maroons, and the Indians for an astonishing variety of purposes: to treat gum problems, as a hypotensive agent, and even to exorcise demons.

**Ku-deh-deh**—*Cecropia sciadophylla* Moraceae: The one hundred species of this genus are restricted to the American tropics. This particular species is one of the few that is not inhabited by aggressive ants.

**Ku-mah-kah**—*Ceiba pentandra* Bombacaceae (Balsa tree family): Commonly known as the kapok tree, the seed hairs of this enormous (over two hundred feet) tree were once used to stuff life vests. Harpy eagles often build their nest in this species, from which they search for sloths in the surrounding forest.

**Ku-mu**—*Oenocarpus bacaba* Palmae: This sixty-foot palm is a common Amazonian species. The fruit produces an oil similar to olive oil.

**Ku-nah-ne-mah**—*Mikania sp.* Compositae: This genus contains 250 species, all but two of which are native to tropical America. The other two species are found in South Africa.

**Ku-neh-beh-beh**—*Marcgravia sp.* Marcgraviaceae (Marcgravia family): There are fifty-five species known from this genus, all restricted to tropical America. The Tirió name for this particular species means "centipede," a reference to this liana's resemblance to the invertebrate as it grows up the bark of a forest tree in search of the canopy.

**Ku-pe-de-yuh**—*Brunfelsia guianensis* Solanaceae: The flowers of this genus often change color as they grow older. I have seen trees in Ecuador with three different-colored flowers growing on them, looking like the results of a genetic engineering experiment.

**Ku-run-yeh**—*Rinorea sp.* Violaceae (Violet family): This graceful six-foot tree is often found growing near creeks in the rain forest of the Guianas.

**Ku-tah-de**—*Swartzia sp.* Leguminosae. *See* KAKABROEKOE.

**Kuwato**—*Caryocar villosum* Caryocaraceae (Caryocar family): This tree sometimes attains a height in excess of 150 feet. The Indians consider the nuts to be much tastier than Brazil nuts.

**Kwatta kama**—*Parkia pendula* Leguminosae: The vernacular name of this large tree means "spider monkey bed," a reference to the broad flat crown that this monkey is supposed to sleep in. The Maroons consider a tea of the bark to be a panacea for stomach ailments. Near some villages almost all the bark up to six feet above the ground has been scraped away—a practice that often kills the tree.

**Kwe-i-ah-ku-wah-nu-puh**—*Gnetum urens* Gnetaceae (Ephedra family): This liana is often found growing near rivers and creeks. The fruit contains an edible seed the size and shape of a half cigarette and that tastes like a walnut when it is roasted.

**Letterwood**—*Helicostylis pedunculata* Moraceae: The bark of this seventy-foot tree is said to be made into a hallucinogenic drink by the Carib Indians of coastal Suriname. Most of the reports, however, are based on secondhand information.

**Lime**—*Citrus aurantifolia* Rutaceae (Lemon family): Citrus fruits had their origin in tropical Asia. Different species and varieties of citrus are now grown in a hundred countries.

**Mace**—*Myristica fragrans* Myristicaceae: Nutmeg and mace are the only spices in commercial trade that are produced by separate parts of the same fruit. Nutmeg is made from the dried seed, while mace is the dried seed cover known botanically as the aril.

**Mahot cochon**—*Sterculia excelsa* Sterculiaceae: This ninety-foot tree is usually found near watercourses in the rain forests of the Guianas.

**Mah-rah-re-uh**—*Geonoma baculifera* Palmae: Widespread in northern South America, this palm thrives in swampy areas.

**Mah-tah-ke**—*Symphonia globulifera* Guttiferae: *See* BUCKWAX.

**Malacca apple**—*Syzygium malaccensis* Myrtaceae: Native to the Malay Peninsula, this species produces a red, pear-shaped fruit with a waxy yet agreeable taste. It often fruits all year round.

**Mammee**—*Mammea americana* Guttiferae: Native to the West Indies, this tree is now cultivated from Florida to Brazil. The fruit can be eaten fresh or made into jam or ice cream.

**Mamukure**—*Strychnos guianensis* Loganiaceae (Logania family): This is one of the most common species of *Strychnos* in Amazonia. In the northeast Amazon, it is used as a component in curare recipes by the Tiriós, the Waiwais, the Wayanas, and the Yanomamo.

**Mandrake**—*Mandragora officinarum* Solanaceae: Rich in the alkaloids atropine and scopolamine, mandrake was long considered a magic plant in medieval Europe. It was considered bad luck to touch a mandrake that was growing, so when the plant was needed for medicinal purposes (such as to kill pain or induce sleep), one end of a string was tied to the plant while the other was tied around the neck of a dog, which was then chased until it had uprooted the mandrake.

**Mango**—*Mangifera indica* Anacardiaceae: Native to Southeast Asia, the mango is now grown around the world. There are hundreds of different varieties.

**Mangosteen**—*Garcinia mangostana* Guttiferae: Native to Southeast Asia, the mangosteen has never been cultivated as widely as the mango. A single mangosteen tree can yield over a thousand fruits in a year.

**Maniballi**—*Moronobea coccinea* Guttiferae: This hundred-foot tree is usually found on rain-forest-covered slopes in the Guianas.

**Manila hemp**—*Musa textilis* Musaceae: Also known as *Abacá*, Manila hemp has been used to make everything from ropes to dollar bills.

**Maracuja**—*Passiflora edulis* Passifloraceae (Passion fruit family): Also known as the purple granadilla, this species produces a delicious fruit. Although native to the Amazon, it is now grown commercially in Kenya and South Africa.

**Marijuana**—*Cannabis sativa* Cannabaceae (Cannabis family): This well-known drug plant is native to the Old World. Although the use of this species has been outlawed in the United States since the 1930s, another species (*C. indica*) is actually more potent. Several cases against pot smokers in the 1960s were lost when the government was unable to prove that the substance seized was *C. sativa* and not one of the other two species.

**Maripa**—*Attalea maripa* Palmae: See ATTALEA.

**Mashohara**—*Justicia pectoralis* Acanthaceae (Acanthus family): The leaves of this aromatic herb are often added to hallucinogenic snuff by the Yanomamo. Whether this species has any particularly potent chemical components or whether the Indians just like the flavor provided by this plant remains unclear.

**Masoesa**—*Renealmia exaltata* Zingiberaceae: See KO-NOY-UH.

**Maveve**—*Solanum surinamense* Solanaceae: This shrub is commonly found growing in disturbed vegetation in Suriname.

**Mayapple**—*Podophyllum peltatum* Berberidaceae (Mayapple family): Native to northeastern North America, the yellow fruit is edible. In pre-Columbian times the Indians used the underground stems both as a purgative and to burn off warts.

**Me-de-bo-no**—*Cymbopetalum sp.* Annonaceae: The eleven species of this genus are found in tropical America. This particular species seems to be fairly common in the rain forests of the Guianas.

**Meh-nu**—*Genipa americana* Rubiaceae: Native to the Amazon, the fruit of this tree is grated and mixed with ashes to produce a blue skin dye popular among Amazonian Indians.

**Mispel**—*Aciotis sp.* Melastomataceae (Melastoma family): The thirty species of this genus are found in tropical America.

**Mokomoko**—*Montrichardia arborescens* Araceae: This species is widespread in Amazonia. The large, heart-shaped leaves are a common sight along Amazonian rivers.

**Montjoly**—*Cordia macrostachya* Boraginaceae (Borage family): This genus contains over two hundred species found throughout the tropics and the subtropics. This particular species is found near rivers in the Guianas.

**Mo-pa**—*Spondias mombin* Anacardiaceae: *See* HOGPLUM.

**Morning glory**—*Ipomoea spp.* Convolvulaceae (Morning glory family): The five hundred species of this genus are found in the tropics and warmer portions of the temperate regions. One species (*I. batatas*) is the sweet potato, while another (*I. pes-caprae*) is a common creeper found on tropical beaches throughout the world. A related species (*Rivea corymbosa*) was employed as a hallucinogen in pre-Columbian Mexico (see Schultes and Hofmann, 1993, in the Recommended Reading section).

**Mu-ru-mu-ru**—*Astrocaryum sciophilum* Palmae: *See* BOEGROE-MAKA.

**Nah-puh-de-ot**—*Heisteria sp.* Olacaceae (Olax famly): The fifty species of this genus are found in both West Africa and tropical America. This particular species thrives near rain forest creeks.

**No-lo-e-muh**—*Piper augustum* Piperaceae: This species is widespread in northern South America.

**Nutmeg**—*Myristica fragrans* Myristicaceae: *See* MACE.

**Nyakwana**—*Virola sp.* Myristicaceae: *See* JEAJEAMADOU.

**O-ko-ne-de-kuh**—*Lacunaria jenmanni* Quiinaceae (Quiina family): The eleven species of this genus are restricted to tropical South America. This particular tree species is common in the Guianas.

**Oncidium**—*Oncidium sp.* Orchidaceae: This huge genus (350 species) of orchids is only found in the New World. Most species are epiphytes and have yellow flowers.

**Opium**—*Papaver somniferum* Papaveraceae (Opium family): Native to central Eurasia, opium has been used for medicinal purposes for thousands of years. This species still provides us with some of our most important therapeutic compounds like codeine and morphine as well as heroin, which is one of our most addictive drugs. Opium is actually the dried latex extracted from unripe fruits.

**Orange**—*Citrus sinensis* Rutaceae: *See* LIME.

**Pacific yew**—*Taxus brevifolia* Taxaceae (Yew family): The ten species of this genus are found only in the temperate zone. In the Middle Ages, the wood of the common yew (*T. baccata*) was used to make bows. Ironically, the wood of the Pacific yew (which is providing the taxol employed in the treatment of ovarian cancer) was until recently considered of no commercial value and was often knocked down in the course of commercial logging and left to rot.

**Pah-nah-ra-pah-nah**—*Phytolacca americana* Phytolaccaceae (Pokeweed family): The leaves of this herbaceous species are boiled and eaten like spinach in both Suriname and Guyana. Research on related species at the University of Texas found that some plants of the genus apparently have antiviral properties.

**Papaya**—*Carica papaya* Caricaceae (Papaya family): Native to South America, the papaya is now grown throughout the tropics. A tree can produce fruit within a year of planting. In Suriname, the unripe papaya is sometimes boiled and eaten as a green vegetable.

**Paprika**—*Capsicum annuum* Solanaceae: This species features many varieties—not only the one that produces paprika, but also all the so-called "sweet" peppers like bell peppers, as well as some of the "hot" varieties. The most famous of the spicy varieties—the Tabasco pepper—is *C. frutescens.*

**Pashiúba**—*Socratea exorrhiza* Palmae: Known as a "stilt palm" because the stem may be six feet off the forest floor, borne aloft by aerial roots, this species and related species of both this genus and the related *Iriartea* must be considered among the Amazon's oddest species.

**Pashiúba barriguda**—*Iriartea ventricosa* Palmae: *See* PASHIUBA.

**Passion fruit**—*Passiflora edulis* Passifloraceae: *See* MARACUJA.

**Peanut**—*Arachis hypogaea* Leguminosae: Native to tropical South America, the peanut exhibits the peculiar habit of ripening its fruit underground. As early as the sixteenth century, Portuguese navigators distributed plants throughout the tropics, hence the appearance of this legume in such "traditional" dishes as west Africa's peanut soup or Thailand's satay sauce. The major use of the peanut crop in the United States is to make peanut butter.

**Pecan**—*Carya illinoinensis* Juglandaceae (Walnut family): Native to North America, the pecan tree can attain a height of over 150 feet. Most pecans are grown in the United States, although plantations have also been established in Australia and South Africa.

**Petrea**—*Petrea bracteata* Verbenaceae (Teak family): Native to the Amazon, this species turns into a six-foot tree with beautiful purple flowers when planted in an urban garden. In the forest, however, this species is a liana that twines through the canopy and is all but impossible to see from the forest floor.

**Peyote**—*Lophophora williamsi* Cacataceae (Cactus family): Native to northern Mexico and southernmost Texas, this little cactus contains over twenty-five alkaloids. Long used for religious purposes by Amerindians, it is considered a sacrament by the Native American Church, whose adherents live in Canada, the United States, and Mexico (See Schultes and Hofmann, 1992, in the Recommended Reading section).

**Philodendron**—*Philodendron sp.* Araceae: The three hundred species of this genus are native to the Neotropics. The name *Philodendron* means "tree loving," a reference to the fact that these climbers are usually found growing on trees.

**Pineapple**—*Ananas comosus* Bromeliaceae (Bromeliad family): Native to Amazonia, pineapples were transplanted by the Portuguese to other parts of the tropics as early as 1502. Thailand is now the world's major producer of pineapples, a title long held by the Hawaiian Islands. Pineapples were originally brought to Hawaii from French Guiana in 1886.

*Piripiri*—*Cyperus* spp.—Cyperaceae (Sedge family): *Piripiri* is a sedge (or possibly several species of sedge) used for birth control and to induce labor.

*Poi-fuh*—*Piper sp.* Piperaceae: *See* AL-LAH-WAH-TAH-WAH-KU.

*Pom-weh*—*Capsicum sp.* Solanaceae: *See* PAPRIKA.

*Po-no*—*Couratari guianensis* Lecythidaceae: This 180-foot rain forest tree is common in the Guianas. The Sranan tongo name is *Ingi pipa*, meaning "Indian's pipe," a reference to the fact that Amerindian shamans sometimes use the conical fruit as a pipe in which they smoke special herbs during curing ceremonies.

**Potato**—*Solanum tuberosum* Solanaceae (Nightshade family): Native to the Andes, this plant was taken in the sixteenth century to Europe, where it became a staple in the diet of local peasants. In 1845 a fungal infestation attacked potatoes in Europe, a tragedy that was particularly devastating in Ireland since this species had become the country's most important crop. The result was large-scale starvation, one of the results of which was large-scale emigration to the United States.

*Pritjari*—*Zanthoxylum rhoifolium* Rutaceae: The one hundred species of this family are found in temperate and tropical Asia and America. This particular species is a small tree with a spiny bark.

*Puh-nah-tah-wah*—*Cassia quinquangulata* Leguminosae: This liana has a very distinctive five-sided stem. It is found in the Guianas in disturbed vegetation.

*Pupunha*—*Bactris gasipaes* Palmae: Also known as peach palm, this species produces a nutritious fruit that tastes like a chestnut. Commercial plantations have been established in Costa Rica and will probably be set up in many other tropical countries in the future, given the high-quality fruit that this palm produces.

**Quinine**—*Cinchona officinalis* Rubiaceae: First discovered by South American Indians, the bark of this tree has long served as our most effective treatment for malaria. Although quinine-resistant strains of malaria have appeared, quinine remains an important drug.

*Rasha*—*Bactris gasipaes* Palmae: *See* PUPUNHA.

**Raspberry**—*Rubus* spp. Rosaceae (Rose family): The 250 species of this genus are native to the northern temperate zones. This genus includes raspberries, blackberries, and loganberries.

**Red peppers**—*Capsicum sp.* Solanaceae: *See* PAPRIKA.

*Rediloksi*—*Hymenaea courbaril* Leguminosae: This hundred-foot tree is common in the Guianas. It produces a resinous gum that is used to make varnishes and as an incense in churches.

**Rice**—*Oryza sativa* Gramineae: Native to Southeast Asia, rice is the world's most important grain. About half of all people on earth eat rice on a daily basis.

**Rosewood**—*Aniba rosaedora* Lauraceae: This hundred-foot tree is the source of commercial rosewood oil. The tree is usually cut down so that the bark can be stripped, and this species has been wiped out in many parts of the Amazon.

**Rosy periwinkle**—*Catharanthus roseus* Apocynaceae: Native to Madagascar, this herb is the source of several major anticancer alkaloids. A related species, *C. coriaceous* from central Madagascar, is on the verge of extinction.

**Rubber**—*Hevea brasiliensis* Euphorbiaceae: Native to the Amazon, this tree produces a latex that remains an industrial raw material of great importance.

**Savanna cashew**—*Curatella americana* Dilleniaceae (Dillenia family): This twelve-foot tree is the most common woody plant on the savannas of the Guianas.

**Selaginella**—*Selaginella sp.* Selaginellaceae (Selaginella family): The seven hundred species of this genus are found mostly in the tropics.

*Sharabe*—*Oenocarpus bacaba* Palmae: See KU-MU.

*She-mah-ne*—*Hymenophyllum sp.* Hymenophyllaceae (Hymenophyllum family): Most of the twenty-five species of this genus of fern are found either in the tropics or in the southern temperate regions.

*Shetebahre*—*Jacaranda copaia* Bignoniaceae: See GOEBAJA.

*Sho*—*Caryocar villosum* Caryocaraceae: See KUWATO.

**Silk-grass**—*Ananas* spp.: Probably not a grass but the fibers of a wild pineapple.

**Snakewood**—*Brosimum sp.* Moraceae: This tree is the species of choice among Amerindians of the Guianas for making bows.

*Sopropo*—*Momordica charantia* Cucurbitaceae: The forty-five species of this genus are native to the Old World tropics. The bitter fruit of this species is an acquired taste that is difficult to acquire.

*Strychnos*—*Strychnos sp.* Loganiaceae: See MAMUKURE.

**Sugarcane**—*Saccharum officinarum* Gramineae: Native to Southeast Asia, sugarcane is a giant grass. Although sugarcane is susceptible to a variety of diseases, none of these diseases is found worldwide, so regional varieties of the plant are bred to resist specific diseases and new varieties are being developed all the time by crossbreeding.

**Sunflower**—*Helianthus annuus* Compositae: Native to North America, the sunflower is an extremely versatile plant in terms of its utility to people. Not only is it a beautiful ornamental, but the seeds contain a high-quality edible oil, the flowers a yellow dye, and the leaves can be used as fodder. Sunflower oil is also employed in the manufacture of paints and lubricants.

*Swartzia* (black bark)—*Swartzia arborescens* Leguminosae: The one hundred species of this genus are found in Africa and the Americas. This species is common in the Guianas and can attain a height of over sixty feet.

**Swartzia** (gray bark)—*Swartzia benthamiana* Leguminosae: *See* KAKA-BROEKOE.

**Sweet potato**—*Ipomoea batatas* Convolvulaceae: *See* MORNING GLORY.

**Tah-mo**—*Coccoloba sp.* Polygonaceae: This genus of 150 species is restricted to tropical and subtropical America. This particular species is either a shrub or a liana and is usually found near creeks and rivers. A related species (*C. uvifera*) is known as the sea grape and is made into a popular jam in Florida.

**Tah-mo-ko-ah-nu**—*Mucuna urens* Leguminosae: The 120 species of this genus are distributed throughout the tropics and subtropics. This particular species is a liana that is common in the Guianas.

**Tamarind**—*Tamarindus indica* Leguminosae: Native to the Old World tropics, this tree produces a fruit that is said to be the secret ingredient in Worcestershire sauce.

**Te-da-te-da**—*Palicourea sp.* Rubiaceae: The two hundred species of this genus are found only in the Americas. In the Guianas, this shrub is most commonly found on forested slopes.

**Tobacco**—*Nicotiana tabacum* Solanaceae: This species, the tobacco of commerce, is native to South America.

**Tomato**—*Lycopersicon esculentum* Solanaceae: The tomato is native to Mexico, although many close relatives are found in South America as well. Before Columbus, the Italians had no tomato sauce. Of course, before Marco Polo returned from China, they didn't have any pasta, either!

**Tonka**—*Dipteryx odorata* Leguminosae: This three-hundred-foot tree is common in the Guianas. The aromatic fruits are made into a shampoo by the Creoles in Suriname.

**Tow-tow**—*Rapatea paludosa* Rapataceae (Rapatea family): The twenty species of this genus are found only in tropical America. This particular species, common in the Guianas, likes to grow on stream banks and extend its roots right into the water.

**Tucúm**—*Astrocaryum tucuma* Palmae: This species produces a high-quality fiber used to weave hammocks in the northwest Amazon.

**Turmeric**—*Cucurma domestica* Zingiberaceae: Native to tropical Asia, turmeric has long been used as a dye, a perfume, and a spice. It is used to both color and flavor both mustard and curry powder.

**Tut-pwa-muh**—*Duroia aquatica* Rubiaceae: *See* DUROIA.

**Uh-pe**—*Bidens sp.* Compositae: The two hundred species of this genus are found in both temperate and tropical regions.

**U-shuh**—*Bixa orellana* Bixaceae (Bixa family): A common tree in the Amazon, this species furnishes a red pigment used by Indians to paint their bodies and dye their breechcloths. Also known as *achiote*, it is used to dye both butter and margarine and is used as a spice in Mexico.

**Vanilla**—*Vanilla planifolia* Orchidaceae: Although there are ninety species in this genus, only two produce commercial vanilla, this one and *V. pompona*. This species, from which we get most of our vanilla, is native to Mexico and is still cultivated by the Totonac Indians, who may have been the people who first domesticated it.

**Vegetable ivory palm**—*Phytelephas macrocarpa* Palmae: Near the turn of the century, a significant proportion of all buttons sold in the United States and Germany were made from the fruit of this palm. The tagua industry was greatly reduced, however, when plastic was invented in the 1930s. Conservation International is trying to resuscitate the tagua industry in order to give local peasants in Colombia and Ecuador the opportunity to earn a living by sustainably utilizing the forest by harvesting tagua fruit and other nontimber products (see Plotkin and Famolare, 1990, in the Recommended Reading section).

**Virola**—*Virola sp.* Myristicaceae: *See* JEAJEAMADOU.

**Wah-kah-gah-mu**—*Macfadyena uncata* Bignoniaceae: The Creoles in Suriname call this species *Fowroefoetoe tite*, which means "bird's foot liana," in reference to the clawlike tendrils that allow this species to climb up other plants.

**Wah-kah-pu**—*Vouacapoua americana* Leguminosae: This hundred-foot tree is common in the Guianas.

**Wah-kah-pwe-mah**—*Vismia sp.* Guttiferae: The yellow sap of this species is used throughout the Guianas to treat fungal infections of the skin. This tree is usually found in disturbed areas.

**Wah-me-do**—*Myrciaria sp.* Myrtaceae: *See* CAMU-CAMU.

**Wah-pu**—*Euterpe oleracea* Palmae: *See* ASSAI.

**Wah-ru-mah**—*Ischnosiphon arouma* Marantaceae (Arrowroot family): This herbaceous species yields a good-quality fiber that is used by many tribes in the Guianas to weave baskets and cassava squeezers.

**Walaba**—*Eperua falcata* Leguminosae: This hundred-foot tree is common in the Guianas. It is often seen growing on the banks of small streams.

**Wan-tah**—*Agave sp.* Amaryllidaceae: Agaves tend to be found in arid portions of the American tropics and subtropics. This particular species grows on the Sipaliwini savannas.

*Wapa*—*Eperua falcata* Leguminosae: See WALABA.

*Weh-da-ka-lu-ah-tuh-pe-lu*—*Bidens sp.* Compositae: The two hundred species of this genus are found in both the tropics and the temperate zone. This particular species thrive in abandoned Amerindian gardens in the northeast Amazon.

**Wheat**—*Triticum* spp. Gramineae: Wheat is native to Eurasia. It has been in cultivation for at least nine thousand years.

*Wih-kah-pu wa-ku*—*Apeiba sp.* Tiliaceae (Linden tree family): This 160-foot tree is often found growing on forested slopes. The Tirió name means "deer belly," a reference to the soft, white wood.

*Wy-a-na-tu-de*—*Talisia sp.* Sapindaceae (Soapberry family): The fifty species of this genus are found only in tropical America.

*Yagé*—*Banisteriopsis caapi* Malpighiaceae: See CAAPI.

*Yam*—*Dioscorea sp.* Dioscoreaceae (Yam family): Yams are mostly native to the tropics. Yam extracts were an important component of early versions of birth-control pills.

Gentle reader, after staying a few months in England, I strayed across the Alps and Apennines, and returned home, but could not tarry. Guiana still whispered in my ear, and seemed to invite me once more to wander through her distant forests. —Charles Waterton, 1825

● ● ● ● ● ● ● ● ● ● ● ● ● ● ● ● ● ● ●

# Index